NUTRITION:

The Healthy Aging Solution

By PAT LAM

Edited by:
Cathy Christensen
Design and Production:
Hon Bannapradist
Amy Gosselink

Allured Publishing Corporation
Carol Stream, Illinois USA

Nutrition: The Healthy Aging Solution
By Pat Lam

ISBN 1-932633-02-2

Note to reader: The information in this book is intended as a source of information guide. The recommendations, strategies and approaches are meant to inform, not to substitute for professional treatment. They are meant to guide more or less healthy individuals and should not be used to treat those who are ill or suffering from skin or body conditions without prior consultation with a qualified health professional.

Allured Publishing Corporation
362 South Schmale Road
Carol Stream, IL 60188-2787 USA
Telephone: 630/653-2155 • Fax: 630/653-2192
www.SkinInc.com

Dedication

This book is dedicated to my loving husband and partner in business for 28 years, and to all the skin care professionals who will make the world a healthier and happier place.

"Education is not a preparation for life, education is life itself."—John Dewey

Table of Contents

Introduction

During the past decade, nutritional education has become recognized as an essential component in all health care professions. This includes physicians, whether dermatologists, cosmetic surgeons or general physicians, naturopaths, chiropractors, massage therapists, nurses or dental hygienists. The mandate for the American Dietetic Association (ADA) for the new millennium is to implement nutritional education as an essential component for all health care professionals.

The phenomenal growth of spas, particularly wellness clinics, has brought physicians and skin care professionals together in a closer working relationship. Physicians now are employing skin care professionals or may work in partnership with them. Within the past few years, a more holistic approach toward skin care is being taken so that lifestyle factors are to be considered in skin and body care making nutrition an integral part in the training of the skin care professional. During the past few years, it has been observed that medicine is leaning toward a preventive approach, rather than the traditional model of health care where the disease is treated only upon detection. It is this author's belief that the skin care industry will adopt a similar mode so that preventive care or anti-aging therapies for the aging skin and body will be adopted.

The changing role of the esthetician

Most occupations do not exist in a vacuum but interact with other social systems. Changes in the social system can impact the skin care profession thus affecting the characteristics of the job. Within the past few years, the role of the esthetician has changed dramatically. The synergistic power of social, economic and political forces have impacted and changed the job characteristics of the profession which now is assuming a more health-oriented role.

Social impact. Changing demographics of aging and new technologies in the workplace during the past decade have had a dramatic impact on all areas of society. Every 7.7 seconds someone turns 50, and it is this burgeoning aging population that has become the driving force behind the economic, social and political trends today. Life expectancy in North America and other industrialized nations such as France, Germany, Italy, Japan and the United Kingdom are at an unprecedented high. Mortality rates are low due to advanced scientific and medical technologies.

The longevity of citizens carries huge implications for society. As baby boomers age, they become more concerned about their health and physical appearance. Health is one of the most popular topics researched on the Internet. The media's ubiquitous coverage of nutrition, fitness and wellness also has spilled over to the younger generation, creating new awareness of preventive health care.

A growing trend in the food industry indicated that consumers, particularly affluent aging baby boomers, increasingly are demanding food that promotes health and wellness. With demographics as one of the key drivers in new food development, the food industry is being forced to improve the quality and functionality of food. According to the *Toronto Star* in October 2003, functional foods, dubbed nutraceuticals or foods with enhanced nutritional properties, now contribute $1–2 billion of the overall food market. The introduction of folic acid in grain products has seen a dramatic reduction in spinal column birth defects in the past five years. The introduction of omega-3 fatty acids in eggs to lower cholesterol levels has led to the possibility of adding it to milk as well in the near future. In the fitness industry, the recent introduction of the holistic approach, integrating the philosophies of yoga and Pilates, has impacted the skin care industry as well. Many skin care centers incorporate wellness centers with yoga and Pilates studios so that the benefits of mind and body treatments can be explored fully.

Economic impact. Aging baby boomers usually have more time and disposable income than their predecessors, and they want to spend it on themselves to look and feel good as long as possible. Their children have left home and these empty nesters now have few financial obligations, so they find more available income for their personal use. Aging always has been associated with negativity, and as their physical appearance begins to deteriorate, baby boomers begin to lose a certain degree of self-esteem.

To increase their confidence, they seek various strategies to improve their skin and body condition. This has led to an explosion of spas focusing on pampering, rejuvenation treatments and stress reduction. Furthermore, the impact of the Internet has made the dot com community quite wealthy and an unprecedented number of young millionaires have evolved, earning much higher incomes than their predecessors. Young professionals work extremely hard with little rest and their lives are highly stressful. Many of them realize the importance of their health and spend time and money to visit spas to relax and rejuvenate their bodies and psyches.

Political impact. During the past decade, several political events have led to the erosion of the public's confidence in the medical system. The present medical care system in the United States does not allow much time for physicians to communicate with their patients because they have to see a huge number of patients on a daily basis to survive in business.

Many individuals, particularly the aging, require more time for personal support during this critical stage of their lives. With physicians' limited time for communication, a great number of people have lost confidence in the medical system and have begun an active search for alternative health care.

Furthermore, the political system of Medicare has had a dramatic impact on the medical profession. Deep cutbacks to medical practitioners have forced physicians to seek alternative means to augment their incomes, which have been dramatically reduced by the health care system. Many physicians, whether general practitioners, plastic surgeons, dermatologists, and even internists or eye surgeons began adding esthetic services to complement their businesses. They view the cosmetic market as a lucrative means of expanding their shrinking income. Many have linked up with estheticians and expanded their practice to medical esthetics.

Because of this partnership, the latest trend is the medical spa which integrates spa services together with conventional and integrative therapies by providing comprehensive medical and wellness care in a relaxing environment. This movement has opened up excellent employment opportunities for skin care professionals. In doing so, it has changed the profile of the esthetician who had to upgrade her education to meet the requirements of working in a medical environment. It became necessary for her to become more knowledgeable in medical terminology and procedures to work in a medical setting, whether cosmetic or dermatology. Estheticians had to become better educated in pre- and post-care procedures, wound healing, nutritional counseling, remedial camouflage and recommending proper home care advice to patients.

In order to understand this holistic perspective, the esthetician must strive to develop a clearer knowledge of the anatomy and physiology of the human body. She must understand that the healthy structure of various parts of the body ultimately depends on dietary intake and bioavailability of nutrients for various tissues, particularly with age.

In the physician's office, the sale of cosmetic products also has proven to be a lucrative source of added revenue, with some physicians investing in their own line of skin care products. Marketing skills are proving to be important criteria in developing successful practices. Most estheticians are well honed in communication skills, an area that typically was lacking between physicians and their patients. This rapport has brought many patients back to the physician's office. However, many estheticians prefer to work autonomously in the medical esthetics role, specializing in getting results for skin problems and wellness—not so much on pampering. Take a look at how these factors have affected the role of the esthetician presently.

The beauty role

Historically, the role of the esthetician has been one of "beautician." The public's perception of an esthetician was that of a female, not necessarily highly educated, performing some type of manual service on a client. As a result, many parents perceived the profession in the context of manual labor and were reluctant to allow their daughters to enter the esthetic field because they believed it was not an admirable profession.

However, over the past 50 years the transgression of the beautician to that of the skin care professional occurred and the term *esthetician* has become well established in North American society. The modern image is that of a neat, attractive individual, usually female, although several males successfully have entered the profession, wearing subtle makeup and uniform performing a face or body treatment. Media coverage and ever-present advertisements in trade magazines have developed this professional image of the esthetician over the past decades raising the credibility of the esthetician in the public eye. The modern image is that of a professional who possesses the skills to improve not only the beauty, but also the health of the skin and body. Aging baby boomers turn toward the esthetician to help recapture the youthful beauty they believe they are losing through the aging process.

The health role

With a significant number of the population turning 50, these aging baby boomers have become more aware of health issues. They are the "young-old" and view themselves as still being youthful. Unlike their predecessors, they are a proactive group. They were the driving force behind the fitness boom in the '80s and continue to be very active, jogging, skiing and working-out in gyms to maintain their youthfulness. In fact, a survey conducted by a professional fitness organization indicated that more than 50% of the membership of most health clubs is comprised of men and women over 40 years of age. A poll published in

U.S. News and World Report on July 29, 1996, indicated that the cosmetic nature of aging is a deep source of anxiety to aging baby boomers. Their main concerns were excess body weight, hair loss, facial wrinkles and gray hair.

In modern society, people live a frenzied lifestyle with so many demands to meet. Despite sociologists' earlier prediction of a more leisurely lifestyle for the future, most of us now constantly are pushed to our limits with stress on a daily basis. Regular high levels of stress activate excessive cortisone hormones into the bloodstream producing high levels of free radicals. Scientific research shows that these molecules can damage the mitochondria and DNA in cells leading to premature skin aging and accelerating age-related diseases. Individuals who constantly experience high levels of stress look older than their chronological age and, if left unchecked, these high levels can lead to heart-related diseases such as high blood pressure and cancer, the leading causes of death today.

During the past few years, the explosion of spas in both urban and rural areas in most industrialized nations has occurred to meet the demand by the public for relaxation, serenity and wellness. The term *wellness* has become synonymous with beauty, health and longevity. People visit spas not only to beautify, but also to unwind and rejuvenate their overworked systems, even on a temporary basis. Various forms of stress reduction therapies leave the client feeling relaxed and rejuvenated with a sense of euphoria or well-being. Estheticians constantly are motivated to seek more knowledge in wellness therapies so that specialized postgraduate courses such as stress therapy massage, ayurvedic therapy, reflexology, massage therapy and similar modalities are sought after in the industry. These changes have led to the present image of the estheticians' role as a health and wellness specialist.

The medical role

Both political and economic factors have caused physicians to turn toward working more with estheticians in expanding their businesses. Estheticians have had to learn how to deal with patients in a medical environment where people may suffer from skin disorders, diseases and other medical conditions. In essence, the role of the skin care professional can incorporate all facets—beauty, health and medical—simultaneously.

The impact of new technology

The advent of new technologies in the esthetic profession has contributed to elevating the present status of the esthetician. New modalities once reserved for physicians now have become more available to skin care professionals. Skin peels such as alpha hydroxyl acids (AHA), chemical peels, and high tech devices for skin resurfacing such as microdermabrasion and various forms of lasers became very popular in the prevention and reversal of premature skin aging. In addition, devices to remove unsightly minor skin growths that appear with aging, such as skin tags, fibromas, hemangiomas and any sebaceous hyperplasia such as milia, cholesterol deposits and pimples have appeared for the esthetician's use. The introduction of sophisticated skin imaging systems to "see inside the skin" and simultaneously document images of clients before, during and after treatments help to boost the high-tech skills of the trade. Other new technologies on the market include sophisticated equipment for cellulite reduction, laser hair removal and ultrasound devices to help products penetrate the skin more efficiently.

Estheticians who continue to update their education and adjust to the changing market tend to be in higher demand than those who do not, and consequently, are more likely to acquire higher earning power. Thus, the impact of political, economic and social systems has influenced greatly the role of the esthetician in the wider social structure.

The ethnic impact

The ease of travel has led people from different countries to settle down far from home. Mass migration from developing countries to industrialized nations has led to the formation of ethnic core enclaves established in large cities. In the new millennium, the world has changed and some cities or towns have become multicultural embracing all cultures whether food, fashion or behavior, while others are a melting pot where individuals assimilate into the major culture and eventually lose their ethnic identities. To be successful in business today, the skin care or health professional must not restrict themselves to one ethnic group, but rather embrace all cultural groups into their clientele. To build an eclectic clientele, it is necessary to learn about cultural differences as much as possible in order to bond with the potential clients.

The changing face of clientele. The ethnic composition of the clientele in many esthetic practices has changed more significantly in urban than rural areas. If you live in a city or country with a more cosmopolitan nature, your clientele probably has changed over the past decade. Knowledge of food practices of various ethnic groups can prove to be very helpful if you are going to cater to clients in a specific geographic location. For example, it is predicted that the Hispanic population will overtake all other ethnic groups in the United States. This means that the face of America will change within the next 50 years.

These demographics have significant implications for all professions, including esthetics. This infers that there will be a higher ratio of more dark-skinned than light-skinned people in America. If this is true, skin care professionals should prepare themselves for the future by learning as much as possible about skin disorders such as hyperpigmentation and skin diseases that are more likely to be prevalent among these ethnic groups. This cultural change also is occurring in other countries such as Europe where migration from third world countries also has changed the face of the population.

Try to learn about the cultures that are dominant in your area, particularly cuisines of the different ethnic groups living in the surrounding areas. Food is an excellent neutral topic that tends to create a closer rapport between the esthetician and the client. Discussion of ethnic foods with the clients can not only help foster closer relationships with these clients, but also can open up a new world of exciting tastes.

If you are going to give nutritional advice to different cultural groups, you need to learn about their foods and eating behaviors. You cannot change a client's cultural eating habits that have been instilled since childhood, but you can modify them with a healthier approach. The cultural impact of food differences has led to nouvelle cuisine such as fusion foods. Many ethnic spices are combined with traditional foods and several eclectic cuisines have evolved. Ignorance of cultural habits can lead to a deep source of embarrassment for both you and your client.

Preventive care

Preventive or *anti-aging* are becoming more important in people's lives as they begin to see their friends, relatives and associates suffering from the diseases associated with aging. A significant number of the population has become more interested in health issues and actively are seeking strategies to prevent or delay deleterious effects of aging.

Anti-aging has become a new sub-specialty of modern medicine where aging is viewed not necessarily as inevitable, but as a disease that can be treated. The hypothesis holds that preventive measures can be taken to avoid or delay the onset of age-associated diseases. It is predicted that the preventive role of medicine will become more defined in society in the very near future. In fact, private health centers already have sprouted up in several large cities to accommodate the needs of those who can afford them. They offer screenings for age-related diseases such as different cancers, osteoporosis, heart-related diseases and counseling on lifestyle behaviors such as nutrition and fitness.

Although it long has been recognized that nutrition is at the core of health and longevity, it only now is being implemented in people's lives. The human body is an incredible system, but in order to maintain its healthy functioning, it needs special care, particularly as it ages. If you take care of priceless items such as a luxurious car, it will stay in good shape longer. The human body probably is the most priceless commodity, and it can be lost if it isn't nurtured. It can be very difficult to replace some parts, so take special care of them by feeding the body with healthy nutrients and loving care. With the emphasis on healthy nutrition, let us attempt to understand how it impacts the skin, body, general health and longevity.

Preface

Knowledge only is powerful if it is used to inform or persuade others to accept and use the information for their benefit. New scientific knowledge evolves every three years—because of this, the basic information contained in my previous book *Practical Nutrition for the Health and Beauty Professional* now is upgraded and expanded for the benefit of those health and skin care professionals who have acquired basic knowledge in nutrition.

Interest in health issues increasingly has become more important among the aging population, many of whom are baby boomers actively seeking information on strategies to maximize good health and longevity, as well as to optimize youthfulness in both face and figure. Without continuing education on health issues, clients will begin to lose confidence in the skin care professional's ability to keep them looking more youthful.

Evolution of the industry

The skin care profession has become very dynamic in recent years with several allied health care professionals implementing skin care into their practices. There is a movement toward wellness that is both physical and psychological. Many estheticians presently are working with physicians, usually dermatologists or plastic surgeons. With this new arm of medical esthetics, it is essential that skin care professionals acquire increased nutritional information to prepare and guide patients in pre- or post-operative care. Furthermore, the rise of obesity during the past decade in most industrialized countries all over the world holds serious implications for our health care systems and society in general.

The esthetician performs various types of body therapies to improve cellulite conditions or rejuvenate the body, and is placed in a unique position to access the health status of the client. This is an ideal opportunity to give advice on positive lifestyle changes such as dietary and fitness guidance. Most people do not visit a nutritionist or dietician unless a medical problem is involved, but they do visit the skin care clinic or spa for their facial or body treatments quite often. The skin care professional must take this wonderful opportunity to encourage the client to change or modify lifestyle behaviors. This involves improving the client's daily nutritional and physical activity as part of an anti-aging approach.

This book provides information for health care professionals and estheticians who are seeking more knowledge in this area.

Chapter content

Chapters 1–3 introduce the reader to the ever-changing role of the skin care professional and give an expanded overview of the basics of nutrition. They also explain how you can use nutrition as a preventive approach for aging and health care. In **Chapter 4**, you can learn how to balance your diet and then make recommendations for a healthy diet. **Chapters 5–8** include probably the most interesting and rewarding information for the skin care professional. It provides both nutrition and lifestyle counseling for various skin and body conditions including a discussion on the effects of free radicals on health. **Chapters 9–11** outline various aspects of nutrition relating to skin allergies, detoxification, sun protection, glycemic index and pre- and post-surgical procedures. In **Chapter 12**, the worldwide epidemic of obesity is covered and very important information is provided for the skin care professional. The different body types are described and how to achieve and manage a healthy body weight. Anti-aging is discussed in **Chapter 13** where you learn strategies on preventing skin and body aging. **Chapter 14** covers the various terminology on food labels so you can make healthier choices when shopping. The active portion of the book is in **Chapter 15** where the various components of physical fitness, including mind fitness, are discussed. **Chapter 16** gives a brief overview of the most common ethnic cuisines found in Westernized societies. Traditional values and diets of various cultures, including ingredients and common foods will enlighten health and skin care professionals in dealing with ethnic clients. Known adaptations to the traditional diets in the United States are noted and the nutritional status is reviewed. Finally, the **Appendices** contain information on updated Dietary Reference Intakes that scientists recommend for use in nutritional counseling for individuals. In addition, you can find various forms and charts that can be photocopied for practical diet assessment as discussed in the book. Schools can use these handy forms for their students' practical workshops. The forms also include the Body Mass Index and an attractive hand-out that can be given to clients to help them make the best choices in common fruits and vegetables when they are shopping.

Conversion Chart

In order to make this book user-friendly, included is the following conversion chart to use throughout when dealing with measurements.

Volume—liters (L)			*Weight—grams (g)*		
1 L	=	100 milliliters (mL)	1 g	=	100 milligrams (mg)
1 mL	=	0.03 ounces (oz)	100 mg	=	0.04 ounces (oz)
250 mL	=	1 cup	1 oz	=	approximately 30 g
			100 g	=	3 1/2 oz
			1 kilogram (kg)	=	1,000 g
			1 kg	=	2.2 lbs
			454 g	=	1 lb

Moving forward

A multidisciplinary approach must be adopted to move this profession forward in this millennium so that it can continue to increase its credibility from the public as an integral part of the wellness team. Your clients expect you to have this knowledge and most of them already know that treatments from the "outside" must be balanced with the "inside," particularly in middle age, the period when the body begins to show signs of degeneration.

Your clients are aging and new clients are young, educated and knowledgeable, therefore, you need to complement treatments with positive healthy lifestyle behaviors to help them achieve or maximize good health and keep them coming back. If you do not engage in this endeavor, you risk the chance of losing clients to the degenerative diseases of aging. Regular mainstream treatments such as facial treatments, manicures and hair removal always will be the industry's forté, but you can wear other hats to strengthen or expand your roles as skin care professionals in the present century.

Those who recognize this change will help move the profession forward while those who resist or negate this philosophy will find it more difficult to survive professionally. You cannot change the aging process, but you can make a significant difference in the way clients age by prolonging youthfulness, not only in physical appearance, but also in strength and vigor as long as possible.

I believe that the information in this book not only will encourage the reader to examine her dietary intake, but also will help skin care professionals work more effectively with various ethnic groups found in modern society in a culturally sensitive manner.

Acknowledgements

I wish to thank several individuals who graciously have given help and support in developing this book. My husband, Hubert Lam, and my children, Lara and Allan, for their continuous encouragement and overwhelming support throughout the computer problems and the stress of meeting deadlines. I wish to extend my deep appreciation to my staff, in particular Martina Kocicka, for her time and patience in helping to proofread and type the difficult charts and tables that always seem to have changes. I am very grateful to Belinda Terzis-Papadatos and Nadine Dundas, true professionals who, despite their busy schedules, donated their precious time to proofread the manuscript. Special thanks to Cathy Christensen, the editor who performed the laborious job of transforming the manuscript into a simpler and more interesting format for the reader. I also would like to acknowledge with appreciation those individuals who gave graciously their permission to use their faces and bodies for illustrations, Lina Bonneau, Robyn Vandermoor and students at the Lam School of Advanced Esthetics. Finally, thanks to the various skin care professionals with whom I consulted for multiple topics that may interest the health and beauty professional.

—Pat Lam

CHAPTER 1

The Basics of Nutrition

The science of nutrition is the study of nutrients in food and how they are utilized by the body. Every living cell needs food to nourish or repair itself, otherwise it dies. While basic nutrition is the same for most people, the daily requirements for each person vary due to age, gender, body size, health status and pregnancy or if the woman is lactating. Sometimes even if sufficient amounts of food are consumed, malnutrition still may occur because of inadequate intake of particular nutrients relative to that person's requirements.

Food is necessary for all life processes from breathing, thinking and digestion to movement. The sun plays a vital role in the origin of food and nutrition. It shines down on the world releasing its energy on inhabitants that absorb it. When **photosynthesis** occurs, plants utilize that energy to convert carbon dioxide and water into carbohydrates and some proteins, releasing oxygen in the process. The rule of survival of the fittest dictates that animals—including fish—and plants are consumed by other animals—including humans—and the ingested food is converted back into carbon dioxide, water and energy.

Most foods contain a mixture of nutrients, although one or two may predominate. For example, foods from plants contain less fat and a higher amount of water, minerals, vitamins and carbohydrates than foods from animals. Six basic nutrients are essential for health, growth and maintenance of body tissues: water, proteins, carbohydrates, fats, vitamins and minerals.

Meat is composed mainly of protein, saturated fats and cholesterol. Like animal tissue, plants also contain different types of proteins, carbohydrates and fats in various proportions. With the exception of palm and coconut oils, most plants contain either **polyunsaturated** (PUFA) or **monounsaturated** (MUFA) **fats**. The type of fats humans consume can affect health status.

In order to fully grasp the impact of food on the body, see **Figure 1-1**, page 2, for a big picture of where food originates.

What is a calorie (kcal)?

Energy from food is expressed in *kcal*—a unit of measurement that equals 1,000-calorie units. **Calories** are used by the body to fuel its physical metabolic activities.

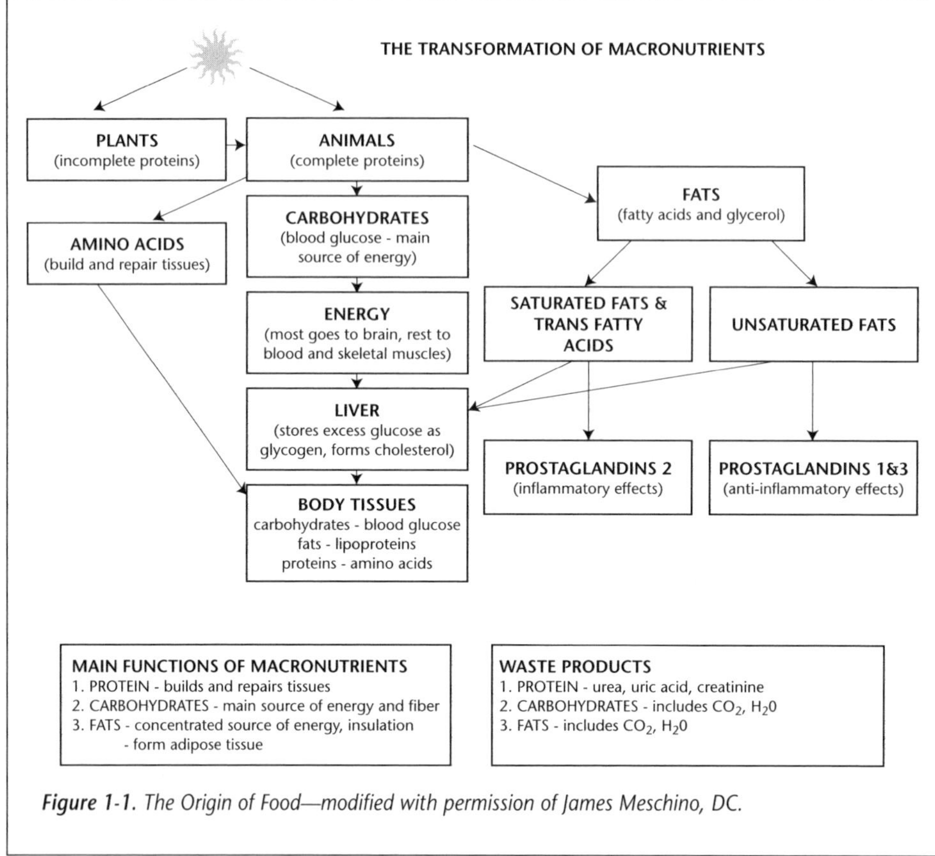

Figure 1-1. *The Origin of Food—modified with permission of James Meschino, DC.*

Metabolism refers to the sum of all physical and chemical processes that occur within living tissues with food intake. This results in the release of energy, the essential component for sustaining life. **Cellular metabolism** is the metabolism that occurs within each living cell, while **basal metabolism** refers to how efficiently the body uses its energy. When excessive food intake is not utilized in metabolic or physical activities, the body converts it to fat and stores it in adipose tissues. This often leads to weight gain. It has been estimated that the brain uses approximately 2/3 of the day's energy. This is why one can feel weak or dizzy if meals are missed. Because of this, it is easy to understand why it is vital to eat breakfast, considered the most important meal of the day.

Metabolism of organic vs. inorganic foods. **Macronutrients** refer to the large amounts of food—proteins, carbohydrates, fats and water—required for health and maintenance of the body. Proteins, carbohydrates and fats are termed **organic** because they contain the element carbon. Although alcohol also provides energy, it is not an essential nutrient and is referred to as empty calories since it does not contribute toward health. Vitamins also are considered organic because they are found in the living tissues of plants and animals. They are not affected by enzymes. Contrary to popular belief, they do not release energy directly, but some vitamins, such as vitamin B, act as **co-enzymes** that help release energy from food. Water is the most important nutrient and is essential for digestion and circulation and, along with minerals, is termed **inorganic**. Both substances also are unaffected by enzymes in the body.

Waste products of metabolism. When macronutrients are oxidized in the tissues, the chemical bonds that bind the various elements are broken down to release the energy. During this process, oxygen is breathed in and combined with the carbon elements from the organic foods to form a carbon dioxide (CO_2) molecule, while hydrogen elements from the metabolized foods combine with oxygen to form water (H_2O) molecules. Therefore, the waste products of metabolism include carbon dioxide and water. Water, in the form of vapor, is eliminated through the nose and mouth, and carbon dioxide is exhaled through the respiratory system while urine and feces are eliminated via the excretory system.

Nutrient components

In order to understand nutrition, it is necessary to know the functions of all nutrients. For review, examine the functions of the essential nutrients for the body.

Water (H_2O)

- An inorganic nutrient.
- The simplest nutrient, composed of two elements, hydrogen (H) and oxygen (O_2). Each molecule of water consists of two atoms of hydrogen and one atom of oxygen (H_2O).

Functions

- Essential to life.
- Comprises approximately two-thirds of the body's weight.
- Main constituent of all body fluids in the circulatory, lymphatic, digestive and excretory systems.
- Acts as shock absorber and lubricant for all tissues.
- Aids in heat regulation through sweat and urine.
- Body needs two-to-three liters daily—eight 8-oz. glasses—to maintain hydric balance.
- The larger the individual, the more water consumption required.

Functions (Water (H_2O) cont'd)

- Water levels in the body are regulated by the anti-diuretic hormone (ADH) in kidneys.
- Thirst is regulated by the hypothalamus, an endocrine gland in brain.
- Caffeinated beverages act as diuretics.

Protein

- The most complex organic nutrient because it consists of at least six elements—carbon, nitrogen, hydrogen, oxygen, phosphorus and sometimes sulfur.
- 1 gram = 4 kcals.

Functions

- Second most abundant substance in the body—approximately 20%.
- Basic building block is amino acid.
- Essential for growth, development and repair of body tissues including bone, muscles, blood, hormones, enzymes, antibodies, plasma proteins, collagen, nails, hair and all cellular structures.
- Source of energy, although the body uses carbohydrates and fats first.
- Blood clotting—manufactures blood proteins such as fibrin.
- Maintains acid/base balance, essential for health.

Carbohydrates

- Organic nutrient composed of carbon, hydrogen and oxygen.
- 1 gram = 4 kcals.

Functions

- Main source of energy.
- Easiest to digest and absorb.
- Required to metabolize fat.
- Broken down into glucose for absorption.

Fats—lipids or triglycerides

- Organic nutrient composed of carbon, hydrogen and oxygen, but a greater amount of carbon and hydrogen in proportion to oxygen.
- 1 gram = 9 kcals; 1 lb = 3,500 kcals.

Functions

- Body heat.
- Formation of phospholipid layer of cell membranes, hormones—steroids, bile and vitamin D.
- Carrier for fat-soluble vitamins.

Functions (Fats—lipids or triglycerides cont'd)

- Gives flavor to food and provides satiety, or the feeling of fullness, quickly.
- Essential for carbohydrate metabolism.
- Takes longer to digest and absorb than other macronutrients.
- Excess fat is stored in adipose tissue.

Vitamins

- Organic substances found in living food—plants and animals.
- Minute amounts required, measured in milligrams (mg) or micrograms (ug).

Functions

- Fat-soluble—vitamins A, D, E and K, and water-soluble—vitamins B, C and P.
- Essential for health and maintenance of tissues.
- Deficiency leads to diseases.
- Can be made synthetically but body absorbs sources from natural foods more readily.
- Some act as antioxidants, such as betacarotene, and vitamins C and E.

Minerals

- Inorganic elements that form electrolytes in solution.
- Minerals sodium, potassium and chloride are essential electrolytes.
- Not affected by enzymes, chemicals or environmental factors such as air or heat.
- Deficiency results in abnormalities or diseases.
- Macrominerals measured in mg, microminerals or trace minerals measured in ug.

Functions

- Role as electrolytes is essential to life by regulating fluid balance in tissues.
- Some, such as selenium and zinc, act as antioxidants.

Social environment's impact on food selection

Although genetics play a strong role in body size and weight, healthy habits instilled in children during their formative years can promote lifestyle habits that may prevent degenerative diseases later in life. The types of food, their preparation and the context in which they are eaten can remain with an individual over a lifetime, despite any changes of environment. For example, a child may have developed a taste for fatty foods during childhood years. Although parents are responsible for establishing proper eating habits at home, the child may be affected by peer group interactions and environmental cues when they enter school, some of which ultimately may override habits from home.

Socioeconomic status also has been found to impact nutritional habits. In low socioeconomic families, insufficient funds as well as lack of education may not only affect the type of foods purchased, but also how they are prepared. However, affordability of cheaper foods does not necessarily mean that nutrient-rich foods are out of reach because many fruits, vegetables and whole grains can be inexpensive, so it may be lack of knowledge that leads to unhealthy choices rather than available income. Wealthier individuals, particularly youth, may have monetary access to better quality foods but do not always purchase healthier foods and may consume the same empty calorie fare as poorer individuals. Thus malnutrition or the lack of essential nutrients can occur in any socioeconomic group. Food choices during youth therefore can have a profound impact on current and future health.

Everyone favors different types of foods for various reasons.

- Personal preference, habit, ethnic/traditional foods, convenience and affordability.
- Social interaction with peer groups, emotional comfort to relieve stress or boredom.
- Values—religious, political, environmental and health.
- Physical appearance.
- Media including peers, magazines, literature, books and the Internet.

The consequence of unwise food selections over a period of time can have a dramatic impact on health and appearance. A healthy diet should consist of the six essential foods in *correct* proportions, limiting the amount of saturated fats, refined sugars, salt and alcohol.

Types of dieting behaviors

As discussed, the eating behaviors of humans and animals vary for different reasons. The following terms describe dieting behaviors among humans.

Carnivores eat primarily all types of meat.
Omnivores eat both plant and animal foods.
Vegetarians:

a. **Semi-vegetarians** avoid red meat but eat poultry, fish and dairy products.
b. **Lacto-vegetarians** avoid meat and eggs but consume dairy products.
c. **Lacto-ovos** avoid meat but eat eggs, milk and milk products.
d. **Ovo-vegetarians** avoid dairy products and meat but eat eggs.
e. **Vegans** are the absolute vegetarians. They consume plant foods only, and absolutely no meat or meat derivatives.

Dietary guidelines

Most countries have established dietary guidelines for essential nutrients to protect and support the health of their citizens. In the United States and Canada, the Food and Nutrition Board of The Institute of Medicine provide **Dietary Reference Intakes** (DRIs), a set of nutrient values based on the dietary intake of healthy people in the two counties. Two international bodies, the Food and Agriculture Organization (FAO) and the World Health Organization (WHO) also provide similar standards with slight differences for many other countries because of the varying food habits and physical activities of their populations. Previous work focused only on essential nutrients that were then known, but in recent years, research on the health benefits of other dietary components such as fiber and **phytochemicals**—chemicals in plants—now have been included in the DRIs. Revised nutrient intakes are updated continuously, not only to protect against nutrient deficiencies, but also to prevent chronic diseases. (See **Important Dietary Terminology**, page 8.)

The RDA. The **Recommended Dietary Allowance** (RDA) was used formerly to refer to the amount of a specific nutrient that was essential to meet the needs of the general population rather than individuals, and for those who were described as "normal and healthy." It originally was intended to provide guidelines for the prevention of certain severe nutritional deficiencies that were prevalent during a specific era—diseases such as **scurvy**, a deficiency of vitamin C; **pellagra**, a deficiency of vitamin B-3 or niacin; and **beri-beri**, a deficiency of vitamin B-1 or thiamin. However, because different diseases exist today, RDA

Important Dietary Terminology

Estimated Average Requirement (EAR) refers to the amount of a nutrient that is estimated to meet the requirement of half of all healthy individuals in a given age and gender group.

Recommended Dietary Allowance (RDA) and Recommended Nutrient Intakes (RNIs) are terms being replaced by the DRIs. They are nutrient values that are defined as sufficient to meet the requirements of nearly all—97–98%—of healthy people and are calculated from the EAR.

Adequate Intake (AI) is a recommended daily intake value based on observed or experimentally determined approximations of nutrient intake by a group or groups of healthy people that are assumed to be adequate and used when an RDA cannot be determined. The AI is not equivalent to an RDA.

Tolerable Upper Intake Level (UL) is the highest level of daily intake that is least likely to pose any risk of adverse health effects to almost all individuals in the general population. As intake increases above the UL, the risks of adverse effects increase. Unless specified otherwise, the UL represents the total intake from food, water and dietary supplements.

was criticized since very few contemporary people fall under its umbrella. It was considered inadequate because modern society nutritionists and dieticians always have relied on the RDA as dietary guidelines for recommending nutrient intakes for their patients and important lifestyle and environmental factors were not considered.

With the new preventive approach in medicine, much higher levels of nutrients have been recommended to ward off age-related diseases and conditions contributing to an anti-aging effect. The effects of alcohol, smoking, eating disorders, heavy metals such as lead and mercury, food additives, carbon monoxide and other chemicals found in modern society need to be considered. Individuals may have habits that require nutrient levels way above the RDA levels to optimize a healthy lifespan. For example, smokers and alcoholics need to have higher levels to compensate for loss of nutrients produced from their lifestyle habits. Modern scientists believe that optimal levels of nutrients, particularly antioxidants, are necessary to optimize the immune system and ultimately extend a healthier lifespan.

DRIs. In recent years, scientists from Canada and the Food and Nutrition Board of the Institute of Medicine in the United States have collaborated and updated their nutrient recommendations to produce new harmonized values called DRIs for micronutrients. These are being released now and the most current information is listed in Appendices I, II and III of this book. Since the process currently is underway, the data presented in these appendices reflect the most current values ranging from 1997 to 2001. The DRIs also replace and expand the 1990 **Recommended Nutrient Intakes** (RNIs) that have been used in Canada as a tool for planning and assessing the diets of healthy people. Different types of reference values, each with different uses, are listed in Appendices I, II and III.

The preventive approach

In **preventive medicine**, the belief is that if one follows certain dietary practices and lives a healthy lifestyle, a wide range of diseases can be prevented, delayed or even reversed in some cases. The principles of the **Recommended Optimal Nutrient Intakes** (RONIs) are based on a preventive approach to aging and the degenerative, debilitating diseases associated with it. A health-promoting diet that focuses on the consumption of fresh, natural foods supplemented by dietary supplements is recommended in an anti-aging program. However, numerous studies show that despite the ubiquitous information by various media, most North Americans continue to follow unhealthy nutritional diets. They tend to compensate for this by taking **dietary supplements**, a phenomenon that has increased by 25% per annum in the past five years. Supplements are not meant to replace diet, but to enhance it, hence the word.

The role of the skin care professional

Although as many as 98% of medical experts and researchers take supplements, they have not endorsed dietary supplementation for the public. Skin care professionals do not need to become nutritionists or dieticians to provide basic nutritional counseling to their clients. A large percentage of clients already are knowledgeable about nutrition information gleaned from media such as magazines and the Internet. In fact, studies show that one in every three people already take supplements. Since they have no guidelines to follow, they tend to purchase supplements through the influence of friends and media.

Estheticians are well positioned to become some of the most influential professionals in guiding their clients to achieve healthier skin and a healthier body through proper nutritional counseling. Unless the client's lifestyle behaviors are considered to treat the underlying principles of cell renewal and repair, the skills of a skin care professional are limited. A more holistic approach to skin and body care must be undertaken to maximize results of treatment.

Let food be your medicine and medicine be your food

A healthy, well-balanced diet should consist of the recommended daily percentage of total daily kcals: carbohydrates, 50–60%; fats, 15–25%, less than 10% saturated; protein, 15–20%; and dietary fiber, 40–50 g.

Primary recommendations for promoting health include a predominantly vegetarian diet made up mainly of fiber-rich foods; reducing fat intake with more plant than animal fats; eliminating refined sugars; avoiding or limiting exposure to pesticides and food allergens; maintaining a low salt/high potassium intake; maintaining adequate daily water intake; and achieving and maintaining a healthy body weight.

Consume plant-based vegetarian diet. Vegetarian diets are healthy because of their low saturated fat and cholesterol content, high levels of essential fatty acids, antioxidants and phytochemicals. This type of diet includes a high intake of fruits, vegetables, legumes and grains that contain high fiber content shown to reduce cancers of the gastrointestinal (GI) tract. Vegetarians are more likely to lead healthier lifestyles because they are more careful about what they do to their bodies. However, plant proteins do not contain all the essential amino acids that the body needs to form good quality body tissue, so different types of protein must be combined carefully to create complete proteins. In recent years, **soy protein**, a plant food, has become recognized as a complete protein since it contains all the essential amino acids. Be sure to check soy foods for varying fat content due to different processing methods.

Reduce fat intake. A diet based on animal foods usually is high in fat content and is more likely to contribute to heart-related diseases. If semi-vegetarian, select lean meats such as whole range skinless poultry, fish and veal. Avoid domesticated animal meats since they possess higher saturated fats and few omega-3 fatty acids. Check for hydrogenated fats—trans fatty acids—that are found in processed foods such as margarine, cakes and biscuits because they have been found to be as harmful as saturated fats.

Reduce refined sugar. More than half of Americans consume huge quantities of sugars found in processed foods in the form of sweeteners. A high intake of simple and refined sugars raises blood sugar levels leading to inflammation within cells. Excess sugar consumption can lead to diseases such as **diabetes**, one of the leading causes of death in the world. Check food labels for clues on various forms of sugar and cut back on them. These forms include sucrose, glucose, maltose, fructose, corn syrup and white grape juice.

Avoid pesticides and food allergens. The use of pesticides, herbicides and other chemicals sprayed on foods has created cause for health concerns. Long-term risks include different types of cancer, diseases and other health-related problems. You can reduce the use of these chemicals by selecting organic foods that are not treated with chemicals or removing and washing the outer leaves. There also are many additives in food that are hidden ingredients in the multitude of commercialized foods. This has led to a rise in food and environmental allergies in the past few decades. People with known allergies must take extra care in selecting foods when shopping in supermarkets or eating out in restaurants.

Maintain low salt/high potassium diet. A high salt intake contributes to high blood pressure. The sodium-potassium pump to maintain a constant osmotic pressure within body cells must be at a specific ratio of 1:2. However, most Americans consume a diet that is too high in sodium with the inverse ratio of 2:1 because of the hidden salt content in most processed foods. Natural sources of high potassium foods are fruits and vegetables. Encourage clients to eat more of these natural foods that also are high in fiber and water content.

Maintain adequate water intake. Inadequate intake of water leads to dehydration and increased levels of toxins in the urinary tract impairing the immune system. Because there are so many chemicals and toxic compounds in water systems such as polychlorinated biphenyls (PCBs), or environmental toxins found in pesticides, paints and more, and heavy metals such as lead and mercury and pesticide residues that can lead to infectious diseases, treated water is recommended. Home treatment programs such as bottled water are the best alternative at this time, but they are only short-term solutions. If you can afford it, try to install water filtration systems in your home and office.

Maintain a healthy body weight. Learning how to achieve and maintain a healthy body weight will help to reduce a high risk of health problems such as obesity, diabetes and heart disease.

CHAPTER 2

Macronutrients

Proteins

After water, **protein** is the second most abundant substance in the body. Protein is derived from both animal and vegetable sources. An **amino acid** is the basic building block of protein. Chemically, each amino acid is a compound consisting of an amino group (NH_2) at one end, an acid group (COOH) at the other end, and a hydrogen (H) atom all bonded to a central carbon atom. (See **Figure 2-1**.) A distinctive molecule or side chain composed of many different elements is bonded to the carbon atom, making protein a more complex molecule than carbohydrates and fats.

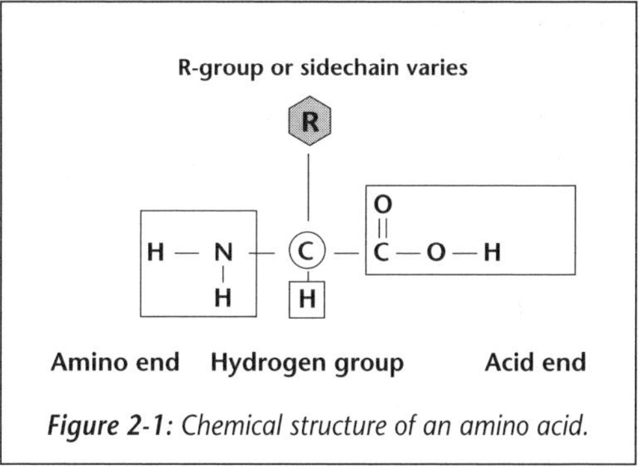

Figure 2-1: Chemical structure of an amino acid.

Amino acids are bonded to one another by chemical bonds forming protein chains of varying lengths called **peptides**. Two amino acids form a **dipeptide**, three, a **tripeptide**, and several peptides form a **polypeptide**, *poly-* meaning "many." Most proteins in the body consist of polypeptides containing 10,000 to 50,000 amino acids. They develop various structural forms of protein such as muscle, skin, nails, hair and collagen. The properties of these polypeptides therefore depend on the length, composition and sequence of the amino acids in the chains. For example, fibrinogen, a blood protein responsible for blood clotting, consists of one polypeptide chain; the hormone insulin consists of two polypeptide chains; and hemoglobin consists of four polypeptide chains.

Every chain of amino acids can twist and fold in a specific sequence to form the various shapes of protein. (See **Figure 2-2**, page 14.) The side chain, or **R-group**, attached to the carbon atom determines the type of protein formed. The varying composition of elements found in this side chain is what makes protein such a complex nutrient. If, for some reason this sequence of protein was affected in any way during its formation in the cell, abnormal protein or mutation will result in some form of illness or disease. For example, in sickle cell

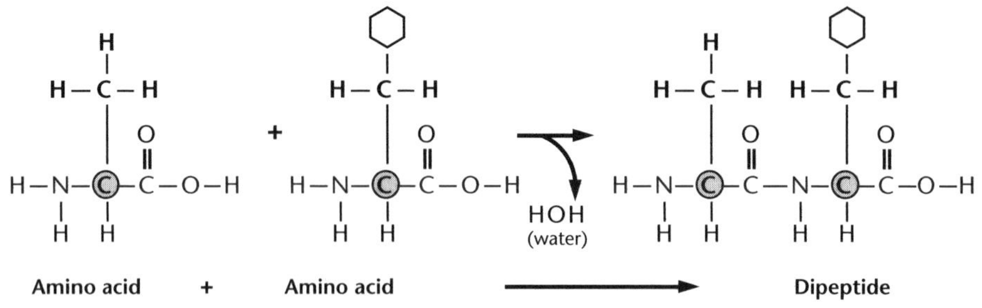

Figure 2-2: *Formation of a dipeptide.*

anemia, a blood disease typically found in people of African descent, the normal position of the amino acid **glutamine** in the chain is replaced by **valine** during its formation. This causes abnormal formation, or **denaturation**, of the disc-shaped cell to a crescent-shaped cell instead. Consequently, the hemoglobin within the cell loses its ability to carry oxygen effectively, resulting in sickle cell anemia.

Essential amino acids. Amino acids are classified as either **essential** or **non-essential**. See **Amino Acids** for a list of approximately 20 amino acids, all of which are essential for protein synthesis. Eleven are synthesized in the body and are termed non-essential amino acids. Those that are not synthesized in the body are called essential amino acids and must be brought into the body through dietary intake.

AMINO ACIDS

Non-essential Amino Acids	***Essential Amino Acids***
Alanine	Histidine
Arginine	Isoleucine
Asparagine	Leucine
Aspartic Acid	Lysine
Cysteine	Methionine
Glumatic Acid	Phenylalanine
Glutamine	Threonine
Glycine	Tryptophan
Proline	Valine
Serine	
Tyrosine	

These essential substrates must be eaten regularly for the manufacture or repair of protein tissues such as blood, bone, muscles and most body tissues. The main sources of protein are meat and dairy products, so a vegan will have to be more selective in choosing the different types of protein that will complement or act as alternatives for these essential amino acids. In many cases, dietary supplements are necessary since B-12 is essential to form red blood cells and perform other metabolic activities. Deficiency can lead to certain diseases including serious anemic conditions.

Complete and incomplete proteins. Protein foods also are classified as complete or incomplete. **Complete proteins** come from animal sources such as meat and dairy products and contain all 20 or more amino acids. **Incomplete proteins** are missing some essential amino acids and are not the best quality protein. Since humans are an animal species, proteins from animal sources contain the essential amino acids that we need to build and repair new animal tissues. Vegetable proteins are incomplete proteins because they do not contain all the essential acids humans need to build new tissue. The latest research suggests that the only complete vegetable protein is soy protein. Egg white is considered a complete protein since it has been found to be one of the most complete and digestible proteins. Therefore, it is used as a standard for measuring protein quality and is assigned a score of 100. The quality of other food proteins is determined based on how they measure up against egg protein. It often is used to measure the quality of other proteins. However, one egg yolk contains approximately 200 mg cholesterol, and nutritionists recommend that consumption should be limited to two-to-three times per week to avoid high cholesterol intake.

Complementary proteins. For the vegan who does not eat meat, the most common deficiencies include nutrients such as iron, zinc, calcium, B-12 and vitamin D. Therefore, it is necessary to carefully select foods that provide essential amino acids. **Complementary proteins** refer to using two or more proteins that balance each other so that the essential amino acids missing from one group will be supplied by the other. Other meat alternatives include beans, nuts, legumes, soy foods, dairy products or eggs to balance the daily protein intake.

Legumes are plants from the bean and pea family and are high quality protein compared to other plant foods. They come in dried or pre-cooked forms and include beans—black, white, kidney, lima, navy, garbanzo; peas—yellow and green split peas; and lentils. They contain high amounts of the amino acids isoleucine and lysine, but are low in methionine and tryptophan. Grains have the opposite strength and weakness, so matching both legumes and grains result in all the essential amino acids needed to support healthy protein synthesis. An example of using complementary proteins is combining whole grains with legumes—eggs with soybeans or rice with beans.

Health benefits of proteins. High protein intake is associated with high fat that, in turn, is positively correlated with heart disease. However, if chosen carefully, a person can eat a healthy high protein and low fat diet. Animal proteins tend to be high in saturated fats while plant proteins generally are low in fat. Recently, soy protein has been accepted by the United States Food and Drug Administration (FDA) as a complete protein, therefore substituting soy or alternative proteins for animal protein can help reduce intake of saturated fats. However, not all soy foods are low fat, so food labels must be checked carefully before making a purchase.

The building blocks of proteins. The amino acids used to build the structure of the body are analogous to cement blocks used in constructing the walls of a building. All essential amino acids are required to build good quality body tissues. The type of protein manufactured is determined by the genetic blueprint—**DNA**—of the cell. Within the cell, the organelle called the **ribosome** can be viewed as the manufacturing plant where the various amino acids are brought by the **tRNA**—messenger cells—to build the desired protein. The sequence of building blocks of amino acids takes place in the ribosomes, and when the peptide or polypeptide chain is built to the specific configuration of that particular protein, it is released in the cytoplasm and transported by the bloodstream that carries it to the tissues in need.

Enzymes

Enzymes are some of the most important proteins produced by living cells and are essential for all chemical reactions within the body. Without them, the human body will not function. They are biological catalysts—speeding up reactions in cells without themselves being affected, and setting off a chain of reactions, or **metabolic effect**. There are thousands of enzymes in every cell, each having a special action—some for digestion, others to release energy from stored supplies and to stimulate the growth and repair of new tissues. Many enzymes can be recognized by the ending *-ase*, such as **lactase**. Lactase acts on lactose, or milk sugar, in the stomach for digestion, and **lipase** breaks down fats into fatty acids and glycerol. The human body needs enzymes to extract energy from nutrients such as carbohydrates for healthy functioning. There are three parts of an enzyme reaction: a **substrate**, the **enzyme** and the resulting **product**. For example, in the digestive process, the substrate can be fats, the enzyme, lipase, and the resulting product, fatty acids and glycerol.

Digestive enzymes. Digestion is one of the most vital processes for good health, and digestive dysfunction can be caused by stress-related diseases such as anxiety and depression. During stress, excessive amounts of hydrochloric acid (HCL) are produced in the stomach which disrupts normal pH. **Proteolytic enzymes** break down proteins into amino acids, each one working on a specific protein. Although enzymes are manufactured in the human body, they also are obtained from food. They are active in raw foods, but cooking kills them. Therefore dietary enzymes from raw vegetables and fruits should be included as part of a healthy diet. As we age, enzyme production is reduced affecting the digestion of nutrients, so regular consumption of digestive enzymatic foods can act as an anti-aging strategy.

Coenzymes. Enzymes need **coenzymes** to help release energy from carbohydrates, proteins and fats and, in many cases, energy cannot be released from any foods unless these coenzymes are present in the body. Most water-soluble vitamins and certain minerals, such as vitamin B and zinc, act as coenzymes.

Enzyme therapy. Eating natural foods rich in enzymes, coenzymes and cofactors can help improve digestion. Their detoxifying effects help to reduce inflammatory conditions and toxins associated with cellulite, rosacea and premenstrual symptoms. However, some people lack certain enzymes or their bodies do not produce them, so many health practitioners advise the use of dietary enzymes in the form of supplements to treat digestive disorders such as bloating, gas or diarrhea. Enzyme supplements such as lactase or **cellulase** now are available in predigested foods to improve digestion and prevent digestive disorders. These supplements should be taken a half hour before or after meals since they may be inactivated by inhibitors in foods that are eaten. Those with medical conditions should check with their physicians before embarking on enzyme supplements.

Enzymes and skin care. In skin analysis, skin congestion is a common disorder that may be noted by the esthetician. One probable cause of skin congestion can be improper digestion. Natural enzymes or dietary skin supplements can help reduce bloating, gas and diarrhea that may be associated with this condition. Enzymes also are used as catalysts in topical applications of skin care products to "digest" the dead superficial cells of the skin. Many skin care manufacturers utilize enzymes in their products from either natural, biological sources such as papain, bromelain and pumpkin, and animal-derived sources such as lactase, or milk acid, and pancreatic enzymes from sheep. Also, chemical peels utilize enzymes to break down the chemical bonds that hold the skin cells together in the strateum corneum. The result is a fresher, smoother, younger-looking skin.

Protein needs

Research indicates that American women consume approximately 60-65 grams of protein instead of the 45–50 grams a day while young males eat about 100 grams instead of the average 60–65 grams per day, dropping to about 75 grams in their older years. Since every individual has different body mass and energy needs, nutritionists recommend that daily protein intake should be approximately 15–20% of total daily calorie intake. However, this equation cannot be applied to those suffering from disease, illness or eating disorders. If the person is an athlete, works out rigorously or suffers from constant stress, that person's body needs a higher supply of energy, or **adenosine triphosphate** (ATP), a compound of high energy, and more protein intake is required to meet the demands of the body. Recommended daily protein intake can be found by converting the weight to kilograms by dividing it by 2.2 and using this simple conversion: weight (in kg) x 0.8.

The excess fat found in high protein foods can lead to obesity. Protein overload can result in **acidosis**, excess acids in blood, dehydration, diarrhea, gout, fever and high urea concentrations in the blood. Deficiencies include growth abnormalities such as stunted growth, poor skin healing or repair, and atrophy of body tissues. Waste products of protein metabolism include urea, uric acid and creatinine.

It would be remiss not to mention the popularity of high protein/low carbohydrate diet fads. While these methods tend to be a quick fix for losing weight, it is recommended that to both lose and maintain a healthy weight, the healthy living lifestyle professed in this book should be followed.

Carbohydrates

Animals and plants rely on the sun for life processes. Plants absorb the sun's energy through a chemical process called photosynthesis, and together with water and carbon dioxide, manufacture carbohydrates, proteins and fats. In the process, oxygen is released in the air. Animals breathe in the oxygen, eat the plants and through the body's metabolic processes, convert plants back into carbon dioxide, water and energy. Most of the world's population relies on carbohydrates as their main food source for energy. Except for milk, the most significant source of carbohydrates in protein foods, carbohydrates are obtained almost exclusively from plants.

Metabolism is the process of life—burning blood sugar to produce energy. In fact, approximately two-thirds of the body's energy comes from glucose, the final breakdown of carbohydrates in the body. The brain needs glucose to function at the beginning of the day. That is one reason why breakfast is the most important meal of the day because without glucose, brain cells are deprived of nutrients. This is why you can feel dizzy, irritable or lacking concentration if breakfast is missed. Carbohydrates are classified as **simple carbohydrates** consisting of sugars, and **complex carbohydrates** composed of starches and fibers.

Simple carbohydrates. When taken into the body, carbohydrates are broken down by enzymes into monosaccharides to be absorbed in the GI tract. Simple carbohydrates appear as monosaccharides and disaccharides. **Monosaccharides** appear in three different forms: glucose, fructose and galactose. (See **Figure 2-3**.)

Although all three monosaccharides have the same chemical formula ($C_6H_{12}O_6$), their atoms are arranged differently, giving rise to various physical and chemical properties such as sweetness. In nature, the most common sugars are **glucose** and **fructose**, the sweetest, found naturally in fruits and honey and appearing as high fructose corn syrup in commercial products. **Galactose** is the sugar from milk. But all carbohydrates are broken down in their final stage to glucose before they are absorbed in the GI tract. In the mouth, simple carbohydrates are broken down into maltose, which consists of two glucose molecules, so they immediately are absorbed into the bloodstream for quick energy.

Disaccharides, or double sugars, contain glucose that is bonded with one of the other monosaccharides. (See **Figure 2-4**.)

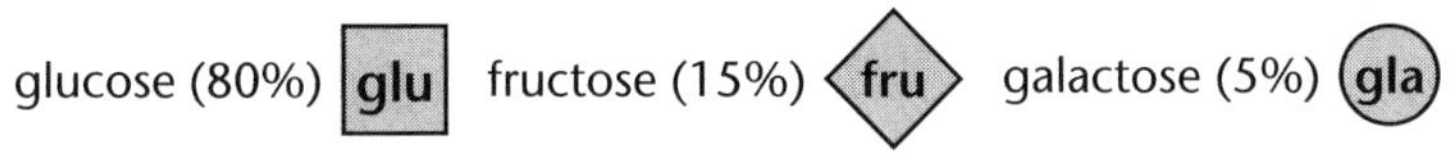

glucose (80%) **glu** fructose (15%) **fru** galactose (5%) **gla**

Figure 2-3: Monosaccharides.

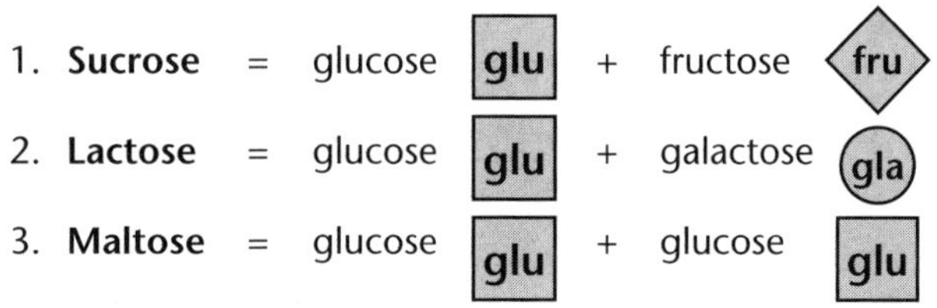

1. **Sucrose** = glucose **glu** + fructose **fru**
2. **Lactose** = glucose **glu** + galactose **gla**
3. **Maltose** = glucose **glu** + glucose **glu**

Figure 2-4: Disaccharides.

Note that glucose is found in every sugar and, during digestion, all carbohydrates in their final form have to be broken down to glucose for absorption into the blood stream. Except for lactose and its component galactose, all other sugars come from plants.

Sucrose—**Sucrose** is the sweetest of the disaccharides because it contains fructose and is found in all fruits, vegetables, grains and most sweets. Depending on how much it is refined, sucrose is produced from the juices of sugar cane and beets, and is further processed to become the familiar brown, white or powdered sugars seen in supermarkets.

Lactose—As the main sugar in milk, **lactose** is split by the enzyme lactase into glucose and galactose during digestion in the stomach. It helps to absorb calcium and promotes the growth of healthy bacteria in the intestines. Lactose is found in breast milk and infants' formulas and provides a simple, easily digestible food for babies. Many people do not digest lactose well, and two common reactions include lactase intolerance and milk allergy.

Lactose intolerance refers to the inability to digest milk sugars resulting in various symptoms such as nausea, bloating, abdominal cramps, diarrhea or excessive gas after drinking or eating any milk products. The enzyme lactase may be lacking or can become dysfunctional among the elderly and certain ethnic groups such as African-Americans, Native-Americans, Asians and some Mediterranean populations. Since milk is a significant source for important nutrients such as calcium, vitamin D and riboflavin, some foods containing predigested enzymes or fermented products have been formulated to reduce discomfort for those suffering from lactase intolerance. This includes acidophilus milk, yogurt and aged cheeses.

Milk allergy is different from lactose intolerance. It is a reaction to milk products resulting in the production of antibodies to increase the body's immunity.

Maltose—**Maltose** consists of two glucose units and is produced from the final breakdown of carbohydrates such as wheat, barley or oats. When fermented, maltose can yield alcohol.

Sugar and health. It has been scientifically proven that foods high in sugar increase insulin blood levels and are harmful to those suffering from diabetes and **hyperglycemia**. It is believe by some scientists that inflamed conditions such as these produce high levels of **free radicals**. Because of this, less free radicals should be produced by reducing the dietary intake of high sugary foods. In recent years, some scientists hypothesize that free radicals, the destructive forces of cells, are first initiated by inflammation that develops within the tissues. In other words, free radicals can be prevented by reducing the dietary intake of sugary foods, particularly in the presence of certain inflammatory conditions such as arthritis and premenstrual syndrome (PMS). Many sugary foods also contain a high proportion of fat and are associated with obesity, heart disease and dental tissue infections.

Sugar and obesity. In recent years, the obesity rate has risen significantly among both adults and children, and scientists are beginning to believe that there is a positive correlation between obesity and high blood sugar levels. Naturally occurring sugars are found in milk and fruits. Data surveys show that high consumption of **added sugars** are correlated to obesity. The body cannot distinguish between naturally occurring sugars and added sugars that are eaten separately or found in processed foods. Commercial forms include white or brown sugar, malt syrup, corn syrup solids, maple syrup, honey and molasses found in soft drinks, pastries and ice cream. The largest source of added sugars in the North American diet is soft drinks, also labeled as "empty calories." Since school children drink soft drinks with many of their meals, health experts are trying to reveal if there is a positive correlation between added dietary sugars and childhood obesity.

When combined with caffeine, sugars can have detrimental effects on mood, PMS and other health-related conditions. It is best to curb strong cravings for sweets with simple sugars such as fruits or unsweetened foods instead of concentrated sweets such as candies, sweet pastries or soft drinks. Furthermore, fruits also contain large amounts of water, fiber, vitamins and minerals, while honey, table sugar and desserts actually have no extra nutrients. Learn to recognize clues for sugar on food labels. For example, if the first words listed on food labels include sucrose, dextrose, fructose or syrup, it indicates high sugar levels. The Dietary Guidelines urge people to choose foods and drinks that limit sugar intake, keeping sugar to no more than 10% of total daily calories.

Artificial sweeteners. After extensive research into sweeteners that don't add extra calories, the FDA approved **saccharin**, **aspartame**, **acesulfame potassium (acesulfame-k)** and **sucralose** to help reduce consumers' intake of sugar. Though helpful, large quantities of artificial sweeteners cannot be consumed either, as excessive intake can have toxic effects. There is still a great deal of controversy about these various sugar alternatives.

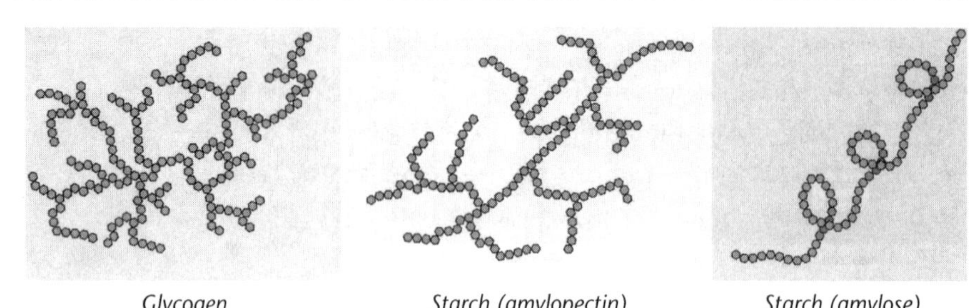

Figure 2-5: The multiple strands of a starch molecule. From Understanding Nutrition (with Dietary Reference Intakes Supplement and InfoTrac) 9th edition by WHITNEY/ROLFES. © 2002. Reprinted with permission of Brooks/Cole, a division of Thomson Learning: www.thomsonrights.com. Fax 800-730-2215.

Complex carbohydrates

Complex carbohydrates are composed of polysaccharides that are broken down by enzymes to monosaccharides for absorption in the GI tract. There are two types—**starch** and **fiber**.

Starch. The starch in plants consists of hundreds of thousands of glucose molecules linked by chemical bonds. For example, one cubic inch of food may consist of a million molecules of starch. When humans consume plants, various enzymes in the GI tract break down the starch molecules into glucose units for absorption. Excess glucose is stored in the liver and skeletal muscles in the form of **glycogen**. When blood sugar levels are low, the stored glycogen is converted back into glucose by certain hormones and shipped to the bloodstream and muscles for immediate use. (See **Figure 2-5**.)

Grains and nutrition. Most of the world's population depends on grains, the richest source of starch. Grains are such a large portion of the daily diet because they are the basis of so many products made from wheat such as bread, cereal and pasta. The staple grains in different countries vary depending on factors such as climate and soil. For example, the major grain grown in North America and Europe is wheat, rice in Asia, corn in Central and South America, and millet, rye, barley and oats in other countries. Common grains include rye, oats, barley and buckwheat. Other significant sources are legumes and tubers—potatoes and yams.

The role of grains in dietary intake often is misunderstood by the health professional. This would be remedied with more understanding on the structure of grains and how the manufacturing process of natural foods affects its

Terminology of Processed Foods

Following are explanations of the terminology of commercially processed foods and their meanings.

Refined—The manufacturing process by which the coarse parts of the food are removed. For example, the refining of wheat involves the removal of the husk, bran and germ, leaving only the endosperm.

Enriched—Vitamins and minerals are added back because the nutrients such as the B vitamins and iron may have been lost during the refining process.

Fortified—Extra nutrients such as vitamin D, calcium and folate are added to prevent the deficiency of a nutrient.

nutrient value. For example, it was discovered in the early twentieth century that the customary practice of removing the germ and the bran in East Asia resulted in the loss of **thiamin**, or vitamin B-1, found in that part of the grain. This deficiency led to a skin disease called beri-beri that damaged the nervous system, heart and muscles. In addition, scientists found that light rays such as ultraviolet or fluorescent lamps can destroy **riboflavin**, or vitamin B-2, in grains. As a result, milk, a rich source of riboflavin, is no longer provided in transparent glass containers in many countries.

Structure of the wheat plant. With the exception of the husk that is used for animal feed and not for human consumption, **whole grain** refers to that which is milled, but not refined. (For definitions, see **Terminology of Processed Foods**.)

A whole grain has four main parts—the germ, endosperm, bran and husk. The **germ** is the nutritious inner part of the grain where cells develop and grow; the **endosperm** is the soft, inner part that is eaten, and contains starch and protein; the **bran** is the fibrous protective part, rich in nutrients and the main source of fiber; and the **husk**, or chaff, is not used for human consumption, only for animal feed. (See **Figure 2-6**.)

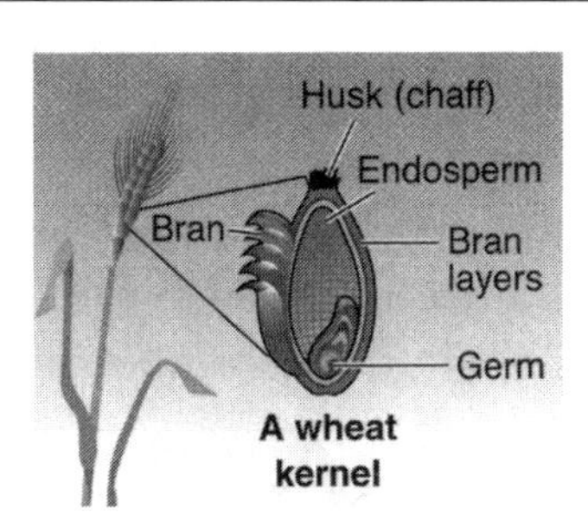

Figure 2-6: *Different parts of a whole grain. From Personal Nutrition (with InfoTrac) 4th Edition by Boyle. © 2001. Reprinted with permission of Brooks/Cole, a division of Thomson Learning: www.thomasonrights.com. Fax 800-730-2215.*

Fiber

Fibers form the structures of plants and are non-starchy and indigestible. Most fibers cannot be broken down by enzymes so they do not contribute energy to the body, but in recent years fiber has become recognized as having significant health benefits.

Benefits. The benefits of fiber include a reduction in high blood cholesterol levels, a feeling of satiety contributing to weight loss, an increase in the regularity of bowel movements, prevention of constipation, and aid in the prevention of colon cancer.

Classification of fibers. Depending on certain properties and their solubility in water, fiber can be classified as either soluble or insoluble. As food enters the GI tract, **soluble fiber** in foods swell with water forming a gelatinous mass. This bulk pushes against the walls of the digestive tract giving a feeling of satiety. Soluble fibers play an important role in reducing high blood cholesterol levels by binding to cholesterol and bile acids in the GI tract eventually leaving the body through feces.

Insoluble fibers are indigestible and increase bulk leading to quick satiety. They soften stools, increase speed and frequency of bowel movements, and reduce the risk of colon cancers. Insoluble fiber helps in preventing constipation, **hemorrhoids**—swollen veins that occur in walls of rectum from forceful expelling of feces—and **diverticulitis**—inflammation of small sacs in intestinal walls that trap feces leading to cancer.

Sufficient fiber intake. A high protein diet often is low in enzymes and fiber that can lead to digestive disorders such as constipation, diarrhea and bloating. These conditions are indicators of a low fiber diet and can lead to hard, painful bowel movements. On the skin's surface, fiber deficiency can appear in the form of a congested, unhealthy skin pallor or complexion. Research indicates that the average American consumes 11–17 grams of fiber instead of the recommended 20–40 grams per day. A good source of fiber can be recognized if it contains at least 2 to 5 grams per serving. Sufficient water must be taken with fiber foods to soften stools for easier passage through the digestive tract. It is recommended to drink an 8-oz. glass of water before and after meals to improve digestion, absorption and elimination of toxins. Eating more raw foods containing natural enzymes to break down food for easier digestion also is recommended. Health care experts highly recommend eating a variety of foods to obtain maximum benefits of both types of fibers.

Different fibers. Fibers have different chemical structures and properties leading to diverse health effects. The most common fibers include the following.

Cellulose—The main constituent of the walls of plant cells, **cellulose** consists of long chains of glucose molecules. They are indigestible and are found in all vegetables, fruits and legumes. Rich sources of cellulose are oats, especially oat bran, barley, apples, pears, cabbage, broccoli, and a variety of legumes and nuts.

Hemicellulose—Mainly found in cereals with branching side chains of monosaccharides, **hemicellulose** can be either soluble or insoluble.

Pectins—Found in skin and rinds of vegetables and fruits, especially apples, carrots and oranges, **pectins**' gel-forming properties help in reducing blood cholesterol and bile acids in the body. Most people are familiar with pectin as a thickener and preservative agent used in the making of jams.

Gums and mucilages—These are gummy parts that exude from plants when cut. Examples include **gum arabic** used as additives in foods and **guar gum** which acts as a stabilizer in the food industry.

Lignin—Tough, woody parts of vegetables and seeds of fruits, the **lignins** found in flaxseed help reduce cholesterol and the risk of colon cancer.

Summary of health benefits of fiber. The typical American diet consists of high intakes of refined carbohydrates, saturated fats, processed foods, salt and cholesterol, and a very low average daily fiber intake of 11–17 grams. The National Cancer Institute recommends an optimal intake of 20–30 grams daily, and anti-aging health practitioners advise even more—25–40 grams a day. Furthermore, many people do not have much knowledge about which foods contain fiber, so advising clients to check the fiber content of the foods they purchase can help educate them. Urge consumers to maintain a daily fiber intake of 20–40 grams to maximize good health and longevity.

Disadvantages of high fiber diet. One disadvantage of a high fiber diet is the risk of losing certain important minerals from the body. A compound called **phytic acid** found in some cereal grains and legumes binds with minerals such as iron, zinc and calcium, excreting them from the body.

RDA for carbohydrates

Health authorities recommend that the daily intake of carbohydrates should be approximately 50–60% of total daily calories and dietary fiber should be 20–40 grams from complex carbohydrates, or unprocessed whole foods.

Deficiencies

Since carbohydrates form the main portion of daily food intake for most people, deficiency only occurs in conditions such as low carbohydrate diets, malnutrition and starvation conditions such as anorexia nervosa. Since the brain uses carbohydrates as its main fuel, the first symptoms of deficiency are dizziness and headaches. Excessive intake leads to the conversion of carbohydrates into fat stored in adipose tissues. Waste products include carbon dioxide and water.

More on fats

The body needs a certain amount of fats to maintain the healthy functioning of cell membranes, fat-soluble vitamins and other tissues including adipotic cells. Fats are broken down by digestive enzymes to fatty acids and glycerol before being absorbed in the intestinal tract. Due to the established positive correlation between dietary fats and chronic diseases, a greater portion on the discussion of fats has been allocated to this section. The type of fats as well as the amount of various types of fats is important to differentiate **triglycerides** which form 95% of fats found in the human body and foods, and **phospholipids** and **sterols** which form the other 5%.

Chemical structure of fatty acids. In order to understand the function of fats in the body, it is important to review briefly the chemical structure of fats. A fatty acid is a unit of fat composed of a number of carbon atoms bonded together with attached hydrogen atoms. It has an acid group (COOH) at one end and a methyl group (CH_2) at the other end.

The simplest and shortest fatty acid is **acetic acid**—a compound containing only two carbons giving vinegar its sour taste. A triglyceride contains one molecule of glycerol (See **Figure 2-7**) and three molecules of fatty acids. (See **Figure 2-8**, page 27.)

3-Carbon Chain Hydroxyl Group

```
      H
      |
  H - C - O - H
      |
  H - C - O - H
      |
  H - C - O - H
      |
      H
```

Figure 2-7: Glycerol molecule.

Fatty acids are hydrocarbon chains of even numbers of carbon atoms, up to 24, but of different lengths—chains range from short and medium to long. (See **Figure 2-9**, page 27.)

A common example of a long chain fatty acid chain, composed of 18 carbons, is **stearic acid** found in all animal fats. It commonly is used as an emulsifier or

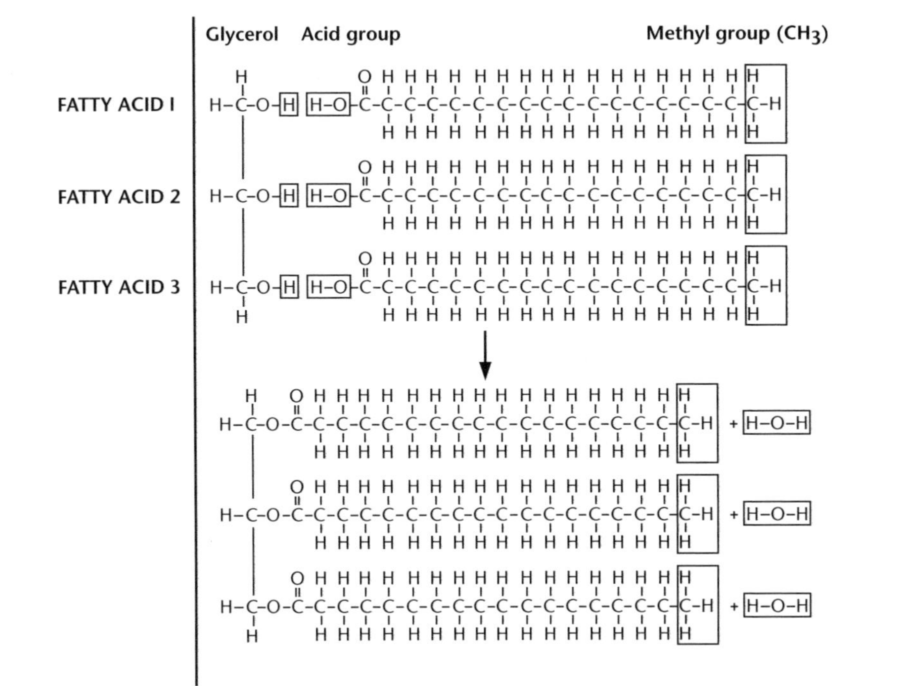

Figure 2-8: A triglyceride: a molecule of glycerol and three fatty acids. From Personal Nutrition (with InfoTrac) 4th Edition by Boyle. © 2001. Reprinted with permission of Brooks/Cole, a division of Thomson Learning: www.thomasonrights.com. Fax 800-730-2215.

stabilizer in the manufacture of cosmetics. (See **Figure 2-10**, page 28.)

Short chains, found in dairy products, are broken down quicker than longer chains, but the longer chains, found in meat and fish, nutritionally are more important because they contain the essential fatty acids omega-3 and omega-6. They are not made in the body and therefore have to be taken into the body.

Saturated and unsaturated fats. Fatty acids either are satu-

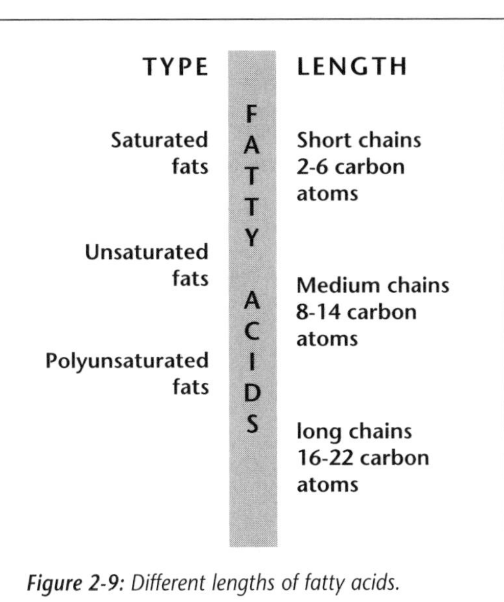

***Figure 2-9:** Different lengths of fatty acids.*

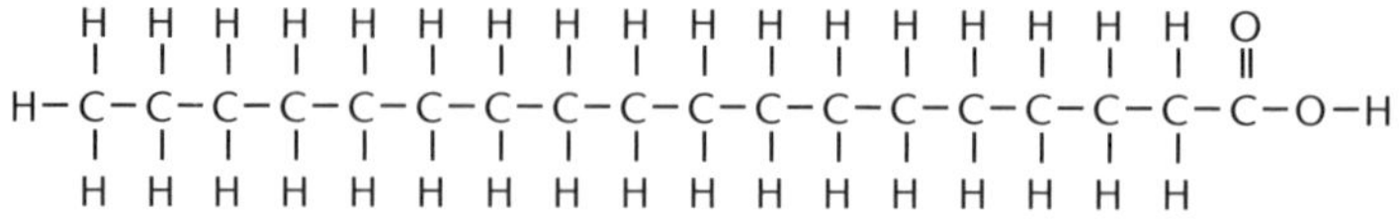

```
    H H H H H H H H H H H H H H H H H O
    | | | | | | | | | | | | | | | | | ‖
  H-C-C-C-C-C-C-C-C-C-C-C-C-C-C-C-C-C-C-O-H
    | | | | | | | | | | | | | | | | |
    H H H H H H H H H H H H H H H H H
```

Figure 2-10: Stearic acid—a long chain fatty acid.

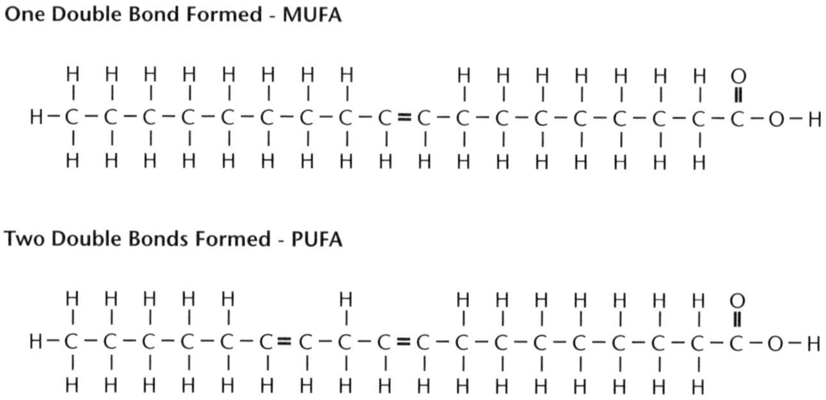

One Double Bond Formed - MUFA

```
    H H H H H H H H     H H H H H H H O
    | | | | | | | |     | | | | | | | ‖
  H-C-C-C-C-C-C-C-C-C=C-C-C-C-C-C-C-C-C-O-H
    | | | | | | | | | | | | | | | | |
    H H H H H H H H H H H H H H H H H
```

Two Double Bonds Formed - PUFA

```
    H H H H H   H     H H H H H H H O
    | | | | |   |     | | | | | | | ‖
  H-C-C-C-C-C-C=C-C-C=C-C-C-C-C-C-C-C-C-O-H
    | | | | | | | | | | | | | | | | |
    H H H H H H H H H H H H H H H H H
```

Figure 2-11: MUFA and PUFA molecule.

rated or unsaturated. (See **Characteristics of Saturated and Unsaturated Fats**, page 29.) Nature requires that every carbon atom must be fully loaded or saturated. The carbon atom has six electrons, two in the first orbit and four in the outer orbit that need to be stabilized or saturated. A **saturated fat** is formed if all carbon atoms in the chain are fully loaded with hydrogen atoms. An **unsaturated fat** results when carbons in the fatty acid have one or more hydrogen atoms missing so that there are points of unsaturation. Single, double or triple bonds develop as a result to stabilize the molecule of fatty acid. (See **Figure 2-11**.)

Trans fatty acids. Trans fatty acids are the result of the chemical process of **hydrogenation** used to convert unsaturated fats to a more solid form in order to reduce susceptibility to rancidity. An example of this is the conversion of vegetable oils to a solid form, such as margarine. The process reduces the number of double bonds making the fats more solid and more resistant to

Characteristics of Saturated and Unsaturated Fats

Characteristics of saturated fats

- Usually hard at room temperature.
- Have a high melting point.
- Bonds are more difficult to break and change physically.
- Mainly derived from animal sources—meat and dairy products.
- Also found in certain vegetable sources such as palm and coconut oils, the only saturated fats from plants that are liquid at room temperature.
- Other than cholesterol, it is the contributing factor in foods that elevates high blood cholesterol.
- Most people tend to eat more saturated fats than unsaturated fats in their diets.

Characteristics of unsaturated fats

- Either *monounsaturated* (MUFA) or *polyunsaturated* (PUFA).
- Low melting point and are liquid at room temperature.
- Mainly are derived from vegetable oils—MUFAs are found in olive, canola and peanut oils, and PUFAs are found in all other vegetable oils.
- MUFA is healthier than PUFA because there is only one double bond in MUFA so it is less likely to oxidize or become rancid. Since PUFA is unstable and thus more susceptible to oxidation, it may contribute in forming free radicals.

oxidation. It has been shown to reduce its nutrient value and change its texture. Studies have indicated that hydrogenated fats are just as harmful as saturated fats to the body's health. Trans fatty acids recently have gained more attention in nutritional circles because health experts are concerned about the increased health risks of these fats, particularly with the obesity epidemic. New regulations for food labels require the manufacturer to now list the trans fatty acids under the saturated fats content.

Cholesterol. Lipids also include sterols, the best known one being **cholesterol**, a sterol fat produced in the liver and found only in animal foods. Although it forms a part of every cell, the amount and type found in the bloodstream either can be beneficial or detrimental to health. **Dietary cholesterol** is found in foods while **blood cholesterol** is the result of the liver manufacturing cholesterol. Blood cholesterol levels also are increased from the dietary intake of saturated fats. It is important to recognize that some cholesterol is essential for good health because it serves as substrates for the manufacture of bile for digestion of fat; manufacture of hormones including most steroids; production of vitamin D in the skin—a derivative of cholesterol reacting with sunlight; and formation of part of the structural lipid component of cell membranes, nerves and the brain. In fact, without cholesterol, the brain's neurotransmitters would not work.

Cholesterol and cardiovascular diseases. **Heart disease** is the leading cause of death today with a strong link to high blood cholesterol levels. It is the number one killer among certain ethnic groups such as African-Americans. Poor lifestyle habits such as heavy smoking and high blood pressure contribute to the damage of the **endothelial cells**, the thin inner layer of arterial walls. **Platelets** in the area become stickier forming clots that grow into arterial walls clogging the width of the artery. Platelets form macrophages that eat the debris and low density lipoprotein cholesterol become overloaded and die forming **foam cells**. They eventually become calcified forming a buildup of plaque, narrowing the width of arterial walls, and preventing oxygen and nutrients from easily passing through. The result of all this buildup is the hardening of the arterial walls, or **artherosclerosis**, which can lead to stroke and heart attacks. This build up of plaque is not visible, so even some young, healthy individuals have died from cardiovascular diseases such as stroke. Blood cannot get to the kidneys leading to kidney failure and other related diseases. This phenomenon is referred to as the "silent killer." It is estimated that every 1% reduction of high blood cholesterol levels reduces the risks of heart attacks by 2–3%.

Therefore, if there is a family history of high blood cholesterol and heart disease, there is a more important reason to practice positive lifestyle behaviors such as a good diet and regular exercise. Reducing risk factors can minimize cardiovascular diseases and contribute toward good health and longevity.

Homocysteine and heart disease. Recent studies have uncovered another biomarker for heart disease. **Homocysteine** is a substance that develops during protein metabolism and high levels have been linked with heart disease, particularly among postmenopausal women. During protein metabolism, sufficient amounts of specific B vitamins, namely B-6, B-12 and folate, must be available for homocysteine to convert to the amino acid methionine. If these co-factors are not present, this conversion cannot take place resulting in high homocysteine levels. Researchers believe that the presence of homocysteine contributes toward the occurrence of strokes and heart attacks. By simply increasing dietary intake of these B vitamins, the risk of heart disease can be removed. Vitamin B-6 is found in meat, whole grains and legumes; B-12 is derived from meat and fortified foods; and folate is found in all green, leafy vegetables and fortified foods. (See **Risk Factors for Heart Disease**, page 31.)

Risk Factors for Heart Disease

- Family history of heart disease.
- Age—men over age 45 and women over 55 who are not using estrogen replacement therapy.
- High blood pressure, or hypertension.
- High blood cholesterol (> 200 mg/dL).
- High LDL cholesterol (>130 mg/dL).
- Low HDL cholesterol (<35 mg/dL).
- Smoking and alcohol consumption.
- Sedentary lifestyle.
- Obesity.
- Diabetes.

Understanding the blood cholesterol test. Significant cholesterol levels are risk factors for heart disease. When getting blood test results from an annual physical examination, the blood profile usually indicates total triglycerides, cholesterol and various lipoproteins. While the total blood cholesterol levels are listed, it does not give important details about the levels of low density lipoprotein and high density lipoprotein blood cholesterol nor the ratio between total blood cholesterol and HDL levels. Blood cholesterol tests are measured differently in the United States, Canada and other countries. It is important to learn how to interpret the test results. Each individual is different; the physician will decide the right individualized levels after taking into account the patient's age, sex and other risk factors. In the United States, the results are expressed in milligrams per deciliter (mg/dL) while in countries using the metric system such as Canada, they are expressed in millimoles per liter (mmol/L). (See **Interpreting Cholesterol Levels**, page 32.)

What does it mean? If your cholesterol levels are normal, congratulations! Try to maintain this level. You probably inherited good genes, but you must reduce any risk factors if you practice any negative lifestyle behaviors. If your personal history includes smoking, high blood pressure, obesity or a sedentary lifestyle, you should adopt or maintain a low fat dietary intake, particularly low saturated fats, exercise regularly and minimize smoking. If you are borderline, you are at risk for a heart attack and need to change your lifestyle behaviors. For many people, simple dietary changes and improving lifestyle behaviors can bring them back to the normal range. The high risk group needs to seek qualified help. For some people, high cholesterol levels are genetic and dietary changes

Interpreting Cholesterol Levels

The table below signifies what is desirable for a healthy blood cholesterol profile.

United States

Age	*Normal*	*Borderline*	*High Risk*
30 years+	**(mg/dL)**	**(mg/dL)**	**(mg/dL)**
Total cholesterol	<200	200-400	400+
LDL cholesterol	<130	130+	
HDL cholesterol	35+	<35	
Triglyceride	<200	200+	
18–29 years			
Total cholesterol	<180	180–220	220+
LDL cholesterol	<115	115+	220+
HDL cholesterol	35+	<35	
Triglyceride	<200	200+	

Canada and other countries

30 years+	**(mmol/L)**	**(mmol/L)**	**(mmol/L)**
Total cholesterol	<5.2	5.2–6.2	6.2+
LDL cholesterol	<2-6	3.4+	
HDL cholesterol	0.9+	<0.9	
Triglyceride	<2-3	2-3+	
18–29 years			
Total cholesterol	<4.7	4.7–5.7	5.7+
LDL cholesterol	<3.0	3.0+	
HDL cholesterol	0.9+	<0.9	
Triglyceride	<2-3	2-3+	

< not less than

> not more than

+ and more

Adapted from Heart and Stroke Foundation, Canada, 1997

will not be effective, so physicians may want to prescribe drug therapy. However, it is far better to control blood cholesterol levels with lifestyle modifications rather than drug therapy. To understand how blood cholesterol levels form, take a closer look at how lipids are processed and absorbed in the body.

Fat distribution and absorption. During the digestive process, fats are emulsified by bile from the liver and broken down by lipase enzymes to monoglycerides and fatty acids for absorption in the intestinal cells. The shorter chains of fatty acids are water soluble to some extent and enter the capillaries going directly to the liver where they are rearranged and sent out to the bloodstream. The larger molecules such as cholesterol, long chain fatty acids and phospholipids are insoluble in water and take longer to digest. They are repackaged in the intestinal cells into special transport vehicles called **lipoproteins** that distribute triglycerides and fatty acids to body tissues via the lymphatic system.

Lipoproteins. These unique carriers are water-soluble proteins with cholesterol arranged on the outside. In this way, they can transport fats in body liquids to all tissue cells. The more lipids they carry, the lower the density; the less lipids, the higher the density. Therefore, **low density lipoprotein** (LDL) vessels carry more lipids and are less dense while **high density lipoprotein** (HDL) vessels carry the least amount of fats and cholesterol. There are four types of lipoproteins, and they are classified by their size as well as the amount of proteins and lipids they carry. (See **Figure 2-12**, page 34.)

Chylomicrons—As the largest and least dense lipoproteins, **chylomicrons** carry a large amount of triglycerides. From the intestinal cells, they bypass the liver carrying the triglycerides directly into the lymphatic system, onward through the heart and finally to body tissues. As the triglycerides are given out, the chylomicrons become smaller and smaller until only little bits of protein and lipids are left in the bloodstream. Their remnants finally are removed by protein receptors in the liver and repackaged into new triglycerides.

Very Low Density Lipoprotein (VLDL)—**Very low density lipoproteins** leave the liver carrying mainly triglycerides packaged by the liver to body tissues where they are needed. As the triglycerides are given out, the lipoprotein becomes denser, carrying more cholesterol than triglycerides, and becomes LDL.

Low Density Lipoprotein (LDL)—LDLs carry high cholesterol made in the liver to build membranes, hormones and other compounds, and delivers them to body cells that have LDL receptors. Any excess cholesterol left in the bloodstream is referred to as **bad cholesterol**. It is susceptible to oxidative processes forming free radicals and contributing to arteriosclerosis.

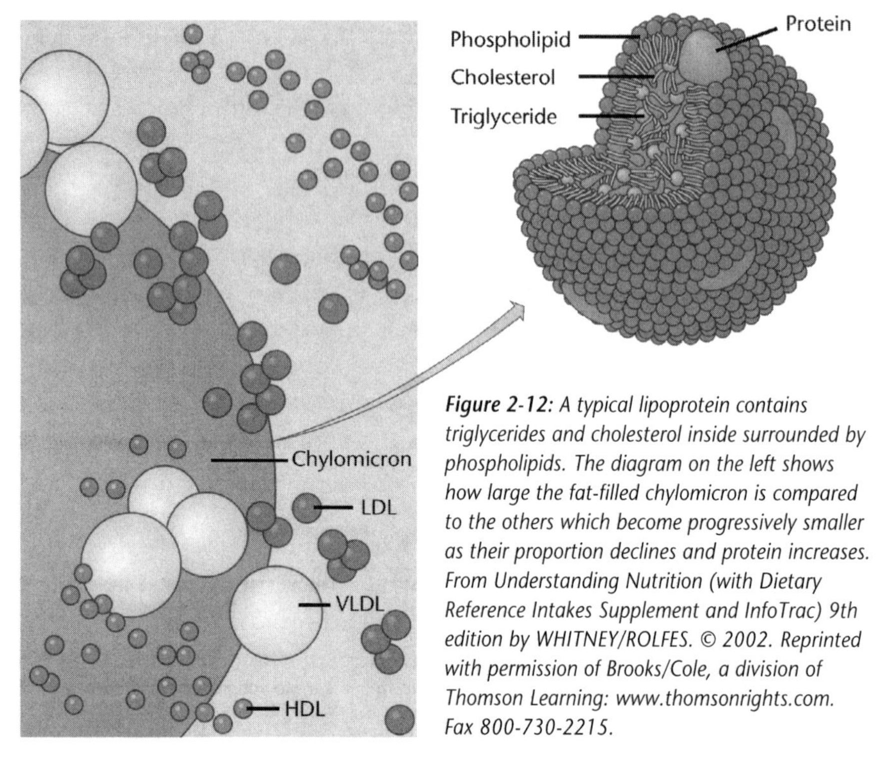

Figure 2-12: *A typical lipoprotein contains triglycerides and cholesterol inside surrounded by phospholipids. The diagram on the left shows how large the fat-filled chylomicron is compared to the others which become progressively smaller as their proportion declines and protein increases. From Understanding Nutrition (with Dietary Reference Intakes Supplement and InfoTrac) 9th edition by WHITNEY/ROLFES. © 2002. Reprinted with permission of Brooks/Cole, a division of Thomson Learning: www.thomsonrights.com. Fax 800-730-2215.*

High Density Lipoprotein (HDL)—Their function is to remove cholesterol or any other lipids left in the bloodstream back to the liver for disposal or recycling. If HDL levels are low, there will be insufficient protein carriers to take the excess LDL cholesterol in the blood back to the liver for disposal increasing the risk of clogging the arteries. Because of this protective function, HDL has acquired the reputation as being the **good cholesterol**. Studies indicate that regular physical exercise also can help raise HDL levels.

The HDL/LDL ratio. The ratio of HDL to LDL blood cholesterol is an important criterion in preventing heart disease. High LDL is linked to heart disease, but higher HDL levels indicate removal of excess cholesterol in the blood for breakdown and excretion, so the lowest risk is to have low LDL and high HDL levels. In the obese, high levels of fatty acids are prone to forming high LDL levels. Women have higher HDL cholesterol levels than men, but during the postmenopausal stage when estrogen levels are low, their HDL level decreases and LDL increases paving the way for higher risks in heart disease. Use preventive strategies to improve the HDL/LDL ratio by maintaining a healthy blood cholesterol profile.

Most foods contain a combination of PUFA, MUFA and saturated fats and are affected by oxidative processes, becoming unstable or rancid. This leads to the formation of excessive free radicals, molecules that lead to cell damage and premature cell aging. Since PUFAs spoil easily, food manufacturers have added certain products, such as chemicals, to prevent spoilage and extend the shelf life of unsaturated fats. These products include *additives*—the most common ones used in processed foods are **butylated hydroxyanisole** (BHA) and **butylated hydroxytoluene** (BHA), antioxidants used to prevent foods from becoming rancid; **antioxidants** such as vitamins A, C and E to combat oxidation; **emulsifiers** such as lecithin, monoglycerides and diglycerides used to stabilize emulsions by binding oil and watery substances together; and **hydrogenation**, a process where liquid fats are chemically and physically altered to a more solid matter, such as when liquid oil is converted to a more solid margarine. (See **Strategies to Improve HDL/LDL Ratio**.)

Essential fatty acids. Except *linoleic acid* and *linolenic acid*, the human body can synthesize all the fatty acids it needs from foods. These PUFAs are called **essential fatty acids** because they have to be taken into the body through diet. Their presence in the body provides protective health benefits and is necessary for the formation of phospholipid layers in cell membranes, as well as the brain and heart. Minimum requirements for essential fatty acids should be no less than 3% of total daily energy intake. Linoleic acid contains omega-6 fatty acids found in plant oils while linolenic acid containing omega-3 fatty acids are obtained mainly from fish oils and flaxseed. Lack of essential fatty acids can result in skin lesions, growth retardation, neurological and visual disorders, skin inflammation, and dry skin and eyes.

Strategies to Improve HDL/LDL Ratio

- Decrease saturated fats and cholesterol dietary intake.
- Eat the better type of fats—essential fatty acids such as MUFAs.
- Consume a variety of antioxidant-rich foods to prevent LDL oxidation.
- Increase physical exercise to increase HDL levels.
- Eat more soluble fibers to lower blood cholesterol levels.
- Strive to achieve or maintain a healthy body weight.

Health benefits of essential fatty acids. *Omega-3 fatty acids* or *linolenic acids*—These essential fatty acids are necessary to manufacture "hormone-like" compounds, eicosapentaenoic acids (EPA) and docosahexaenoic acids (DHA) important for the healthy function of the body. **Omega-3 fatty acids** give protective elements by strengthening the immune system, regulating blood cholesterol levels and blood pressure, and reducing blood clot formation. The protective factor extends to reducing certain cancers and tissue inflammation. Omega-3 fatty acids may be lacking in some diets because many people do not like fish or even know how to cook it. Researchers found that although indigenous Alaskan people's diet was high in fat, their incidence of heart disease was low, and studies indicated that the omega-3 fatty acids found in the abundant fish diet produced substances that had beneficial effects on cardiovascular diseases. They reduced blood cholesterol and triglyceride levels, lowered blood pressure and helped to dissolve blood clots. Studies suggest that their immune system became stronger due to reduced tissue inflammation. Health experts recommend a healthier balance of fats would include a higher ratio of omega-3 to omega-6.

Significant sources—Eating fish two or three times a week will have beneficial health effects. Sources include fish oils from cold water fish such as salmon, sardines, herrings, mackerel and other marine life. For those who dislike fish, fish oil supplements can be taken instead. Other excellent sources include flax seed oil, borage oil, black currant and soy foods. Commercial sources include evening primrose oil, the least expensive fatty acid.

Omega-6 fatty acids or linoleic acid. **Omega-6 fatty acids** manufacture the longer 20-carbon chains of **arachidonic acid** that help to maintain the function and structure of the cell membranes. Arachidonic acid is found in animal products such as meat and from vegetable oils that would build these longer chains of arachidonic acid even though the process takes longer. Most people consume a sufficient amount of vegetable oils, so omega-6 is not deficient in most diets.

Significant sources—These include vegetable oils, seeds such as corn, safflower and sunflower, wheat germ and walnuts.

Fats and inflammatory conditions

Scientists have found that consuming certain types of fats either can increase or decrease cellular inflammation. Prostaglandins are small hormone-like substances formed in the body from dietary fats, and they can be classified as prostaglandins derived from unsaturated fats such as vegetable oils, or PG1; derived from saturated fats from animal foods such as meat, or PG2; or derived from unsaturated fats such as fish, beans and flax seed oil, or PG3.

Although most fats contain a combination of all the prostaglandins, certain fats contain more of one than the other. PG1 and PG3 have been shown to produce anti-inflammatory effects while PG2 are associated with inflammation. When any inflammatory conditions such as acne, rosacea, psoriasis, eczema, arthritis, tendonitis and colitis occur, the intake of PG1 and PG3 foods should be increased while avoiding or reducing the inflammatory foods of the PG2 group. Other inflammatory stimulants such as alcohol, steroids and stress also should be minimized. Unfortunately, most people tend to eat an excess of PG2 foods that exacerbate inflammation. Increasing the intake of PG1 and PG3 foods also is very beneficial if you wish to reduce or avoid the use of anti-inflammatory drugs. The use of dietary supplements such as omega-3 fatty acids is an alternative recourse for those who do not like fish.

It is important to know that certain vitamins such as C, E, B-3 and B-6, and minerals such as zinc and calcium, must be present in the body in order for linoleic acid and alpha linolenic acid to convert to gamma linolenic acid and eicosapenteanoic acid respectively, and then into PG1 and PG3.

The better fats. The longer chains of fatty acids (18+) are harder and firmer than the shorter carbon chains, and the bonds holding them take longer to break down or digest. Butter is saturated and harder while margarine is unsaturated and softer. Since one should avoid saturated fats, which unsaturated fats are healthier? Chemically, MUFAs have only one unsaturated point while PUFAs have several, leaving them more vulnerable to oxidative processes. Health experts believe that MUFAs, including olive, canola and peanut oils, should be consumed in a higher ratio to PUFAs because they are more stable. Compare the health effects of different kinds of fats:

Saturated fats and trans fatty acids = ↑ LDL and HDL
Polyunsaturated fats = ↓ both LDL and HDL
Monounsaturated fats = ↓ LDL but maintains HDL

The best oils. The best oil for everyday use is extra virgin olive oil extracted from the cold pressing of olives. The first pressing gives the best flavor. When cooking with olive oil, use the lowest temperature and the least amount of time to avoid losing flavor. With the vast array of olive oils on supermarket shelves, it is difficult to decide which one is the best. Generally, you get what you pay for. Following are classifications for imported oils.

Extra virgin olive oil—This oil has the best quality, taste, stability and is the most expensive with less than 1% natural acid. It has the best flavor and is an excellent healthy alternative for use on breads and salads.

Virgin olive oil—This is a good cooking oil. It contains 1–3.3% acid that affects taste.

Pure—This oil's acidity is neutralized with chemicals resulting in a higher pH than 3.3%. It is the lowest and cheapest grade with the least flavor. Sometimes a little extra virgin oil may be added back to give more flavor.

Olive oils from the United States are rated differently from imported oils and generally don't have the variation and taste of imported oils.

Virgin—Oil from the first pressing, best quality and most expensive in the U.S. Lacks flavor of imported oils.

Refined—Oil from the second pressing with added chemicals to reduce acidity. Lacks taste.

Fat substitutes and replacements. Fat replacers reduce fat and calorie content while maintaining the flavor and texture of fat. They are based on carbohydrates, protein or fat-based substances. Several fat-free foods have been introduced in the market to give dieters some happy alternatives to eating the fat they love with fewer calories. The FDA has approved a number of fat substitutes that include thickeners and stabilizers that already are used in foods for other purposes. Olestra was the first artificial fat substitute, approved since 1996 and used in many products such as potato chips, crackers and other savory snacks. It looks good, taste like real fat, provides no extra fat or calories, is indigestible, non-toxic and is not absorbed by the body. It has a long shelf life and is resistant to high temperatures such as those that occur during frying. Isn't this simply too good to be true? Well, almost.

Fat replacers—**Fat replacers** are found in a large variety of foods such as dairy products, sauces, frozen desserts, baked goods and salad dressings. They provide less than half of the nine calories per gram of regular fat with the exception of olestra, which has no calories.

Carbohydrate substitutes—**Carbohydrate substitutes** include dextrins, fiber, gums and starches that are used as emulsifiers and stabilizers.

Protein replacers—**Protein replacers** include *Simplesse** made from whey, milk or egg protein. They contain only 1–2 calories and taste like the real thing.

Side effects. Few side effects have been reported except for abdominal

**Simplesse is a trademark of CP Kelco, Wilmington, DE*

Healthier Fats Substitutes

Choose more often	*Choose less often*
• Low fat milk products	• Whole milk, high fat cheeses, sour cream and ice cream
• Lean beef such as round and flank steaks as well as lean ground beef	• Prime rib, regular ground beef and spareribs.
• Lean cuts such as pork and lamb	• Luncheon meats, sausage and hot dogs
• Fish, free range meats such as skinless chicken, turkey and brown meat	• Duck, goose, bacon, white meat and fried meats
• Tuna and other fish packed in water	• Tuna packed in oil
• Plain cookies and dried fruits	• Processed carbohydrates such as rich cakes, pastries, pies and croissants
• Granola bars, saltless pretzels and light popcorn	• Chips
• Light mayonnaise, light salad dressing	• Regular mayonnaise and salad dressing
• Olive oil on bread	• Butter, hard margarine, shortening and trans fatty acids
• Olive, canola, sunflower and safflower oils	• Palm, coconut oils and hydrogenated vegetable oils

Heart and Stroke Foundation Canada, 1997.

cramping or diarrhea in some people, possibly preventing fat-soluble vitamins from being absorbed. However, vitamins A, D, E and K now have been added to foods such as milk, cereal and packaged foods, and it is mandatory to list the additives on the food labels. Other fat substitutes waiting to be approved by the FDA are Salatrim, short- and long-chain triglycerides, and Caprenin, a fat substitute for cocoa butter. *The Women's Health Study* found that for most people, the most difficult dietary change was giving up fats as flavorings, especially eating bread without butter or margarine. A few studies also indicated that some people used the fat substitutes as an excuse to eat more calories from other sources thus increasing more caloric intake. Consumers must learn to read and understand the nutrition facts on food labels when using food replacers. (See **Healthier Fat Substitutes**.)

Healthy fat intake. Health professionals recommend that fat intake should be less than 30% of total daily calorie intake and less than 10% of total fat should be saturated fat. Waste products of fats include carbon dioxide and water. (See **Strategies for Reducing Fat Intake**.)

Water. Water is the most important nutrient for the body since it forms part of every cell: 75% in muscles, and the rest in dry bone and teeth. Water is lost through water vapor via the nose, sweat, urine and feces, and must be replenished to prevent dehydration. It is found in liquids and foods such as fruits and vegetables, which contain 85–90% water, while meat contains much less. Health experts recommend that you drink approximately eight 8-oz. glasses of water daily, one before and after meals to aid digestion, absorption and elimination processes.

Tap or bottled. The rising awareness of health issues, thanks in part to media attention and dissatisfaction with tap water, has led consumers to buy a commodity that once was free. Because of the popular notion that tap water is contaminated and unhealthy, an explosion in the popularity of bottled water in the past decades recently has occurred. People want assurance that they are drinking pure, uncontaminated water and surveys have shown that people perceive bottled water as being pure, free from contaminants, and drink it for health and safety. (See **Water Terminology**, page 41.) This is a fallacy since 25–

Strategies for Reducing Fat Intake

- Focus more on reducing dietary saturated fats than on reducing cholesterol.
- Choose low fat alternatives such as more fish, lean meat and low fat dairy products.
- Vegans can try flax seed, an alternative to fish and an excellent source of omega-3.
- Use olive oils instead of butter and margarine on breads.
- Avoid hydrogenated fats typically found in snack foods.
- Minimize cholesterol-rich foods such as eggs and dairy products—try soy food alternatives.
- Use low fat versions of creamy dressings or try vinegar-based dressings instead.
- Eat egg whites or non-cholesterol egg substitutes instead of egg yolks.
- Learn to recognize hidden fats by checking the percentage of saturated fats and total fat intake on food labels.
- Maintain a healthy body weight by combining healthy eating with a regular exercise program.

Water Terminology

What do all these terms about water mean? Following are explanations of terms commonly used in the water industry.

Artesian water—**Artesian water** contains high mineral concentration—comes from a well that taps into a rock formation.

Purified water—Otherwise known as *soft water, demineralized, distilled, deionized* or *reverse osmosis,* **purified water** denotes that all minerals have been removed.

Spring water—**Spring water** has been collected from an underground spring that flows to the Earth's surface. No minerals have been added to its natural mineral state. Usually there is no added information about whether it was obtained near any area that is contaminated with pesticides or sewage.

Mineral water—Otherwise known as hard water, **mineral water** is drawn from an underground source and contains at least 250 parts per million of dissolved solid mineral salts such as calcium, iron and sodium. These tend to crystallize within the arterial walls forming parts of plaque that contribute toward arteriosclerosis. Mineral water with carbonation is known as **sparkling water** and is not a good choice of bottled water because it contains gas and is considered a soft drink. Gas is not a nutrient that is necessary for the body's health.

Various Water Filters and Purifiers

Activated carbon, carbon block and Halogen Reduction Media (HRM)—Carbon filters remove the bad taste and odor such as chlorine and organic compounds in the water. However, heavy metals such as aluminum are not removed. The better systems are the combination of carbon with HRM or the carbon block that removes the taste of chlorine and other odors simultaneously filtering any parasites.

Water softeners—These remove hard minerals from water, but do not get rid of chlorine and bacteria.

Distillers—These remove sodium and other salts found in water, but are ineffective in removing industrial chemicals. They also are expensive to maintain because the elements have to be cleaned or replaced constantly.

Reverse Osmosis (RO)—RO uses faucet pressure to force water through a semi-permeable membrane to remove heavy metals except for organic mercury, most microparticles and parasites. The system is self-cleaning, and when combined with a carbon filter, removes the taste of chlorine. It is considered the most effective, but also is the most expensive method for purifying water.

40% of bottled water is derived from municipal tap water which could contain varying concentrations of minerals, bacteria, microganisms, heavy metals and sometimes sewage. Moreover, some bottled water even lacks sufficient fluoride to fight cavities. One of the main reasons for its popularity is its good taste and effective marketing strategies using a variety of terms such as *pure*, *sparkling* and *mineral* inferring that bottled water is better than tap water. The bottled water industry has become a billion dollar industry with unparalleled marketing by creating a new taste for water throughout the world.

The most common methods for obtaining clean water include the usage of filters and purifiers. (See **Various Water Filters and Purifiers**, page 41.)

Vitamins

Vitamins are minute organic substances found in living foods, both plants and animal. They are essential for the good health and maintenance of the body. Deficiency results in certain diseases. Although vitamins proliferate as dietary supplements, they are absorbed from natural foods more readily than their synthetic forms. Natural foods also have the additional advantage of other nutrients such as fiber and minerals.

Since early on, when vitamins B and C first were discovered to eradicate **pellagra**, a skin rash, and **scurvy**, a disease marked by spongy gums and bleeding into the skin due to a lack of vitamin C, many scientists have recognized that vitamins are potent compounds necessary for the healthy functioning of the body. The onset of preventive health care in modern society has led to current intense research of the role of vitamins as antioxidants, and how they can help prevent the onset of disease. The deep interest shown by the public in vitamin therapy to optimize good health was spurred by ubiquitous media information, generated in part by the burgeoning aging population in their quest for longevity, and the consumer's increasing awareness of health issues.

Functions. Vitamins play several roles in the body. They are essential for good health; some act as coenzymes to help to release energy from foods indirectly, and some act as antioxidants and free radical scavengers.

People who consume generous amounts of natural fresh fruits and vegetables are more likely to receive sufficient vitamins and minerals than those who do not. However, several environmental factors such as food processing can remove the nutrients. Because of this, some are enriched or fortified after processing with nutrients such as folate, and vitamins C and D. Although the general purpose of the vitamin B complex is for proper functioning of the nervous system, each B vitamin has a specific role in itself. Several of them act as coenzymes to assist enzymes in liberating energy for metabolic functions in the cells. That is perhaps why some people feel more energetic when they take vitamin B supplements. Antioxidants such as beta-carotene, and vitamins C and E help to defend the body against harmful free radicals generated from oxidative stress reactions in tissues. Antioxidants have been shown to protect against cardiovascular diseases, various forms of cancer and other chronic diseases.

Types of vitamins. Vitamins are water-soluble or fat-soluble. Since they only are needed in small doses, vitamins are measured either in milligrams (mg) or in tiny doses, micrograms (ug). Many of them were given a letter or a number as they were discovered, and then assigned a name so the various names given to some of them can become quite confusing at times. Although **Appendices I** and **II** list brief and concise summaries of both water- and fat-soluble vitamins, they are described here in somewhat more detail for better comprehension of their functions.

Differences Between Water- and Fat-soluble Vitamins

Water-soluble (B, C, P)	*Fat-soluble (A, D, E, K)*
Hydrophilic—soluble in water	Hydrophobic—insoluble in water
Not stored in the body—little risk of toxicity	Stored in the body so higher risk toxicity from animal sources
Can be taken more regularly	Travel in lymphatic system
Vulnerable to environment—heat and light	Need protein carriers (LDL) for transportation
Affected by food preparation and storage	Excess stored in liver and adipose tissue

Provitamins are precursors or substrates that undergo chemical reactions in the body before being converted to active vitamins. They include:

Precursors	***Vitamins produced***
Beta-carotene (yellow/orange fruits and vegetables)	Vitamin A
1,25-OH vitamin D (in presence of sunlight)	Vitamin D
Tryptophan (amino acid)	Vitamin B
Intestinal bacteria act on precursor	Vitamin K

Water-soluble vitamins. Many vitamins carry multiple names, so it is beneficial to be able to recognize them by their different names (see **Appendices I** and **II**). The large family of B vitamins includes thiamin (B-1), riboflavin (B-2), niacin (B-3), pyridoxine (B-6), cobalamin (B-12), biotin, folate and pantothenic acid. In general, the B vitamin complex is essential for the healthy functioning of the nervous system, clear skin, nails and hair. Many of them act as coenzymes and without them, energy cannot be released from energy-yielding foods—carbohydrates, fats and proteins.

Many B vitamins are of particular importance for females. Of these, adequate daily intake of 400 ug of folate is essential in the diet of childbearing females before and during the first few months of pregnancy when the nervous system is being developed in the embryo. Deficiency results in **spina bifida**, a neurological disorder found in babies where the brain and spine that forms from the neural tube becomes defective. To help prevent deficiency, the FDA has mandated that many products such as fruit juices and milk should be fortified with this important nutrient for women.

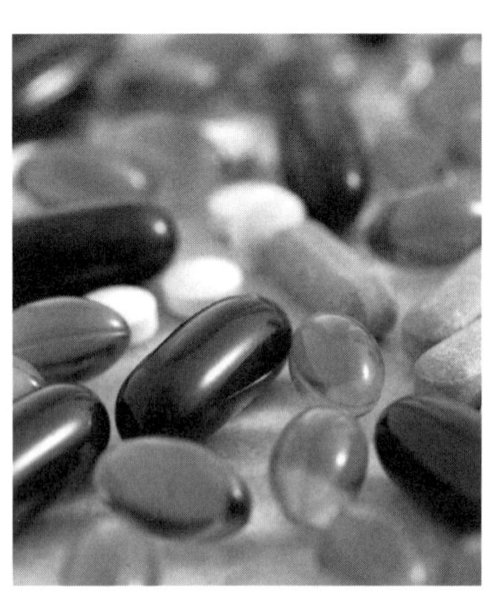

Vitamins are essential for the good health and maintenance of the body.

Vitamin B-12 and folate depend on each other for activation. B-12 is found primarily in animal foods, so vegans are typically at high risk of B-12 deficiency. Deficiency of folate and vitamin B-12 results in large immature red blood cells, or *pernicious anemia.* As covered earlier in the text, a low dietary intake of folate, vitamins B-6 and B-12 also is linked with a high levels of homocysteine, a risk factor for heart disease since the presence of these vitamins are necessary to convert homocysteine into the amino acid methionine.

Following are descriptions of the roles vitamin C holds:

Collagen formation—Vitamin C is essential for the formation of collagen and elastic fibers, the protein matrix of connective tissue, skin, nails, hair, teeth, bones, and the elasticity of the walls of arteries.

Antioxidant—Increased amounts of vitamin C are needed during physical or physiological stress to fight free radicals.

Immunity—Vitamin C is used to fight infections such as the common cold or burns. Researchers believe that vitamin C also plays an important role in preventing heart diseases and various forms of cancer. Deficiency results in reduced immunity leading to various infections such as the common cold, slow healing, particularly after surgery, and increased susceptibility to weakened blood vessels and capillaries.

Fat-soluble vitamins. *Vitamin A* was the first fat-soluble vitamin to be recognized. It is found in animal sources and brightly colored vegetables and fruits. Vitamin A is lost during food processing so it is fortified in fat-free milk. There are two forms of vitamin A—**carotenoids** and **retinoids**.

Carotenoids—As pigments commonly found in plants and animals, some of them act as precursors for vitamin A. After absorption in the body, they are then converted to the active form of vitamin A. Beta-carotene is a well-known precursor of vitamin A and has the greatest vitamin A activity. Carotenoids commonly are found in brightly colored yellow, red and orange vegetables such as carrots, tomatoes, sweet potatoes and dark, leafy greens such as broccoli.

Retinoids—This is a collective term for the three active forms of vitamin A—*retinol, retinal* and *retinoic acid*, each having specific functions in the body. For example, the retinoids in the eyes allow the viewing of the brightly colored carotenoids in the plants. Significant sources of retinoids are animal-derived such as liver, fish oils and dairy products.

Each form of vitamin A has specific functions. The alcohol form of retinol is the active form and acts as the main transport and storage form of vitamin A. It is essential for protein synthesis, particularly for the growth and repair of all epithelial cells such as the skin, nails, hair and mucous membranes of the body. Special protein carriers carry retinol to cells that have special protein receptors. Vitamin A's retinoic acid functions as a hormone and regulates cell growth and reproduction. Also, it acts as an antioxidant—the precursor betacarotene fights the formation of free radicals. Retinal, the aldehyde form, improves vision and can be converted to retinoic acid if required by the body.

Measurements of vitamin A. **International units** or **IU** was the old measurement for vitamin A activity before chemical analysis was developed. The more recent term **retinol equivalents (RE)** now commonly is used. The RE or IU equivalent of retinol derived from food depends on whether from animals or other precursors such as beta carotene. The RE is easier to work with than the IU since it carries whole numbers. The following indicates the differences between RE and IU measurements of retinol.

1 RE (retinol equivalent) = 1 ug retinol or 12 ug beta-carotene or 24 ug from other precursors of carotenoids

1 IU (international unit) = 0.3 ug retinol or 3.6 ug beta-carotene or 7.2 ug from other precursors from carotenoids

The DRIs for vitamin A vary for different age groups and are listed in **Appendix I.**

Additional vitamins. Vitamin D in the body is formed from the chemical reaction of sunlight on a precursor, cholesterol made by the liver. The final active vitamin D is a compound known as 1,25,dihydroxycholecalciferol, or **calciferol**. Vitamin D forms strong bones and teeth in early child development. Deficiency leads to bowed legs. Also, it is a hormone that helps absorb calcium in the intestines.

Excessive sun exposure can lead to premature skin aging and various forms of skin cancer. As a result of media's extensive coverage, the use of sunscreens and sun blocks has been become overused in several instances. In some cases, this over education has led to excessive use of these products, resulting instead in the prevention of vitamin D synthesis. The media's constant warning about excessive sun exposure also has led the elderly to avoid the sun, and this practice can increase the risk of weak, brittle bones, or osteoporosis. The best advice is to have early morning or late evening sun exposure and avoid direct sun exposure at midday. As a preventive measure, the FDA now has set a mandate that foods such as milk products be fortified with vitamin D. Consumers should check food labels for this information.

There are several components of vitamin E, but the one that has the most biological activity is *alpha-tocopherol*. Values of vitamin E in food are expressed as mg of tocopherol equivalents. Vitamin E is one of the most important antioxidants in fighting heart disease and cancer, preventing oxidation of LDL cholesterol and PUFA fats. Although the adult DRIs for vitamin E is very low (15 mg/d), most anti-aging health practitioners recommend a minimum of 400 mg with the upper levels of 1,000 mg for critical diseases. Vitamin E is destroyed by heat processing, or deep frying. Significant sources of this vitamin are vegetable oils, especially wheat germ oils, nuts and seeds

Since most people consume vegetable oils, deficiency is rare.

Vitamin K is a necessary component in blood clotting. It must be present in order for **prothrombin**, an inactive protein, to convert to the active **thrombin** that leads to the formation of **fibrin**, a blood clotting protein. (See **Figure 2-13.**)

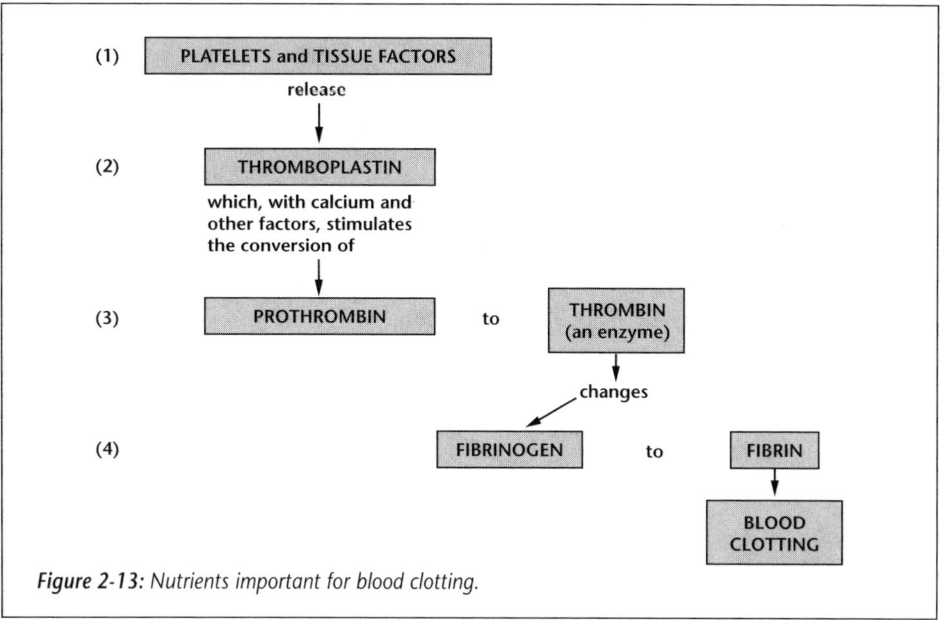

Figure 2-13: *Nutrients important for blood clotting.*

Minerals or trace elements

Minerals are essentially inorganic elements found mainly in plants, the major ones found in larger amounts, larger than 5 g in the body while the **trace elements** occur in tiny doses. When taken into the body, minerals are not acted upon by enzymes but remain in the same form until they are excreted. Some act as co-factors with vitamins for special functions and excess minerals in the body can be toxic. Certain ones such as sodium, potassium and chloride are important to form electrolytes and maintain the body's fluid balance. Calcium, phosphorus and magnesium are the three minerals that are important for healthy growth and maintenance of bone. However, excess minerals in the body can be toxic. The above minerals will be discussed briefly here, but a summarized table can be found in **Appendix III**.

Sodium, or salt. Sodium is the main **cation**, or positively charged ion, in the extracellular fluid located outside the cell and helps to maintain acid-base balance. It is essential for transmitting nerve impulses and muscle contraction. Processed foods such as fast foods use sodium as a preservative and contain excessive amounts not needed by the body. When salty foods are eaten, the sodium in the blood rises signaling the brain to drink until the appropriate sodium-to-water ratio is reached. Then the kidneys excrete not only the excess salt but the water as well. The DRI of sodium is 2,400 mg daily, but most people's salt intake is much higher due to high sodium levels found in processed foods. Those suffering from hypertension need to cut down salt intake by cooking with little or no added salt and preparing foods with spices instead; tasting foods before adding salt; reading food labels for sodium content; selecting low-salt or salt-free foods if available; and using minimal amounts of heavy sodium foods such as pickles, salted or smoked meats, salty snack items, processed cheese, and canned or instant soups. Excess intake of sodium can result in hypertension or edema. Deficiency is rare except in vomiting, diarrhea and heavy sweating such as athletes experience during endurance activities. In this case, drinking beverages with sodium and glucose for recovery is beneficial.

Potassium. This is the main cation found *inside* the cell. A cation is a positive—an atom with a positive charge. This electrolyte activity maintains blood pressure and keeps tissues healthy and alive. Potassium is found abundantly in all living cells—the richest sources are in all fresh foods, either plant or animal. Potassium-rich fruits and vegetables help to reduce blood pressure. There is no toxicity with excessive intake of potassium if they are from foods. Concern only lies with dietary supplements. Deficiency usually is caused from excessive loss rather than by deficiency. This occurs in diabetic acidosis, dehydration, prolonged vomiting, diarrhea and regular use of certain drugs.

Chloride. This trace element is composed of two atoms of chlorine gas (Cl_2) and when it reacts with sodium or hydrogen, it forms a negative chloride ion (Cl-). It is the main **anion** of the extracellular fluids, and like sodium and potassium, helps to maintain fluid balance in the body. Chloride is abundant in foods, especially processed foods, as part of sodium chloride and other salts. Detrimental reactions with excessive intake and deficiency are rare.

Calcium. This is the most abundant mineral in the body with 99% found in the bones and teeth. Various hormones are responsible for maintaining constant levels of calcium in the blood. **Parathormone** from the parathyroid gland increases calcium when levels are low in the blood; **calcitonin** from the thyroid gland inhibits the release of calcium from bone; and vitamin D, which also acts as a hormone, promotes calcium absorption in the intestines. The DRI for calcium varies according to age, pregnancy, whether a woman is lactating and postmenopausal status. The absorption of calcium is reduced by certain dietary fibers and enhanced by vitamin D, stomach acid and lactose in the stomach. Excess intake can cause stiffness, constipation and urinary stones. Deficiency can cause **tetany**, stunted growth in children, **osteomalacia**, soft bones in adults, and **osteoporosis**.

Phosphorus. It is the second most abundant mineral in the body and works with calcium. It is found not only in bones and teeth, but also in all body cells and is essential in energy metabolism.

Magnesium. Over half of the body's magnesium is found in the bones, the rest in muscles and soft tissues and a little in the extracellular fluid. Magnesium is essential for release of ATP, heart function, muscular contraction, blood clotting and many other functions. Legumes, seeds, nuts and leafy green vegetables are significant sources. Issues due to excess intake and deficiency are rare.

CHAPTER 3

Preventive Health Care

Aside from antioxidants, active research in other plant compounds is creating widespread interest among those who are seeking preventive health care to improve quality of life. The aging population, particularly those who have experienced diseases of aging such as cardiovascular or cancer, are seeking ways to prevent these diseases and simultaneously retain independence and functionality. Traditional therapies including acupuncture, massage therapy and naturopathy are being revived. Disease prevention has accelerated new discoveries and product innovation in the health care market. Following are some terms that continue to crop up regularly in today's literature regarding health.

Phytotherapy. Plants have been used for medicinal purposes for many centuries, and about 80% of the world's population depends primarily on botanicals as medicine. Phytotherapy commonly is used in Europe, and it is predicted that herbal remedies will proliferate dramatically in North America during the 21st century. The terms **phytochemicals, nutraceuticals, functional foods** and **phytosterols** are used interchangeably by many people, but there are very slight differences between them. The terminology used depends on who is using it. There currently is no legal definition for the different terms. For instance, there is a preference for the food industry to use the term *functional foods* while *nutraceuticals* are being increasingly associated with dietary supplements. The resurgent interest in preventive health care has spurred relatively new scientific discoveries of other substances found in traditional foods that are beyond that food's established health benefits. Although these substances aim to treat, cure and prevent specific illnesses or diseases, they target two different groups of people. They not only are marketed to those who already are suffering from diseases, but also to healthy people to enhance their health or possibly prevent disease.

Phytochemicals are specific compounds in plants that are not necessarily nutrients but have been found to possess healthy properties that prevent certain diseases. Some have been shown to have even more powerful antioxidant properties than traditional antioxidants and include anti-inflammatory, anti-allergic, anti-viral and anti-cancer abilities.

Functional foods are described as any modified food or food ingredient that may provide health benefits beyond the traditional nutrients it contains, such as orange juice with added fiber or calcium.

Nutraceuticals often are used to describe the biological activity of an ingredient in food that can deliver health benefits such as the active ingredients of so-called functional foods. They are not necessarily nutrients, but clinical studies show that when isolated from other nutrients, they give protective medicinal benefits. An excellent example is lycopene, found in tomatoes, which has been recognized as the most effective antioxidant in maintaining prostate health and preventing heart diseases. Nutraceuticals are found in pill, powder or capsule forms, as well as in certain foods and beverages.

Phytosterols refer to steroids in plant seeds, such as pumpkin seeds.

Health benefits of phytochemicals. Many phytochemicals give bright colors to plants and absorb light in the visible spectrum. Think of bright colors and phytochemicals together so that by using a color code, consumers easily can make healthier choices when selecting various sources of phytochemicals. Researchers have grouped phytonutrients according to their specific effects in preventing certain diseases. The National Cancer Institute and American Institute for Cancer Research recommend that one serving of each of the following groups should be eaten daily for preventive health care. See **Phytochemicals and their Health Benefits.**

More on flavonoids. These are a large group of compounds found ubiquitously in plants, and more than 4,000 flavonoids have been researched and documented. Like all phytochemicals, they are powerful antioxidants and exhibit anti-viral and anti-cancer effects by inhibiting tumor formation. **Flavonoids** have been found to help in the long-term care of diabetes by improving blood flow to tissues. Plant flavonoids also are known as **proanthocyanidins** or **procyanidins**. One of the most beneficial ones is **quercetin**, considered the most active flavonoid. Good dietary sources are all berries, rutin, onions, parsley, legumes and red wine.

Skin care and citrus flavonoids. **Bioflavonoids** found in citrus fruits and green tea have specific benefits on the skin. Besides preventing free radical attacks, they have anti-inflammatory effects by inhibiting the production or release of histamine and other allergic mediators produced by mast cells in the dermis. They prevent the release of harmful prostaglandins that instigate inflammatory reactions. In addition, they prevent the breakdown of the collagen matrix improving the skin's tone. The endothelial cells lining blood vessels are

Phytochemicals and their Health Benefits

Food Components and Colors	*Potential Health Benefits*	*Significant Sources*
Carotenoids		
Beta-carotene (orange)	Antioxidant	Carrots, mangoes, pumpkins and sweet potatoes
Lutein zeaxanthin	Healthy vision (yellow-green)	Eggs, citrus, corn and green vegetables
Lycopene (red)	May reduce risk of prostate cancer	Tomatoes, tomato products
Flavonoids		
Anthocyanidins and proanthocyanidins (red/purple colors)	Antioxidant, may reduce risk of cancer, cardiovascular diseases, and improve urinary tract health	All berries and red wine, apples, cocoa and chocolate
Polyphenols (catechins)	Antioxidant, may reduce risk of cancer	Green or black tea
Flavonoids (yellow-orange)	Antioxidant; improves capillary function; reduce edema, bruising and varicosity	Citrus fruits such as oranges, tangerines, lemons and peaches
Dietary fiber		
Beta glucan	Reduce risk of cardiovascular psyllium disease	Oat bran, wheat bran
Whole grains	Reduce risk of cardiovascular disease	Cereal grains
Phytoestrogens		
Isoflavones (diadzein, genistein)	May reduce hormonal symptoms and may reduce breast cancer	Soy beans, soy-based foods
Lignans	May protect against heart disease, some cancers; reduce LDL cholesterol, total cholesterol and triglycerides	Flaxseed, rye, legumes

Phytochemicals and their Health Benefits *(cont.)*

Food Components and Colors	***Potential Health Benefits***	***Significant Sources***
Saponis		
Saponis	May lower LDL cholesterol, anti-cancer properties	Soy beans, soy foods
Sulfides/thiols		
Allylic sulfides	Lowers LDL cholesterol, strengthens immune system	Onion family, including leeks, scallions, chives and garlic
Glucosinolates, indoles	Antioxidant, anti-cancer properties	Cruceriferous vegetables, such as cauliflower, brussel sprouts, kale, bok choy

International Food Information Council, Washington, DC, 2000, and 11th Annual Research Conference on Diet, Nutrition and Cancer, Washington, July 2001. Sponsored by American Institute for Cancer Research.

strengthened preventing capillary breakage, varicosity and cellulite conditions. A good example is rutin which helps in reducing skin bruising, edema, broken capillaries, varicosity and hemorrhoids.

Herbs and disease prevention

Herbs have been used in food flavoring for centuries and also have been known to deliver health benefits. Many western drugs such as aspirin also are derived from plants. In recent years, many consumers have become dissatisfied with traditional medicine and conventional drug therapy. They find them expensive and impersonal with side effects, but perceive herbs and botanicals to be more natural and less expensive with little or no side effects. Heart and cancer patients often seek information on complementary or alternative therapies as an adjunct to traditional medicine. Many people educate themselves about nutrition from various sources such as books, articles and the Internet, becoming quite sophisticated and discriminating consumers over a period of time. The sense of empowerment that develops in being able to treat oneself in health concerns has attracted many people to alternative medicine. A survey conducted in 1999 showed that 49% of all adult Americans used at least one herbal medicine in the past year and 24% use herbs regularly, often along with conventional drugs. There is sufficient evidence that herbal drugs are well suited for preventive medicine. Some include botanicals and herbals such as echinacea, evening primrose oil and biological supplements such as melatonin, CoQ10 and shark cartilage. Using small amounts of herbs in cooking reduces the likelihood of using salt. Like fruits and vegetables, popular herbs such as basil, cumin and rosemary also contain phytochemicals such as flavonoids, saponins and carotenoids, however, it must be noted that excessive use of herbs can result in toxicity. The following herbal remedies are well-known and traditionally have been used for potential health benefits in treating various skin disorders and diseases. See **Herbal Aids.**

Herbal Aids

Herbal Aids for Skin Afflictions

Herbs	*Potential health benefits*
Chamomile	Anti-inflammatory, anti-bacterial, reduces surface skin inflammation
Rutin	Reduces skin bruising, edema, capillary breakage, varicosity, hemorrhoids
Horse chestnut	Active ingredient increases venous flow, strengthens capillary walls, reduces edema, bruising and varicosity
Grapeseed extracts	Commercial extracts of anthocyanins, strengthen capillary walls, reduces vascularity—edema and bruising
Green tea	Antioxidant, helps to prevent skin cancer
Bioflavonoids	Antioxidant, strengthens capillary walls
Aloe vera	Emollient, anti-inflammatory, healing properties
Witch hazel	Extracts from hammellis plant, topical astringent, anti-inflammatory effects on skin
Tea tree oil	Topical germicidal
Lemon balm	Topical anti-bacterial, germicidal

Herbal Aids *(cont.)*

Herbal Aids for Cardiovascular Diseases

Psyllium	Reduces high blood cholesterol levels
Hawthorn	Increases blood flow in heart, beneficial in angina
Garlic	Contains sulfur compounds that reduce blood pressure in cardiovascular diseases, antioxidant, anti-cancer properties, improves immunity
Flaxseed	Oils from linseeds contain significant sources of omega-3, reduces high blood cholesterol levels

Herbal Aids for Digestive Disorders

Chamomile	Internal effects—anti-inflammatory, anti-bacterial, reduces menstrual cramps and digestive spasms
Ginger	Aids in digestion, nausea, dizziness, motion sickness
Licorice	Anti-ulcer, anti-inflammatory, anti-allergic, blocks formation of inflammatory prostaglandins (PG2)
Milk thistle	Contains silymarin which helps in liver toxicity
Peppermint	Reduces inflammation of GI tract
Psyllium	High fiber reduces high blood cholesterol levels

Anti-cancer Herbs

Green and black teas	Contains *tannins* that helps reduce cancer in lungs, colon, skin
Tumeric	Gives yellow color to foods, anti-inflammatory, anti-microbial, anti-tumor properties
Isoflavones (daidzen, geinstein)	Helps in reducing breast cancer
Allylic sulfide (garlic and onion family)	Helps reduce cancers in lung, colon, GI tract
Flavonoids	Helps reduce colon and skin cancers

Herbal Aids *(cont.)*

Herbal Aids for High Blood Sugar Levels

Fenugreek	Helps diabetic conditions
Bitter lemon	Helps to reduce high sugar levels

Herbal Aids for Nervous System Disorders

St. John's wort	Leaves and flowers of plant reduces anxiety, treats mild to moderate depression without side effects
Valerian	Acts as a mild sedative, reduces anxiety, improves quality of sleep
Kava Kava	Roots of shrub from South Pacific—relaxes nerves, increases tranquility, helps inhibit uptake of serotonin
Passion flower	Treats sleep disorders, reduces anxiety
Willow bark	Reduces mild headaches
Mixed essential oils	Creates relaxation

Herbal Aids for Aging Diseases

Ginseng	Contains ginsenoisides believed to possess anti-cancer properties, reduce fatigue, improve stamina and concentration
Gingko biloba	Improves memory by increasing blood flow to brain, anti-depressant effects.

Herbal Aids for Endocrine/Hormonal Disorders

Black cohosh	Contains triterpenes used to relieve hormonal dysfunctions such as vaginitis, hot flashes, depression
Chaste tree berry	Extracts of ripe dried fruits reduces symptoms of PMS and dysmen orrheal, or painful menses
Evening primrose oil	Contains gamma linoleic acid the precursor to prostaglandins 1 and 3; has anti-inflammatory effects
Black currant	The seeds contain linoleic acid that has anti-inflammatory effects
Red clover	Rich in phytoestrogens, used as alternative therapy to estrogen replacement therapy

Herbal Aids *(cont.)*

Herbal Aids for Endocrine/Hormonal Disorders (cont.)

Soya	Significant source of phytoestrogens
Licorice	Anti-inflammatory, reduces menopausal symptoms
Gingko biloba	Improves memory in aging by increasing blood flow to brain, helps relieve depression

Herbal Aids for Detoxification

Milk thistle	Contains silymarin for removing toxins from liver

Herbals Aids for the Immune System

Echinacea	Treats infection—anti-inflammatory, improves immunity, helps fight flu symptoms
Cat's claw	Contains flavonoids to improve immunity
Allyl sulfur	Strengthens immune system

Herbal Aids for Kidney/Prostate/Urinary Tract Disorders

Saw palmetto	From palm tree, treats benign enlarged prostate gland, improves urinary flow and frequency
Cranberry	Rich in flavonoids, contains ellagic acid with anti-cancer properties, anti-inflammatory, anti-bacterial
Golden rod	Anti-inflammatory, anti-bacterial effect in urinary tract, diuretic
Licorice	Blocks formation of inflammatory prostaglandins (PG2), anti-allergic, anti-ulcer effects
Pumpkin seeds	Contains phytosterols believed to relieve difficulty of enlarged prostate gland
Pygeum africanum	Bark helps to reduce enlarged prostate gland

Modified from "Nutraceuticals: the Link between Nutrition and Medicine." 2000, pp.8-10.

Precautions with phytochemicals and herbs

The current data on phytochemicals is overwhelming and prompts many people to take them. Many clients of health care practitioners already may be taking some of the above phytochemicals, so it is important to know the benefits and potential risks of these natural products and, at the same time, increase professional credibility. One should exercise caution in taking high doses, particularly by cancer patients, since research still is ongoing. There are many unknown interactions that may lead to adverse effects, and herbs are not strictly regulated in terms of accuracy and safety for the public. For instance, the recent death of some individuals who were using ephedra, a cardiac stimulant, led the FDA to issue a strong warning to remove this herb from stores. It is safer to consume fresh fruits and vegetables that are rich in phytochemicals rather than isolated, concentrated supplements due to possible contamination, inaccuracy and mislabeling of substances. If you have a medical problem, consult a professional health care practitioner before you purchase any supplements, and use standardized products whenever possible.

CHAPTER 4

Diet Planning

After reading this chapter, you should be able to plan a healthy, balanced diet for individuals according to their weight, body size and physical activity. Research studies show a positive correlation between diet, body weight and longevity. Clients with chronic or severe medical problems such as heart disease, diabetes, extreme obesity or gastrointestinal problems should be referred to a certified nutritionist or dietitian.

A healthy diet should include a limited intake of fats, refined sugar, salt and alcohol. Energy in foods is described as the amount of heat produced from foods after they have been absorbed and transformed by the body. Energy is measured in kcals, or 1,000-calorie units:

1 g protein = 4 kcals
1 g carbohydrate = 4 kcals
1g fat = 9 kcals
1 g alcohol = 7 kcals

How much should you eat?

Daily energy intake should correlate with energy needs defined by body weight *plus* a percentage of daily activity levels. In general:

To maintain weight—daily energy input (kcals) = energy of physical activity
To lose weight—less energy input (kcals) + increased physical activity
To gain weight—increase energy input (kcals)

Regular intake of excess kcals causes them to become stored in the body as fat leading to an unhealthy body weight over time. Although alcohol provides kcals, it is not considered a nutrient since it does not help in the manufacture or repair of tissues.

There are five basic principles to be considered in planning a nutritious diet:

1. ***Adequacy.*** Daily consumption of essential nutrients, including sufficient kcals according to an individual's age, gender, whether she is pregnant or lactating, body mass and physical activity.
2. ***Balance.*** This ensures that one food type containing more of certain nutrients will not create an imbalance of another essential nutrient and

instead, will be supported by another food group to balance nutrient values. For example, foods rich in calcium such as milk products provide little or no iron—this should be supplemented by iron-rich foods such as lean red meat, soy foods, legumes or whole grains.

3. ***Moderation.*** It is better to eat some forbidden foods in moderation rather than completely abstaining from them, which promotes cravings. For example, if you give in to eating chocolates one day, cut back on foods rich in fats the next day. Learn to control these forbidden urges more effectively.
4. ***Nutrient-dense foods.*** These are foods containing optimal nutrients—protein, vitamins and minerals—with relatively low kcal values and fat. For example, a cup of non-fat milk contains 12 grams of protein and traces of fat with only 90 kcals, while whole milk has the same amount of proteins but contains 8 grams of fat with 150 kcals—60 kcals more.
5. ***Variety.*** Since different foods contain varying amounts of nutrients, try eating a wide array of foods within each food group to not only have a balanced diet, but also acquire new tastes and make eating more fun and interesting. Trying ethnic cuisine can open a cornucopia of incredible tastes and can help foster bonds between yourself and others, including clients.

Diet planning guides

In nutritional counseling, food group plans and exchange systems are used by many nutritionists to help guide clients to obtain adequate essential nutrients through their daily food intake. In the following food group plans, foods are placed in groups according to similar nutrient content. For example, bread and whole grains are grouped together, while milk and milk products are placed in the same category. The food group plan helps to ensure that sufficient servings of the essential nutrients are taken from each food group daily. The required daily servings for each food group are listed below.

Milk group. Cheese, milk and yogurt; 2–3 servings; one serving = 1 cup milk; 2-oz. processed cheese or 1 1/2-oz. cheese.

Meat and meat alternatives. Beef, veal, chicken, eggs, fish, beans or soy foods; 2–3 servings; one serving = 2–3-oz. cooked, lean meat, 1 egg, 1/2 cup legumes or 2 tablespoons peanut butter.

Fruits. Apple, grapefruit, fruit juice, chopped or canned fruit, dried fruit; 2–3 servings; one serving = 1 medium apple, 1/2 grapefruit, 3/4 cup juice, 1/2 cup chopped or canned fruit or 1/4 cup dried fruit.

Bread, cereals/whole grains. Bread, cooked cereal, rice or pasta, bun or bagel, crackers; 6–11 servings; one serving = 1 slice bread, 1/2 cup cooked cereal, rice or pasta, 1/2 bun or bagel or 2 large crackers.

Vegetables. Raw vegetables, vegetable juice, legumes; 3–5 servings; one serving = 1/2 cup cooked or raw vegetables, 3/4 cup vegetable juice, 1 cup leafy raw vegetables or 1/2 cup cooked legumes.

The Daily Food Guide. One of the most familiar food guides is the Daily Food Guide. This can be viewed as a pyramid comprised of either a five group or four group plan. Most countries, including the United States, use a five group plan while Canada uses a four group plan. The Daily Food Guide outlines the daily requirements for each food group, and is based on nutrient density as well as varying factors such as age, gender and level of physical activity. For example, males have a larger body mass and need more kcals than females, although during pregnancy, needs are greater; and active individuals need more kcals than sedentary people. Growing children need the lesser number of servings and in smaller amounts than adults.

A personal analysis—self-evaluation

Do you think you eat healthy? Try evaluating your diet. You may be surprised or even shocked at what you discover with the results. This research process can make you aware of the quality of foods you eat and enjoy regularly, and probably will motivate you to look more carefully at food labels when shopping. In doing this simple exercise, your knowledge of nutrition will expand enormously and you will be able to recommend healthier choices of foods to clients, friends and family. The forms for recording your daily food intake or 3-Day Food Diary are found in **Appendix V** where they can be photocopied for use.

Recording your 3-Day Food Diary. In order to assess diet, first begin to think of the foods eaten in terms of serving sizes as given above. Using the 3-Day Food Diary, list the foods eaten each day for three days—account for two weekdays and one weekend day. Remember to include snacks or drinks. Do not forget to list teaspoons or tablespoons of sugar or milk that you use in your drinks, such as coffee or tea, and condiments or spices such as mustard and ketchup. You may want to carry your record sheet around with you. This simple exercise may seem

How to Record a Daily Food Diary

Day of the week (circle): Mon Tue Wed Thur Fri Sat Sun Date: Oct. 1 Day of Record: 1

Quantity	Type of food	How Prepared
1	egg	boiled
1 slice	bread	toasted
2 cups	coffee	2 tbs. 2% milk

time-consuming but it will help to expand or reinforce your knowledge about the foods you choose to eat. See **How to Record a Daily Food Diary**.

For accuracy, you should record what you ate immediately after consumption. Research studies have shown that trying to remember what food and how much you ate is an inaccurate method, and this is reflected when using food recalls to record food diaries. It is important to record the portion sizes accurately in terms of standard measurements such as slices, cups, ounces and small versus large fruit. For example, a small banana contains less nutrients and kcals than a medium one, while a large banana is 1 1/2 servings and contains more kcals and nutrients. In recording a complex meal such a soup, try to list the ingredients of the soup and estimate the average amount of each ingredient in it such as 1 cup carrots, 2-oz. chicken and 2 teaspoons spices. Soup can be difficult to estimate unless it is homemade. Canned foods, such as soups, usually give kcals and ingredients on the label. The miscellaneous column should record any foods that do not fall under the four or five food groups. This includes all beverages, additives such as ketchup, mustard, salt, soy sauce, sugar, dressings such as mayonnaise and butter, and snacks. See

Sample of a 3-Day Dietary Intake

Food Group:	*Bread/ whole grains*	*Meat Products*	*Vegetables*	*Milk Products*	*Fruits*	*Misc.*	*Water*
Servings:	6-11	2-3	3-5	2-3	2-4	tbs.	8 g/d
Example							
Wed.	1+1+2+1+1= 6	1+1=2	2+1+1=4	1+1=2	1+1=2	1+1/2+1/2=2	1+1=2
Fri.	2+1+2+2=7	1+1+1=3	1+1=2	1+1/2=1 1/2	1	1+1+1/2=2 1/2	1+1+1=3
Sun.	3+2+2+3=10	3+1=4	2+1=3	1	1+1+1=3	2+2+2=6	1+1+1+1=4
Total	**23**	**9**	**9**	**4 1/2**	**6**	**10 1/2**	**9**
Avg.	8	3	3	1 1/2	2	3 1/2	3

Sample of a 3-Day Dietary Intake, on page 64, for a sample of a recorded daily food group plan for dietary analysis.

Balancing your diet. When you have finished recording your 3-Day Food Diary, transfer your servings to **Daily Food Guide Chart**, found in **Appendix V**.

Use the appropriate four or five food group plan for the correct country. Now, average daily servings can be compared with the daily food guide plan to see if a diet is balanced in each food group. The example shown in **Sample of a 3-Day Diary Intake**, on page 64, indicates that the total number of servings for the three days for bread or whole grains is 23. To get an average daily serving, divide by three. Since the average daily intake of bread/whole grains should be 6–11 servings, this is adequate for this food group. Do the same for each food group to see if your diet is balanced according to the food group plan.

Analyzing your diet

This exercise allows you to analyze the eating patterns of an individual and give advice on modifications for a healthier diet. Check the following:

Do your servings comply with each of the food groups?
Are you eating too many meat servings?
Are your milk or dairy products, and fruits and vegetables servings adequate?
Is there adequate daily water intake?
Look at the miscellaneous column for the snacks and additives. Are there excess hidden fats or sodium?

Some individuals eat too many snacks and not enough nutritious food, resulting in "hidden fats" contributing to unwanted kcals and unhealthy nutrients. Saturated fats and trans fatty acids commonly are hidden as hydrogenated fats, palm oils or coconut oils on food labels. If one has a habit of adding salt or sugar to foods, then make recommendations for healthier substitutes or to simply avoid them. Changes should be gradual and not forced. For example, most people have difficulty giving up certain tastes in their favorite foods, such as two teaspoons of sugar in their coffee. It may be wise to change this habit gradually by reducing the amount to half of a teaspoon of sugar instead of a full spoon, slowly reducing the amount until no sugar is used. Hidden sources of additives such as salt, soy sauce and mustard should be limited and substituted by spices when an individual is suffering from premenstrual symptoms or hypertensive conditions. Diabetic and weight loss plans should reduce hidden sugar intake especially in beverages such as sodas and baked goods. If cream is used in coffee, try recommending using whole milk first and gradually switch to low fat and finally to skim or non fat milk if tolerable.

Check how food is prepared, as well. If it is fried, the food contains higher amounts of kcals than grilled or steamed meats. Finally, if your diet conforms to the Daily Food Guide, it will be adequate, balanced, moderate, nutrient-dense and varied. If not, it can be rectified. The next step is to evaluate your daily kcal intake to control body weight using The Healthy Exchange System.

The Healthy Exchange System

Now that the daily food intake is balanced, the kcal value of foods must be considered. This is when the incorporation of the Healthy Exchange System will help to control imbalance. This system promotes healthy eating by focusing on exchanging unhealthy foods for natural, unprocessed foods. Developed by the American Dietetic Association, American Diabetes Association and other organizations, it provides a quick calculation of nutrients and kcal values in your daily diet. Carbohydrates, proteins, fats and kcals are grouped by their similarity in content. The exchanges are arranged in six groups—milk, vegetable, fruit, bread, meat and fat. You can substitute any food listed for another food item in the same list. Because of its emphasis on macronutrient and kcal content, this system is most effective for weight loss and diabetics. This research process promotes awareness to control energy intake by making a person more aware of the composition of favorite foods, particularly those high in fat, kcals and salt content. For example, milk can be thought as *non fat, low fat or whole,* while meat can be classified as *lean, medium fat or high fat*. You also will increase awareness of foods containing excessive sugar or salt. With the The Healthy Exchange System, lower kcal foods can be substituted for higher kcal foods while still maintaining the healthy, nutrient-dense quality of the foods you enjoy. Substitution should be done gradually and not be forced.

Try to think of the following foods in these measurements. As they become internalized, you will find that selecting healthy, low kcal foods will become automatic.

Starch/bread—1 slice of bread or 1/3 cup cooked rice or pasta = 80 kcals
Meat—1-oz. lean beef = 90 kcals; 1 egg = 75 kcal; 1-oz. cheddar cheese/1 tablespoon peanut butter/1 small hot dog = 100 kcal
Vegetables—1/2 cup cooked vegetables or one large tomato = 25 kcal
Fruits—1/2 banana or small fruit, 1/2 grapefruit or 15 small grapes = 60 kcal
Milk—1 cup non fat milk = 90 kcal; 1 cup low fat 2% milk = 120 kcal; 1 cup whole milk = 150 kcal
Fats—1 tablespoon butter/oil, 1 slice bacon, 10 large peanuts = 45 kcals

Source: U.S. Exchange System

The Healthy Exchange System can be used to make an average estimate of energy in foods. First convert the foods into exchanges then add the kcal values for each exchange. With practice, you eventually will become very aware and "see" the number of kcals in foods, thus controlling energy intake. Hopefully, this habit will become internalized, allowing you to form healthy choices all the time and without restraint. After practicing a few times, you will develop a lower tolerance for high fat, excessively sweet and salty foods, and will see foods through different eyes, always aware of their healthy or unhealthy composition. For example, the taste of cream in coffee or salt in foods becomes intolerable. You will begin to choose less salty, less sweet foods and begin to enjoy them just as much as you previously did with the unhealthier food choices.

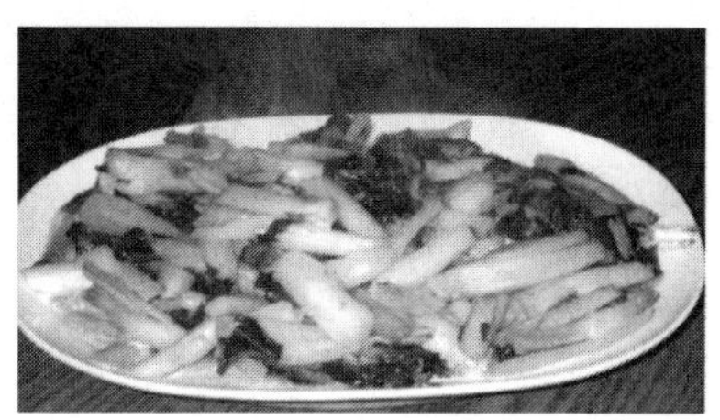

Bok Choy is a good source of calcium, iron and vitamins.

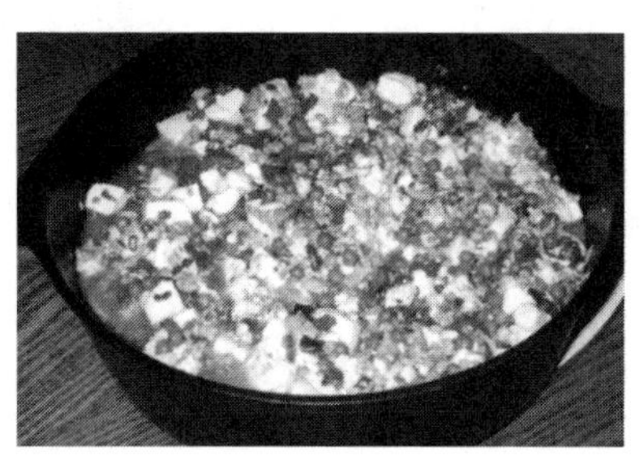

Cooking in ironware enhances iron absorption.

Although the daily food group plan ensures that adequate servings from each food group are consumed daily, The Healthy Exchange System allows you to control the kcal values of foods by substituting lower kcal foods in your diet. Food guides help to promote healthy eating—they guide you to eating a wider variety of foods that will allow you to obtain necessary nutrients without rigidity. What is important is not what is found in a single food or meal but rather how you balance your average intake of nutrients and calories over a few days. The total energy values for a sample meal using The Healthy Exchange System are shown as follows.

Lunch

2 slices turkey (2 meat exchanges, 55 x 2)	= 110 kcal
2 slices whole grain bread (2 starch exchanges, 80 x 2)	= 160 kcal
1 tablespoon mayonnaise (1 fat exchange)	= 45 kcal
1 cup non fat milk	= 90 kcal
15 small grapes	= 60 kcal
Total energy intake	**= 465 kcal**

Calculating Your Daily Nutrient Intake

Day: Wednesday (use one form for each day)

Approximate measure for...

							Fat Breakdown			
Food	**Weight**	*Energy* (kcal)	*Protein* (g)	*Carbo.* (g)	*Fiber* (g)	*Fat* (g)	*Sat* (g)	*Mono* (g)	*Poly* (g)	*Chol.* (mg)
Milk (whole)	1 cup	149	8	11	0	8	5.1	2.3	0.3	.12
White bread	4 slices	212	8	40	4	0.4	0.8	1.2	0.8	.0
Total		**361**	**16**	**51**	**4**	**8.4**	**5.9**	**3.5**	**1.1**	**.12**

Calculating nutrient values

Macronutrients are foods required in large amounts—proteins, carbohydrates and fats—and usually are measured in grams or ounces. In order to calculate the nutrient values of foods eaten, take the number of servings or portion sizes from the recorded 3-Day Food Diary and transfer them onto a Daily Nutrient Intake form found in **Appendix V**. This can be photocopied and used to calculate the nutrient values of macronutrients and micronutrients.

Next, obtain a Food Composition Index Chart from a recognized nutrition authority such as the Food and Drug Administration in the United States or the Ministry of Food and Agriculture in Canada. This index usually lists the nutrient values of one serving of most common foods including fast and convenience foods. If you had two servings of one food, you have to remember to *multiply* the nutrient values of all the macronutrients and micronutrients found in that food given in the Food Composition Index. For example, if one slice of whole grain bread is given at 64 kcals, two slices will be 128 kcals, and the values of all the macronutrients and micronutrients also have to be doubled. To find an average daily intake of each nutrient, add and total each column then divide by three. (See **Calculating Your Daily Nutrient Intake**.)

Calculating percentage of daily intake of nutrients. The next step is to find out if the macronutrients fall within the recommended percentages of total daily macronutrient intake. The following sample shows how to work out parameters of proteins, carbohydrates, fats and saturated fats. Remember, the lower end of proteins (15%) and carbohydrates (55%) are recommended for smaller individuals and the upper levels are for larger individuals.

Recommended Percentage of Macronutrients: Daily Intake

Protein	*Carbohydrates*	*Total Fats*
15–20%	55–60%	<30% <10% saturated fats

Recommended percentage of daily protein intake. Nutritionists recommend that daily protein intake should be 15–20% of total daily energy intake. To calculate if your protein intake falls within the realm of this recommendation, use the following formula:

% protein intake =
daily protein intake (grams x 4 kcals) / total daily energy intake (kcals) x 100

Recommended percentage of daily carbohydrates intake. To calculate if your carbohydrates fall within the parameters of the recommended 55–60% of total daily energy intake, use this formula:

% carbohydrates intake =
daily carbohydrates intake (grams x 4 kcals) / total daily energy intake (kcals) x 100

Recommended percentage of daily fat intake. To find out if your total daily intake of fats falls within the range of less than 30%, use the following formula:

% fats intake =
daily fats intake (grams x 9 kcals) / total daily energy intake (kcals) x 100

For example: if your total daily fat intake is 100 grams and your total daily intake is 2,700 kcals:

(100 g x 9 kcals) = 900 kcals / 2700 kcals x 100 = 33%

This is more than the recommended fat percentage of 30%. Therefore, if you scrutinized your food diary and the Food Composition Index that gives nutrient values, you can trace the food that contains the highest fat content and use The Healthy Exchange System to choose healthier substitutions to reduce your fat intake.

Recommended percentage of daily saturated fat intake. To find out if your total saturated fat intake is acceptable, use the following formula:

% daily saturated fat =
daily saturated fats (grams x 9 kcals) / total daily fat intake x 100

For example, if the total daily saturated fats intake is 20 g:

(20 g x 9 kcals) = 180 / 900 kcals x 100 = 20%

Calculating % of Daily Intake of Macronutrients

Day	*Energy* (kcal)	*Protein* (g)	*Carbo.* (g)	*Fiber* (g)	*Fat* (g)	*Sat Fat* (g)	*Mono Unsat. Fat* (g)	*Poly Unsat. Fat* (g)	*Chol.* (mg)	*Water* (g/d)
1	2300	89	293	19	93	19	50	12	146	2
2	2417	55	361	24	101	32	46	21	335	3
3	2840	130	352	21	104	32	46	21	335	4
Total	**7557**	**274**	**1006**	**64**	**298**	**83**	**142**	**4**	**816**	**9**
Average Daily Intake	2519	91	335	21	99	22	47	19	176	3
% Daily Intake	n/a	**14%**	**53%**	**n/a**	**36%**	**8%**	**17%**	**7%**	**n/a**	**n/a**
Comparison with DRIs/RDA of similar age, gender, weight, height, physical activity										
DRIs/RDA	n/a	15-20%	>50%	25-35	<30%	<10%	<10%	<10%	<300%	8 g/d

This is far above the level of 10% recommended by nutritionists. Remember, it is the saturated fat content in foods that contain cholesterol that forms plaque in the walls of blood vessels leading to heart disease. It is more important to qualify the *type* of fat and not just the total amount of fat consumed. **Calculating % of Daily Intake of Macronutrients** shows a sample diet of the average daily intake of three days of macronutrients. The percentage of the daily intake of proteins, fats, carbohydrates, cholesterol, vitamins and minerals are indicated. The breakdown of fats into saturated, monounsaturated, polyunsaturated and cholesterol also are listed. These figures can be compared against the RDA/DRI or a similar standardized guide in your country. Except for kcals, fiber and cholesterol, the DRIs of vitamins and minerals according to age and gender are given in **Appendix I**. From this comparison, you can determine if there is a deficiency or excessive intake of these nutrients. Anti-aging health practitioners recommend that 30–40 grams of fiber act as a preventive measure for health—this can be compared against the total daily intake of fiber.

Too many kcals?

To find out if you are eating too many or too few kcals, check your average daily kcal intake with your daily energy output in the next section. If this figure shows that your daily energy intake is more than your daily energy output, or activity, then weight gain will occur. Conversely, weight loss will occur if the energy intake is less than energy output. If energy input is equal to energy output, weight will be maintained. **Calculating % of Daily Intake of Macronutrients** shows the average daily intake of macronutrients from foods recorded in the 3-Day Food Diary. A comparison of the RDA/DRIs of individuals with similar age, gender, height, weight and physical activity also is shown at the bottom of the table and compared with your daily macronutrient intake.

The example shown in **Calculating % of Daily Intake of Macronutrients** on page 70, indicates that the daily percentage of proteins and carbohydrates were adequate but the percentage of fats was a little excessive. However, the percentage of saturated fats was below 10% of total fats and this is good as indicated by low cholesterol intake levels. However, fiber needs to be increased by eating more complex carbohydrates such as fruits, vegetables and whole grains.

Now that you have determined your daily energy intake, the next step is to work out your basal energy need, or BEN.

How to determine daily energy output needs. Before the BEN can be determined, the Basic Metabolic Rate (BMR) must be worked out. The BMR refers to the amount of energy output (kcals) required when the body is at complete rest, but not asleep, 12 hours after a meal so no digestion is taking place, in a warm room so no energy is used keeping warm. Men and women differ in their expenditures of energy. Since men possess more muscle mass, they burn more energy per kilogram than women: men = 1 kcal/kg/hour, women = 0.0 kcal/kg/hour.

However, humans must move to conduct their daily activities and the BEN is the daily energy intake required to do this. This is seen as the BMR multiplied by the activity level.

Choose the appropriate factor according to your activity level from the following chart. See **Activity Levels**, page 72.

Find out the BMR by converting your weight to kilograms using the following formula: 2.2 lb = 1 kg. If your body weight is 130 lb = 130 divided by 2.2 = 59 kg

BMR = kcal/kg/hr (gender) x weight (kg) x 24 (hours/day)

Therefore, a woman weighing 59 kg = 0.9 x 59 x 24 = 1,274 kcal/d. Work out the BEN by choosing the appropriate factor from the Activity Level Chart according to activity level.

BEN = BMR x activity level. For example, 1,274 x 1.6 = 2,038 kcal/d.

Therefore, a 59 kg individual with a moderate activity level will require 2,038 kcal/d to maintain their body weight. If weight loss is desired, the kcal input can be reduced or physical activity can be increased to a higher level. The average woman and man need about 2,000 and 2,500 kcal/d, respectively. This data now can be used to compare with the actual daily energy values that already have been worked out. This analysis will reveal whether the actual daily intake of

Activity Levels

Type of Activity	*Activity Level*	*% Activity Factor*
Sitting, standing, driving, typing, light-household duties such as cooking, cleaning, light gardening	Sedentary (female) Sedentary (male)	30% or 1.3 30% or 1.3
Slow walking, carpentry, golf, table tennis, doubles tennis, heavier house duties such as vacuuming	Light active (female) Light active (male)	50% or 1.5 60% or 1.6
Brisk walking, jogging, singles tennis, dancing, cycling, aerobics or treadmill 3–4 times per week, skiing	Moderately active (female) Moderately active (male)	60% or 1.6 70% or 1.7
Aerobics 5–6 times per week, heavy gardening, swimming, climbing, soccer	Very active (female) Very active (male)	90% or 1.0 n/a

Reprinted with permission from Recommended Dietary Allowances: 10th Edition *by the National Academy of Sciences, courtesy of the National Academics Press, Washington, D.C.*

Calculating Daily Micronutrient Intake

Day	**Calc** (mg)	**Iron** (mg)	**Magn** (mg)	**Phos** (mg)	**Potas** (mg)	**Sodium** (mg)	**Zinc** (mg)
1	1104	17	425	1365	3902	2635	9
2	739	16	362	975	4546	1288	6
3	712	20	371	1529	2821	5192	12
Total	**2555**	**53**	**1158**	**3869**	**11269**	**9115**	**27**
Average Daily Intake	852	18	386	1290	3756	3038	9
Comparison with DRIs of similar age, gender, weight, height, physical activity							
DRIs female (19-50 yrs)	1200	18	310-20	700	2000	<2400	8
Upper Levels	2500		350	4000			40

kcals, proteins, carbohydrates, fats and saturated fats are sufficiently relative to the BEN. This figure is more accurate than the DRIs, which is more generalized. The following example shows how to calculate the percentage of macronutrients that you actually have consumed and compare it with the BEN.

Comparing actual energy intake (kcals) with BEN. If your energy output is 2,038 kcal/d and the actual energy intake, calculated from the 3-Day Food Diary, is 2,638 kcals/d, you are consuming 600 kcals more than your BEN (2,638–2,038). This may lead to weight gain if no physical exercise is performed. Since fats contain the highest amount of kcals, check the 3-Day Food Diary to trace the foods containing the highest fat content and choose healthier substitutions with a lower fat content. The miscellaneous column should be checked closely because the additives including salad dressings and snacks, and food preparatory methods may contain hidden fats. Make the same comparison for all the micronutrients against the DRIs relative to age, gender, weight, and physical activity as shown in **Calculating Daily Intake of Micronutrients**. Note any deficiencies in each nutrient and suggest alternative foods for them that are nutrient-dense and healthier choices and somewhat similar in taste. It is difficult for people to give up their favorite foods and switch to a completely new taste, so doing it slowly is best.

By performing this self-study exercise, you will become increasingly aware of the nutrient values of foods that you eat regularly. You will find out if you are meeting the recommended percentage of total daily intake of proteins, carbohydrates, fats, fiber, iron and other nutrients. You also will note that some foods which you thought were very nutritious are not, and begin to search for other foods in the same category that also are nutrient-dense but contain less fat and

Vit. A (ug)	Vit. B1 (mg)	Vit. B2 (mg)	Vit. B3 (mg)	Vit. B6 (mg)	Vit. B12 (mg)	Folate (mg)	Vit. C (mg)	Vit. E (mg)
969	21	3	19	2	1	271	217	5
526	2	2	23	2	1	243	629	10
1439	2	2	45	3	2	215	120	12
2934	**25**	**7**	**87**	**7**	**4**	**729**	**966**	**27**
978	8	2	29	2	1	243	322	9
700	1.1	1.1	14	1.5	2.4	400	75	15
3000			35	100		1000	2000	1000

sodium, more fiber and other nutrients such as calcium and iron that may be lacking in your daily diet. It is a learning experience. Therefore, it is possible to analyze an individual's average daily intake to determine their total nutritional status and give guidance to help improve eating patterns.

Summary

Health experts recommend that no more than 30% of total daily calories should be derived from fats. Each gram of fat is equal to 9 kcals, therefore the average amount of daily fat consumption for a female who consumes an average of 2,000 kcals/d will be about 2,000 x .30 = 666 kcals from fats. The average man needs about 2,500 kcals, and this works out to 833 kcals from fats (2,500 x .30). Few people fit exactly into the mold, but this can be used as a guideline. Younger and more active people require more kcals, and a few extra grams of fat would not harm them. However, older, less active people should consume less fats and kcals.

If there is an imbalance of nutrients, the body becomes malnourished often leading to diseases or abnormalities. For example, a deficiency of fiber can lead to constipation, excess vitamin A can lead to toxic effects such as headaches and dry, peeling skin, while excess fat intake results in weight gain. **Appendix II** lists the DRIs giving more information on deficiencies or excessive intakes of micronutrients. Ultimately, it is important to remember that proper nutrition must be combined with regular exercise for good health and longevity.

CHAPTER 5

Dietary Supplements and Their Role in Esthetics

In the **preventive approach** to medicine, the belief is that if one follows certain dietary practices and lives a healthy lifestyle, a wide range of diseases can be prevented, delayed or in some cases, even reversed. The principles of the upper level of DRIs are based on a preventive approach to aging and the degenerative diseases associated with it. A healthy diet focusing on the consumption of fresh, natural foods and complemented by dietary supplements is recommended in an anti-aging program. However, numerous studies show that despite the ubiquitous information by various media, most North Americans still have inadequate nutritional diets and tend to compensate for their eating habits by taking dietary supplements, a phenomenon that has grown by 25% per annum in the past five years.

Supplements are not meant to replace diet, but to enhance it, hence the word "supplement." Several studies show that one in every three people already take supplements. Since they have no guidelines to follow, they tend to purchase supplements through the influence of friends, physicians and the media. Although almost 98% of medical experts and researchers also take supplements, they have not endorsed dietary supplementation for the public. Skin care professionals do not need to become nutritionists or dieticians to provide basic nutritional counseling to their clients. With such a high percentage of people taking dietary supplements, acquiring some knowledge of the most common dietary supplements can help to understand their benefits and the reasons why people take them.

Why do people take supplements?

Studies show that the media plays a very powerful role in influencing people's decision to take dietary supplements. Although many people can derive their nutrient needs from natural foods, they still prefer to take food supplements. Some feel reassured that supplements will overcome or prevent any nutrient deficiencies that they may be suffering, while others take them simply because it is trendy, and many are influenced by friends or relatives. Results of a study on women suggested that one of the reasons they took dietary supplements was that it gave them some degree of control over their health. It is interesting to note that supplement users were found to be most common among Caucasians, women, older people, those with higher incomes and higher education, non-smokers—especially former smokers, those who don't consume large amounts of alcohol and those who live in the western United States.

It has been found that supplements taken by prescription contain higher nutrient content than self-prescribed ones, particularly vitamin B complex. Many supplements are sold in drug-like formulations even though government authorities have not approved them. This can lead to serious problems due to varying levels of natural constituents in herbs. For example, the concentration of a constituent varies according to the part of the plant from which it is derived, the harvesting stage, processing and dilution during manufacture. Furthermore, some herbal products naturally contain harmful chemicals such as certain alkaloids.

Who needs supplements?

According to many major medical organizations such as the American Dietetic Association (ADA), supplements are essential among the following populations.

- Women who suffer from heavy menstrual flow.
- Pregnant or lactating women.
- Post-menopausal women—especially calcium and vitamin D to protect against osteoporosis.
- Those on low-kcal or special diets such as vegans who need vitamin B-12, only found in meat.
- Individuals whose nutritional status may be affected by surgery, disease or medication and may suffer from impaired absorption of certain nutrients.
- Those over the age of 65. Health problems may contribute to a poor diet so dietary supplements may help ensure adequate vitamin and mineral intake.
- Those who excessively smoke or drink alcohol suffer impaired nutrient absorption. Alcoholics are likely to substitute alcohol for food.
- Those who do not eat a balanced diet—less than the recommended five servings of fruits and vegetables—need to take multivitamin supplements, but it is best to adopt better eating habits.

Calcium supplements. Calcium supplements are very beneficial to women during menopausal years, even though results may be slow and bone loss still may occur. However, they should not be used as a substitute for estrogen. Several calcium supplements have been discovered to contain some lead and have had to be reformulated. Others contained excess levels of vitamin D that can become toxic in the body.

Calcium supplements are available in three forms:

- Purified calcium compounds such as calcium carbonate, citrate, gluconate, lactate, maltate or phosphate. Calcium carbonate contains 40% calcium while calcium gluconate has only 9%.
- Amino acid chelates—compounds with amino acids.
- Calcium compounds mixed with other minerals, such as calcium carbonate with magnesium carbonate, vitamin B or aluminum salts.

Calcium supplements also come in powder forms such as bone meal, dolomite or limestone, but these are more likely to cause adverse reactions. They are not absorbed as well as the other compounds, and it is recommended that low doses be taken several times a day instead of one large dose at a time. This strategy can help to increase total daily absorption.

Health risks of calcium supplements. Several problems may be associated in taking calcium supplements and include impaired iron absorption where high calcium intakes can interfere with iron absorption; milk alkali syndrome, an alkaline state that occurs from excessive milk intake; drug interactions—excessive calcium intakes may have adverse effects with certain drugs; constipation which can occur when excessive consumption of milk and vitamin D toxicity or excess—vitamin D in the body can have an adverse effect on the body's health such as calcification of soft tissues such as kidney stones.

Regulations of dietary supplements

The Dietary Supplement Health and Education Act 1994 (DSHEA) has deregulated the marketing of dietary supplements making manufacturers more responsible for the safety of supplements as long as certain statements of nutritional support were indicated on food labels. Most vitamin and mineral supplements pose little or no danger to the general population since they usually are labeled accurately. However, other products such as amino acids, herbs and botanicals that make health claims may pose unsubstantiated safety risks since little research has been done on them. This neglect can lead to an increased development of more untested products in the industry.

While the FDA is the controlling body for dietary supplements, they are regulated as foods and not as drugs. Except for safety reasons, this restricts it from limiting potency and composition of most multi-nutrient products. Although there is a wide safety limit for most nutrients, there are very narrow limits for certain minerals such as selenium. It is therefore recommended that consumers take precaution in consuming dietary supplements of high potency unless they are prescribed by knowledgeable people such as nutritionists or medical practitioners.

Dietary supplements and fitness

Exercise in moderation is a healthy but slow way to lose body fat. The fitness media, particularly magazines, tend to use nutrition advertisements to sell or market substances and products that are depicted to enhance athletic performance, otherwise known as **ergogenic.** Some advertisements use scientific data to support their health claims in order to impress readers. However, although they sound good, the majority of these claims are not supported by research findings.

Many fit individuals already have healthy diets and do not need supplements because they are careful about what they eat. It is important to consume a high intake of complex carbohydrates to promote physical performance.

Nutrition after workouts. If active people need to quench their thirst after a workout, they usually reach for diet beverages, but nutritious juices are better choices since carbohydrates help to refuel the muscles. Glucose provides more energy for the body when compared with amino acids, so eating fruits, or drinking juices or a glass of non fat milk, is very beneficial. Most sports diets tend to lack sufficient carbohydrates. Consuming low glycemic index foods before exercising can sustain blood glucose levels leading to duration and improved exercise performance. After a workout, an athlete who burns off 4,000 kcals per day (kcals/d) easily can recover the lost calories with two cans of sugar-sweetened soda drinks—not something that is recommended.

Why and when to eat breakfast. Without question, breakfast is the most important meal of the day, and yet many people use the excuse of having "no time for breakfast." In fact, eating breakfast actually may help to control weight by avoiding that ravenous feeling in the middle of the morning, reducing the temptation to indulge in a high-fat treat. It is more beneficial to start off with a large healthy breakfast and lunch followed by a smaller dinner. People who exercise early in the morning may feel uncomfortable with

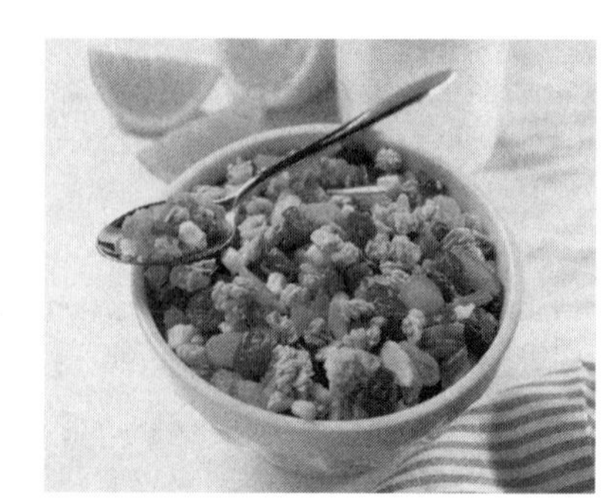

Fig. 5-1: *A healthy breakfast.*

a large breakfast. A small breakfast that includes half a whole grain bagel or slice of multigrain toast with fruit or a glass of juice is excellent because it helps to increase body metabolism for the day. Liquid breakfasts such as a glass of juice or low fat milk are good and take no preparation. (See ***Figure 5-1***, page 78.)

An evening athlete can consume a hearty breakfast of 600–700 kcals to fuel their workout. Since most individuals who work out regularly are very concerned about their shape and body weight, they should eat a decent breakfast to prevent binging on junk foods later in the day. Moreover, it will provide more energy for working out. Most fitness enthusiasts should consume at least 400–600 kcals for breakfast.

The adage of a "good" American breakfast of fried eggs, bacon, hash browns and toast was discarded a long time ago. It contains too many calories from fat and can clog up the arteries leading to the development of heart diseases. Oatmeal is a good choice if you have the time to prepare it. Cold cereal is faster and can be eaten on the run with fruit or small carton of low fat milk. Choose a cereal with 3–5 grams of fiber and make sure that sugar is not one of the first three ingredients on the food label.

A hearty, wholesome breakfast should include:

Grains—Enriched breakfast cereals, whole grains such as bagels, melba toast or low fat bran muffins.

Dairy—Cheese, yogurt or a glass of low fat milk.

Protein—Hard boiled or poached eggs, peanut butter, lean slices of meat, poultry or fish.

Fruits and vegetables—A fresh fruit or vegetable or 100% fruit juice without added sugar.

Alternatives—A smoothie blended from exotic fruits; some low fat yogurt and a spoonful of wheat germ or flaxseed; vegetable pizza; or vegetables, salsa and low fat shredded cheeses wrapped in a whole wheat tortilla.

Unless you have high cholesterol, you can consume up to 3–4 eggs per week. Eggs are the best source of protein and are full of nutrients. In fact, several types of eggs are available today for the health conscious such as omega-3 and cholesterol-free eggs. If you eat at fast food restaurants, choose whole grain bagels, rolls and English muffins over fat-filled doughnuts, scones and croissants.

Popular supplements

Research has indicated that approximately 1/3 of populations in modern cities use some form of nutrient supplements regularly, particularly vitamins and minerals. Dietary supplements appear in various forms such as capsules, tablets, liquids and powders. Others are botanicals such as ginseng, fish oils, fibers such as guar gum, enzymes and herbal mixtures. Dietary supplements found in supermarkets include vitamins, minerals, proteins, amino acids and calcium—the most common ones were single nutrient products containing vitamins A, B-12, C, E and the rest of the vitamin B complex. Other popular ones include those containing more than one nutrient, or multi-nutrients, followed in the order of calcium, iron, zinc, potassium, magnesium, fluorine, iodine and copper. Multi-nutrient products primarily are marketed to children in chewable forms. Although some products are advertised as single nutrient supplements, they actually contain varying amounts of other nutrients. For example, some calcium supplements made from calcium phosphate compounds and other chemicals contain, in addition to calcium, other nutrients such as phosphorus, iron, magnesium, zinc or vitamin D. Vitamins C and D usually are included in calcium supplements in order to enhance absorption.

Choosing and using supplements

It should be stressed that supplements are not to be substitutes for whole fresh foods because they cannot replace the numerous nutrients found in foods. However, if you do decide to take supplements, consider the following factors.

- Avoid supplements with "mega doses." Choose a multivitamin/mineral supplement that provides 100% daily values of all the nutrients instead of one that supplies an overdose such as 500% of one vitamin and only 20% of another. (See **Chapter 7** for more information on daily values.)
- Look for the United States Pharmacopeia (USP) label that ensures standardized quality needs have been met by the testing organization. Dietary supplements should be manufactured at an FDA licensed facility in accordance to Good Manufacturing Practice (GMP) guidelines.
- Do not be taken in by gimmicks such as added herbs, enzymes and amino acids.
- Check for expiration dates.
- Store supplements in a cool, dry place.
- If you are on medication or have some medical problems, check with your physician before purchasing dietary supplements, especially if they contain more than 100% of dietary values because supplements can interfere with medications. For example, individuals taking anticoagulants, or blood-thinners, should not take vitamins E and K. High doses of niacin also can result in liver problems.

Become a resource

The food supplement industry has become a lucrative market for many health care companies that have capitalized on those individuals who depend on food supplements as a form of "insurance" for their health. In 1993, the United Kingdom exported sales of dietary supplements was $238 million, according to Benn Publications, 1994. Skin care professionals can become credible resources for their clients. They already are providing treatments for their client's skin and body, and by recommending dietary supplements, they can enhance the results and improve their client's health status. With more knowledge about dietary supplements, estheticians can influence their clients to purchase some of their dietary supplements at the spa instead of mass market retailers.

CHAPTER 6

Nutritional Issues among Women

The role of nutrition in women's health and disease must be emphasized throughout their life cycles. For example, the hormonal changes that occur during major life events such as menstruation, contraception, pregnancy, lactation, menopause and aging affect women deeply. The risk of gaining excess weight and developing breast cancer and chronic diseases tends to increase with age. In addition, the pursuit of beauty and the "ideal" physical figure of a young, slim and fit body has had a dramatic psychological and social impact on the eating behavior of women in modern society.

This ideal image has been created and perpetuated by the media that constantly stresses the importance of being slim and attractive. Women in particular are more susceptible to these standards starting from early childhood when they tend to affect a female's self-perception and self-esteem, sometimes culminating in various eating disorders such as anorexia nervosa and bulimia. Other major industries such as fashion, cosmetics, fitness and cosmetic surgery also have contributed to the support of this ongoing quest for youth and beauty. Studies conducted between 1988 and 1991 indicate that, in general, females of all ages and all ethnic groups exceeded the current dietary guidelines for fat and were below DRIs for dietary fiber. Females were more likely to be deficient in certain nutrients such as calcium, iron and folate, or folic acid. In many cases, dietary supplements may be necessary to correct these inadequacies.

Older women. As women age, the state of their health becomes increasingly important. They become more interested in nutrition relating to prevention and treatment of chronic diseases such as osteoporosis. They also become concerned about body weight, but place more emphasis on health rather than appearance. Some are unsure of which guidelines they ought to follow and eventually, many of them begin to use supplements, but not regularly. With the vast number of aging baby boomers, women were shown to outlive men according to *www.unescape.org*. As a result, more research is being conducted on women than ever before.

The Anti-aging Theory of Calorie Restriction has been proven. (See **Chapter 13**.) It holds that reduced consumption of calories in aging will result in reduced formation of free radicals. Research studies indicate that older women need a

High Risk Factors for Osteoporosis

Low calcium and low protein intake—During youth, this can lead to decreased bone and body mass.

Gender—Females lose estrogen hormones, the main cause of reduced bone mass, during menopause. Dense body mass is considered to be a protective factor in osteoporosis. Because males have greater skeletal mass and body weight than females, they suffer less from osteoporosis.

Race—Osteoporosis is more common among small-boned individuals, particularly Causcasian and Asian females than women of African descent who tend to have a larger body mass.

Lifestyle factors—Lack of physical activity, smoking and alcoholism can increase the risk of developing osteoporosis.

Prolonged use of antacids and steroid therapy—This may impair the absorption of calcium in the body.

Certain population groups—Some population groups are more prone to osteoporosis in later life. They include those who have experienced anorexia nervosa and young athletes such as gymnasts and ballet dancers, particularly those who do not get their menses. This finding was attributed to their poor eating habits even though they were very physically active. This may infer that both nutrition and exercise are essential to offset osteoporosis.

higher amount of protein, vitamins B-6, B-12 and D, calcium and zinc, but lower levels of iron, than younger people due to the cease of menstruation. However, requirements for the rest of vitamin B complex remain the same.

Common deficiencies

Calcium. The DRIs for calcium among females 19–25 years is 800 milligrams per day (mg/d) while menopausal, post-menopausal, pregnant and lactating women require 1,200–1,500 mg/d. **Osteoporosis** is a health problem that affects both women and men later in life, but is more prevalent among women. Surveys indicate that there are about 50 million postmenopausal women during this first decade of the new millennium which will result in a significant rise in osteoporosis increasing public health costs. In addition, this health hazard reduces the quality of life for the elderly resulting in many debilitating disorders such as hip and spinal fractures. Osteoporosis is a brittle bone disease that can be hereditary or can occur as a result of lifestyle. Symptoms are seen in 25% of women after menopause and are associated with a decline in estrogen hormones which leads to loss of skeletal bone mass. (See **High Risk Factors for Osteoporosis**, page 84.)

In normal, healthy bones, worn out cells are continuously removed by **osteoclast** bone cells and replaced by the action of **osteoblast** cells. Porous bone develops when the activity of the osteoblasts is reduced by various factors such as deficiency of estrogen, but the osteoclasts keep working so that the bone cells are removed faster than they are built. This imbalance of bone formation results in brittle, porous bones susceptible to bone fractures, even after a minor fall or injury, particularly in the wrists and hips. Spontaneous compression fractures can occur in the vertebrae, particularly dorsal bones, and they become wedge-shaped giving rise to the typical Dowager's hump that can be extremely painful and unsightly, often causing an overall reduction in height. (See **Figure 6-1**.)

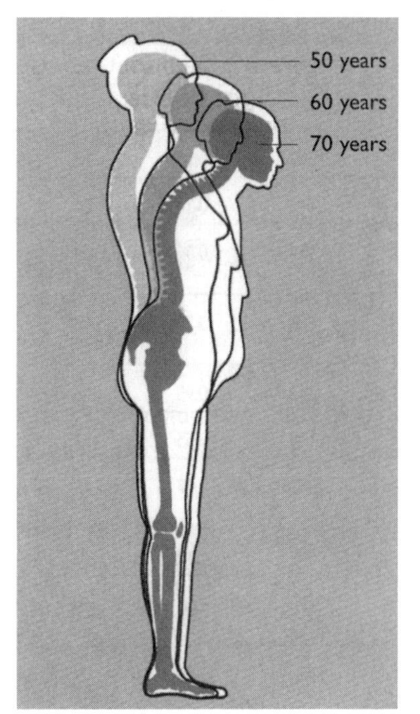

Figure 6-1: *Dowagers' hump. From Understanding Nutrition (with Dietary Reference Intakes Supplement and InfoTrac) 9th edition by WHITNEY/ROLFES. © 2002. Reprinted with permission of Brooks/Cole, a division of Thomson Learning: www.thomsonrights.com. Fax 800-730-2215.*

Bone breakdown and rebuilding processes occur continuously during a person's lifetime with bones reaching their maximum mass and strength potential around age 35, after which they begin to deteriorate. Much of what will happen to bones later in life depends on the quality of the bones developed up to this age, especially between 10 to 20 years old when bone growth is most rapid. The consequences of inevitable bone loss in later years will be less severe if you can start out with a dense bone structure that has been built up with a high calcium intake.

Building strong bones. Exercise and diet are the two most important ingredients in building strong bones. A minimum of three hours a week of weight-bearing exercises such as walking, running and weight training can increase the quality of bone mass. The DRIs for calcium in the average individual is 1,000 mg/d—the most significant sources are found in milk and milk products. Since one glass of milk contains 300 mg, drinking at least three 8-oz. glasses of milk daily will help young women to reach their DRI levels. However, many studies show that females of all ages do not have sufficient milk intake. Some reasons include the belief that they will gain weight because milk is fattening, while others simply do not like the taste. Women need to be educated about other sources of calcium, such as low fat milk and cheese, yogurt, tofu and dark green leafy vegetables.

A study showed that drinking more than three cups of coffee daily increased bone loss in women with low calcium intake, while healthy postmenopausal women who consumed sufficient calcium were unaffected.

Other nutrients needed for strong bone formation include vitamin C and D, copper, magnesium and fluoride. Recent studies show that the elderly tend to shun sunlight, and this can have a crucial effect on the formation of osteoporosis since vitamin D is necessary for the absorption of calcium in the intestines. The elderly should be encouraged to have sun exposure early in the morning or late in the evening to obtain the necessary vitamin D.

Iron. Iron deficiency, or anemia, is a worldwide problem. Women need 10–15 mg of iron daily and are especially prone to iron deficiency because of heavy menstrual flow or menstrual blood loss, particularly those who suffer from **amenorrhea**. Anemia can be detected in an individual by pale eyes and skin pallor. In a dark skinned person, the inside of the eyes, which usually is pink, will be very pale or even white. Other symptoms include fatigue, headaches and poor cold tolerance. Excellent sources of iron are red meat, legumes and green vegetables. Other factors that affect iron absorption include calcium and phosphorus in milk, and tannic acid in tea and coffee. Because of this, only drink these beverages about half an hour after meals.

Vegetarians are more likely to suffer from iron deficiency because of absence of red meat. However, they can obtain their DRIs from legumes, soy products and green vegetables, such as spinach, and enriched foods. Iron from animal foods, or **heme**, is better absorbed than iron from plants, **non-heme**. Contamination iron may help to increase dietary iron, so cooking foods in iron cookware is highly recommended. The more acidic the food and the longer it is cooked in iron cookware, the higher the iron contamination. It also is important to eat foods rich in vitamin C together with iron-rich foods because they enhance iron absorption. An example would be eating meat with potatoes or squash. It should be noted that iron in dietary supplementary form is not absorbed as efficiently as iron from natural foods.

Folate, or folic acid. Folate is a B vitamin that is especially important for young females of childbearing age. Several research studies have confirmed the importance of folate in reducing the risks of neural tube defects such as **spina bifida** that affects the development of the brain and spinal cord, particularly during the first trimester of pregnancy. As a result, it is highly recommended that young females, particularly those who are likely to become pregnant, consume a diet containing high amounts of folate in order to offset the possibility of producing a child born with neural defects. In addition to a folate-rich diet, they should take a multivitamin containing at least 0.4 mg of folic acid daily. Foods containing brewer's yeast, and green leafy vegetables, are high sources of folate. In North America, many foods now are enriched with folate to help offset deficiency of this important vitamin for young females who do not eat many fruits and vegetables.

Nutrition and women's health

As people are beginning to turn away from conventional medicine and drugs, they are seeking more natural alternative strategies. Women are becoming more aware that nutritional factors can help alleviate the symptoms of both premenstrual syndrome (PMS) and menopause without taking medications. In addition, dietary supplements are increasingly used to combat these discomforting symptoms without any side effects. Some nutritional factors include the following.

Soy and soy products. The daily intake of soy and soy products as well as dietary supplements is highly recommended for both premenstrual and menopausal women to combat cancer and heart disease. When compared to the United States, the lower incidence of heart disease and female reproductive cancers in Asia have been attributed to the traditional dietary practice of daily soy consumption. It is believed that **soy isoflavones**, or phytoestrogens, are responsible for this protective influence.

Research studies suggest that the chemical structure of soy isoflavones is similar to that of estrogen, allowing them to act as estrogen receptors blocking estrogen from entering into breast cells and giving a protective influence against the formation of breast cancer. In PMS, the levels of estrogen are higher than progesterone, and the similar action of isoflavones in mimicking estrogen also can help to reduce PMS symptoms. One cup of soybeans provides approximately 300 mg of isoflavones.

While hormone replacement therapy may increase the risk for cancer, scientists have found that consumption of soy foods containing phytoestrogens is associated with reduction of the risk of cancer.

Another useful effect of soy is its protection against LDL oxidation, a significant factor in reducing heart disease. Soy foods contain less fat and are a better source of protein for women during PMS and menopause. Tofu made from soybean curd is low in fat, cholesterol-free and rich in protein. It also is an excellent source of essential fatty acids—linolenic and oleic, iron, thiamin, phosphorus and potassium.

The two most common types of tofu available in North America are cotton and silken. The silken form is smoother and more suited for desserts, drinks and dips while the cotton type is water-packed and is best for cooking. (See **Figure 6-2**.) Tofu appears in many different forms in the supermarkets today, and Asian markets carry soy products such as tempeh and miso.

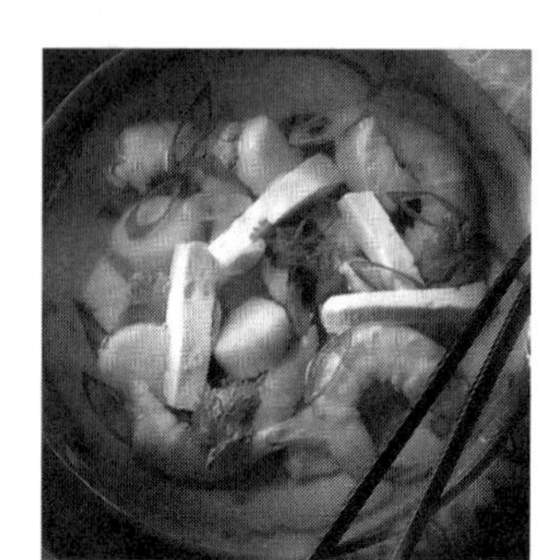

Figure 6-2: Delicious tofu.

Silken tofu is vacuum-packed and has a long shelf life of several months. It contains more solidifier and is not drained of water. Cotton tofu is produced by placing soybean milk that has been mixed with a solidifier in a cotton-lined container with tiny holes. The cloth is folded over this curd, and a weight is used to press out the liquid. Always check the expiration date on tofu packages when shopping.

Black cohosh extract. This herbal extract has been used to relieve PMS cramps, depression, hot flashes and to reduce vaginal atrophy in menopause.

Caffeine. Lower consumption of caffeine is highly recommended to reduce mood swings, especially irritability, depression and anxiety symptoms, particularly in PMS.

Salt. Reduced consumption of salt and salty foods lowers the incidence of high blood pressure in postmenopausal women, bloating, water retention and breast tenderness during PMS.

Essential fatty acids. Reducing the intake of inflammatory foods such as animal-derived foods—PG2, and increasing the consumption of anti-inflammatory foods—PG1 and PG3, are highly recommended during these periods of a woman's life.

Zinc. Because immunity is low during PMS, zinc is beneficial to strengthen the immune system during this time.

Vegetarian diet. There is a positive correlation between the risk of breast cancer and saturated fat intake in postmenopausal women. Those suffering from PMS tend to have food cravings and eat a poor diet high in refined carbohydrates and sugars. Eating more plant foods and reducing fats and trans fatty acids will increase the intake of dietary fiber helping to remove built-up toxins in the body.

Vitamin C and hesperidin. These combined flavonoids help improve vascular integrity and increase capillary permeability, particularly during hot flashes.

Female hormonal issues

Premenstrual Syndrome (PMS). This topic is of significant interest to the health and beauty professional because of its psychological and physical effects on females. PMS is characterized by debilitating mood and behavioral changes that affect the ability to function normally with varying degrees of severity. Women experience emotional symptoms that last from several days to several weeks before the onset of their menstrual flow. However, they do not normally disrupt a women's life. Emotional symptoms include depression, hypersensitive skin, irritability, mood swings, tension and confusion while physiological symptoms include bloating, body aches, breast tenderness, food cravings and feeling heavy.

Menopause. The cessation of the menses is both a blessing and a curse at the same time. For some, it is a sad reflection of the end of a woman's ability to reproduce, but is a blessing not to have the symptoms of monthly menses anymore. Menopause usually occurs in women over age 45 and is associated with the decline of estrogen production.

There are four stages: pre-menopause—the period before irregular menses begins; peri-menopause—irregular ovulation occurring for approximately two years before menses ceases, accompanied by menopausal symptoms; menopause—menses ceases completely; and postmenopause—five years after last period.

Menopausal symptoms affect every woman differently and they vary from mild to severe. Physiological symptoms include hot flashes, profuse sweating, headaches, vertigo, heart palpitations, sleep disturbances, atrophy of sex organs and depression. Psychological symptoms include mood swings, irritability, loss of concentration and loss of feelings of femininity.

Because most women suffer from hot flashes that have a marked effect on their skins, a better understanding of the physiological action may be appreciated. Hot flashes mainly are caused by hormonal changes but also can be affected by lifestyle and medication. The lowered levels of estrogen affects the hypothalamus, an endocrine gland that controls the body's drives for body temperature, sex, thirst, sleep and food. The body temperature is read as being too hot, and the body responds by increasing the heartbeat, blood circulation and action of the nervous system to remove the heat resulting in dilated capillaries and increased sweat to cool the body. Thin women may experience more severe hot flashes than larger sized women because their bodies produce less estrone, one of the natural estrogens by fat and muscle cells.

Those women who smoke also may suffer worst hot flashes because smoking causes the blood vessels to lose some ability to radiate heat. Instead of hormone replacement therapy, natural alternatives include diet modifications such as low fat diet, soy foods, herbal remedies and regular exercise to alleviate symptoms of hot flashes and avoid triggers such as alcohol, smoking, hot spicy foods, caffeine, and hot showers and baths. Practice stress reduction techniques such as deep breathing, yoga, massage and mediation.

In addition, three health concerns facing the postmenopausal woman are heart disease, osteoporosis and breast cancer. With a prolonged life span, a woman can expect to spend at least 1/3 of her lifetime in postmenopausal phase. Hormonal replacement therapy (HRT) has been used by millions of post-menopausal women for decades, but several recent studies have indicated that this therapy poses a high risk of heart disease and cancer.

Nutritional support for menopausal women includes the following:

- Reduce animal foods because they contain high hormonal levels, increase consumption of fresh, natural fruit and vegetables.
- Consume phytoestrogen-rich plants such as soy foods. Soy consumption in menopause has been shown to reduce hot flashes, vaginal dryness, prevent cardiovascular diseases, reduce depression and is beneficial for other diseases.
- Other nutrients that help to reduce symptoms of menopause include essential fatty acids—omega-3 and omega-6—richest sources are salmon and mackerel, and flaxseed and evening primrose oils.

Nutritional supplements include:

- *Vitamin E* for relief of hot flashes. Topical application of vitamin E creams reduce dryness and inflammation of atrophic vaginitis.
- *Black cohosh and licorice root* are herbal extracts that support female reproductive systems.
- *Ginkgo biloba* extracts increase circulation in limbs and in the brain leading to improved memory and concentration; the longer they are taken, the more obvious and long-lasting the results.

Health benefits of exercise in menopause include relief from hot flashes, increased bone mass to prevent osteoporosis, reduced blood pressure, decreased stress, improved cardiovascular function, decreased body fat, increased lean body mass for improved muscular strength, and improved body image leading to increased self-esteem.

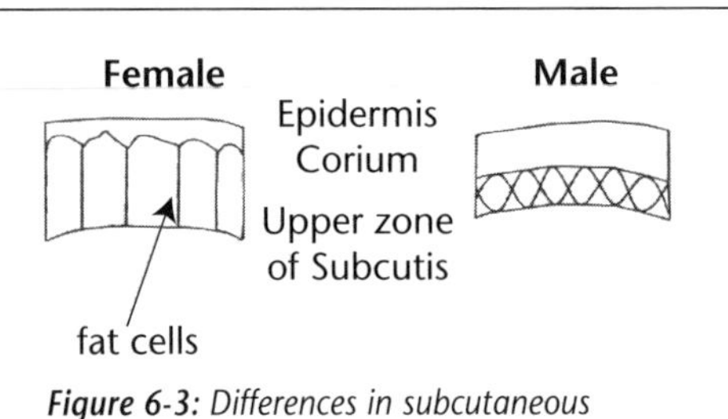

Figure 6-3: Differences in subcutaneous tissue in men and women.

Cellulite

Cellulite is not a disease but a cosmetic disorder caused from anatomical changes in cellular structure. It commonly is found in women—even some slim women—and is closely associated with obesity. While there is no conclusive evidence that cellulite is a hormonal disorder, anatomically it is believed to occur from loss of integrity of supportive connective tissue:

Characteristics. Characteristics include a "mattress" look—bulging, pitting, deformed skin tissues, accompanied by tightness, heaviness—especially on the thighs; the buttocks tender when pinched, pressed or massaged vigorously; and often accompanied by varicosity.

Histology. The subcutaneous layers in women and men differ as shown in **Figure 6-3**. The differences include:

Women. The subcutaneous tissues in the thighs are composed of three layers of fat with two planes of connective tissues between them. The subcutaneous layer in women consists of large "fat cell chambers" separated by arched dividing walls of connective tissue that are anchored to the overlying connective tissue of skin, the corium. As the female body ages, the corium becomes thinner and looser, allowing fat cells to enter this layer, and the walls between fat cell chambers become thinner, allowing fat cell chambers to hypertrophy and project. This results in alternating depressions and protrusions in the upper subcutaneous layer giving the appearance of a "mattress look". In obese individuals, the pressure is heavier and increases the bulging effect.

Men. The top layer is thicker with a network of criss-crossing connective tissue walls. Cellulite in men is uncommon because men have more lean muscle mass than females.

Stages of formation

Stage 0—when standing or lying down, there are no bulges or pitting. This is normal among slim people.

Stage 1—this is considered the ideal stage. When standing or lying down, the skin appears smooth but shows up in pinch test.

Stage 2—when lying down, the skin is smooth, but when standing, shows pitting and bulging.

Stage 3—shows whether standing or lying down, common after menopause or obesity. (**See Figure 6-4.**)

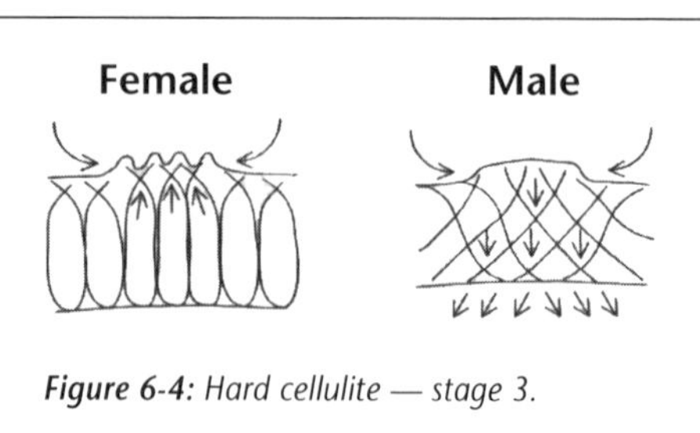

Figure 6-4: *Hard cellulite — stage 3.*

Best approach is preventive

- Practice a healthy diet with adequate fiber and dietary supplements for detoxification.
- Achieve or maintain a healthy body weight relevant to your height (body mass index).
- If overweight, lose weight gradually thus avoiding formation of stretch marks, or vergetures.
- Exercise regularly throughout life to control body weight—a minimum of three times per week for at least 30 minutes per session.
- Have regular massages to improve lymphatic flow. Manual lymphatic drainage is an effective form of preventive care for cellulite.

Nutritional support

Eat more wholesome fresh, natural foods and minimize refined foods, especially starches and sugars, and consume high dietary fiber, including whole grains, vegetables.

Some herbal extracts that claim to help improve cellulite conditions, reduce edema, increase lymphatic flow and reduce varicosity include:

- *Centella Asiatica*, a triterpenoid compound containing 70% triterpenic acids, essential oils such as camphor, and flavonoids; it acts directly on fibroblasts to increase cellular metabolism by enhancing the structure of connective tissue without overstimulating collagen synthesis.
- *Escin*, seeds of horse chestnut, gives an anti-flammatory effect and an anti-edema effect that improve better permeability of capillaries thus allowing better blood circulation.
- *Bladderwrack*, a topical application of seaweed extracts, contains high iodine content to stimulate metabolism and help soothe, soften and improve tone of connective tissue.

CHAPTER 7

Nutritional Support for Skin and Body Conditions

The skin is the largest organ of the body, covering it from head to toe. Together with its appendages, the nails and hair, the skin acts as a biomarker for a person's health status. The human skin continuously is subjected to both internal and external stressors, and this ultimately affects its condition and function. External changes include various skin disorders such as photoaging, pH imbalance and inflammation, while internal effects include dysfunction of the immune system.

The skin is composed of three main layers—epidermis, dermis and hypodermis, or subcutaneous layer. The uppermost layer, the **epidermis**, also is composed of several layers, the deepest being the basal layer where new cells are fed by the underlying dermal layer. Pigment-producing cells, melanocytes, also are found here, and it is estimated that one in every ten cells in this layer produces the pigment melanin that progresses upward to the top layers of the epidermis where it protects the skin from the damaging UV rays of the sun.

As these basal cells move upward toward the stratum corneum, they lose water, become dry, flattened, and tightly packed and eventually are shed. This process of keratinization takes approximately 3–4 weeks. The **dermis** lies between the epidermis and the subcutaneous layers. The top layer contains a highly vascular network that projects into the basal layers of the epidermis to feed the newly born cells. The dermis also contains a nerve plexus that gives sensation to the skin and all the glands within it such as the sebaceous and sweat glands that lubricate the skin and hair. The dermis is composed of connective tissue containing collagen and elastin fibers, the proteins that make the skin supple and elastic. The **subcutaneous layer** is composed of adipose tissue that cushions the bony skeletal structure and provides heat for the body's organs.

Functions of the skin

The skin performs many important functions, but the main one is protection. It protects underlying tissues from bacteria invasion, and the melanin pigment helps to protect the skin from the sun's harmful rays. The skin also regulates body temperature by dilating the blood capillaries at the skin's surface and releasing heat. Conversely, in cool temperatures or when one is frightened, the capillaries constrict to maintain a constant homeostasis of 37°C or 98.6°F. The thickness of the skin varies on different parts of the body, and the thicker skin on the joints helps cushion bones and organs from damage. When the skin's function is impaired, the complexion is affected resulting in skin lesions.

Nutrition and the skin

One of the most important and popular services in the spa is the enhancement of the texture and health of the client's skin. During a skin examination under a magnifying lamp, it may be possible to detect some nutritional deficiencies, stress or disease since the skin receives nutrients from underlying blood vessels. Many individuals suffer psychological effects when they experience minor skin abnormalities, hyperpigmentation, wrinkles or any other esthetic disorder. This is particularly upsetting to those suffering from acne or when a woman notices her first superficial wrinkles in her early 30s and the impact of aging becomes a reality. Although the skin care professional may possess the practical knowledge and skills to enhance the external appearance of the skin using various peels, ampoules, creams, lotions and masks, the results are limited or short-term unless the underlying principles of cell renewal or skin repair are considered. The skin cannot appear clear, smooth or healthy unless the client's lifestyle behaviors are not evaluated. Therefore, it is important that some time is taken to find out more about lifestyle behaviors such as dietary intake, exercise, stress and sleep disorders that contribute to the skin's appearance. In other words, a more holistic approach to skin care is essential for the esthetician to cater to today's knowledgeable clients.

Skin diagnosis

Most skin care professionals don't make a direct correlation between nutrition and the skin's condition immediately during the skin analysis. They tend to focus more on external manipulations of skin tissues such as cleansing, moisturizing and massage of the skin. However, the formulation of new cells is contingent on the raw materials taken into the body. This includes cells, enzymes, hormones, blood vessels, blood, nails and hair. Almost 75% of the protein in the skin is collagen, the major structural protein—50% is present in bone, 40% in skin and 10% in other internal or external tissues such as blood. Because of this, a protein or vitamin intake deficiency will result in impaired formation of skin tissue.

First class proteins found in meat, dairy products or alternative proteins such as soy foods and legumes are necessary for cell renewal or repair, particularly in acne or photodamaged skin. Nutrient deficiencies lead to unhealthy skin conditions and poor health, and many visual symptoms may be indicative of basic nutritional needs. Digestive disorders play a major role in skin complexion. High stress levels, excessive sun exposure, smoking and alcohol generate excessive free radicals leading to premature aging and skin disorders.

Nutritional skin care

Nutritional skin care uses nutritional regimens augmented by dietary supplementation to enhance the results of skin treatments and prevent skin disorders. The holistic notion of treating "inside" and "outside" is becoming a reality in health care, and skin care specialists, including estheticians, are beginning to incorporate a nutritional approach in their skin care practices.

A great number of clients already are using dietary supplements such as vitamins, minerals, enzymes, herbs and pre-digested proteins in their daily lives to optimize the health of the skin and body. They are beginning to realize that, in addition to regular facial treatments, healthy skin needs a diet with adequate supplies of both macronutrients and micronutrients in the correct proportions.

In the clinic, the skin care prescription form also should include a brief listing of some pertinent medical history and other lifestyle behaviors that would help the skin and body care therapist determine some of the more obvious nutritional deficiencies. Questions on daily food intake can reveal hidden eating disorders, impaired absorption of nutrients due to medication, drugs, improper food selection, preparation and storage. Most medical practitioners, including dentists, also require similar information because they are aware of the impact of nutrition. Many people do not eat properly due to lack of knowledge, dental problems, chronic diseases, excessive use of laxatives or drugs, infections, or physical and mental stress. The skin acts as a mirror for the health of the body. See **Personal Lifestyle Questionnaire**, page 96.

Several nutritional deficiencies can be related to complexion and the skin care professional should have the knowledge and skills to recognize certain underlying nutritional deficiencies. For example, skin congestion may indicate a digestive problem, or a pale complexion can infer iron deficiency and excessive dehydration.

The following considerations can be applied toward specific skin disorders, and the skin therapist can recommend behavioral lifestyle modifications to the client to improve the condition of the skin and body. Skin care professionals do not have to be nutritionists or dieticians to recommend basic nutritional guidelines to a client. **Nutritional Support for Skin Conditions** (pages 98-115), lists various skin types, their appearance, possible causes, treatments recommended and home care advice that includes both nutritional advice and lifestyle modifi-

Personal Lifestyle Questionnaire

A helpful strategy to determine the basic nutritional needs of the client is to have each client fill out a simple questionnaire:

Please answer yes or no to the following questions:

1. Eat absolutely no meat or meat derivatives?
2. Eat breakfast daily?
3. Eat less than 2 servings of milk/milk products daily?
4. Eat less than 2 servings of meat/alternative products daily?
5. Eat less than 3-5 servings of fruits/vegetables daily?
6. Eat brightly colored fruits/vegetables?
7. Eat fish at least once/twice a week?
8. Eat convenience or highly processed foods regularly?
9. Drink less than eight 8-oz.glasses of water daily?
10. Add salt or sugar in your foods?
11. Do you suffer regularly from digestive problems such as constipation and bloating?
12. Drink more than 1glass of alcohol daily?
13. Smoke more than 1 pack daily?
14. Bruise easily?
15. Suffer from colds or infections easily?
16. Have soft nails?
17. Exercise two or three times per week?
18. Suffer from high stress levels regularly?

The answers to the above questions can help you determine basic strategies in recommending changes in lifestyle behaviors, primarily dietary changes. For example, insufficient consumption of fruits and vegetables will indicate deficiencies in vitamins, minerals and fiber leading to constipation, high stress levels may lead to "skin breakouts" or red flushes on the skin's surface, bruising easily suggests weak capillary walls and therefore deficiency of vitamin C and bioflavonoids, smoking indicates insufficient oxygen availability to skin tissues while insufficient water intake will lead to a dry, dehydrated skin and body.

cations. In the spa, proper nutrition can be viewed from two perspectives—facial care and body care. For facial care, nutritional advice should concentrate on cell renewal to produce clear, healthy, glowing skin and should be related to the quality of daily nutrient intake. This includes adequate intake of organic nutrients such as protein, essential fatty acids, and inorganic nutrients such as antioxidants A, C and E, selenium, iron, copper and sulfur. Not to be forgotten is sufficient intake of pure water, at least eight 8-oz. glasses daily.

Cell tissues are composed of protein and fatty acids. Vitamins and minerals act as antioxidants to combat the destructive free radicals that cause cell damage and contribute to skin aging. Dietary supplements can be recommended along with fresh natural foods. For example, frozen vegetables have 25% less vitamins than fresh vegetables, while canned vegetables contain 2–3 times fewer vitamins than frozen ones. Exposure to oxygen, carbon dioxide, cold, moisture, light and poor food preparation all have detrimental effects on fresh foods. Antioxidant supplements lower these nutrient deficiencies and help fight free radical formation and other environmental toxins.

Skin conditions and interpretations

The superficial appearance of the facial area may be indicative of various internal disorders caused by genetics or, more often, unhealthy lifestyles. For example:

- A very pale skin accompanied by pale insides of eyes may be indicative of iron deficiency. This probably is more likely if the client is underweight or suffers from heavy menstrual loss.
- Congested skin conditions may reflect the presence of some circulatory disorders such as high blood pressure, digestive problems such as constipation, or food allergies. Avoidance of the most congesting foods such as fats, fried foods, dairy products, refined foods and sugars is recommended. Eat lighter foods such as fresh fruits and vegetables, and drink plenty of water.
- Uneven skin texture suggests poor cell turnover and can be a sign of a vitamin deficiency such as vitamin A or B.
- A red, splotchy skin accompanied by extreme telangiestacia in middle-aged individuals may indicate the skin condition rosacea that is exacerbated by excess intake of alcohol, particularly among men. Another indication of this skin condition is excessive sun exposure.

Text continues on page 116.

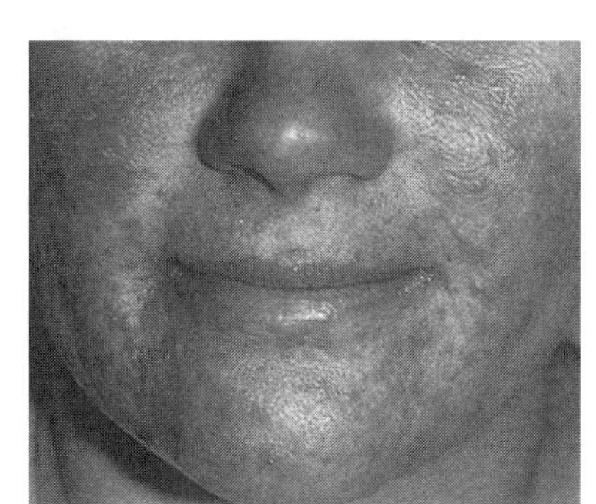

A red, splotchy skin accompanied by extreme telangiestacia in middle-aged individuals may indicate the skin condition rosacea.

Nutritional Support for Skin Conditions

Skin	*Appearance*	*Possible Causes*
Normal	• T-area can be a little oily at certain times, including during menstration, but this is normal. • No excess oil secretions. • No dryness. • Pink, healthy-looking complexion. • Normal sized pores, good tone.	• Heredity. • Good skin care routine. • Good diet. treatments.
Sensitive	• Usually thin skin, but also can be thick. • Blotchy, hot to the touch. • Easily stimulated. • Telangiestacia, or broken capillaries. • Fragile, translucent-looking. • Oily and dehydrated skin becomes sensitive.	• Heredity. • Medication. • Allergies. • Improper cleansing. • Photodamaged skin. • Very dry skin. • No protective creams. • Stress and nerves. • Improper diet.

Treatment Recommended	*Nutritional Advice*	*Home Care Advice*
• Maintain moisture content and good tone. • Anti-aging treatments.	• Eat a balanced diet. • Drink eight 8-oz. glasses of pure water daily. • Omega-3 fatty acids. • Continue good eating habits. • Take anti-aging dietary supplements.	• Use proper products for skin type. • Regular exercise. • Wear sunscreens. • Avoid smoking. • Practice stress management.
• Decongest. • Strengthen. • If oily/dehydrated, use moisturizing treatments.	• Increase vitamins C and P (bioflavonoids) for collagen formation and strengthening of capillary walls. • Take vitamin B complex to reduce stress. • Take antioxidant supplements such as beta carotene, vitamins C and E, and selenium. • Take omega-3 fatty acids to reduce inflamation. • Drink eight 8-oz. glasses of pure water daily.	• Use proper products. • Sufficient sleep. • Stress management. • Avoid sun exposure. • Wear high SPF sun blocks. • Use cool to lukewarm water to clean skin and body. • Use light pressure on face. • Avoid scrubs, hot baths, steam/saunas.

Nutritional Support for Skin Conditions *(cont.)*

Skin	*Appearance*	*Possible Causes*
Blotchy	• Redness, hot to touch. • Skin appears congested. • Can be thin or thick skin. • Thin skin is stimulated easily and remains blotchy for longer time. • Prone to broken capillaries.	• Excessive blood circulation on skin's surface caused by various factors: • Allergies. • Extreme sun exposure. • High blood pressure. • Diet–spicy foods, hot drinks, alcohol • Strong emotions. • Acne rosacea.

Treatment Recommended	*Nutritional Advice*	*Home Care Advice*
• Decongest. • Strengthen–thin skin must be treated delicately while thicker skin can be treated normally.	• Increase antioxidants and phytochemicals. • Drink eight 8-oz. glasses of pure water daily. • Increase fiber. • Avoid alcohol. • Avoid stimulants. • Ingest flavonoids. • Reduce animal-derived food intake. • Consume omega-3 fatty acids. • Minimize inflammatory food intake.	• Avoid sun exposure. • Use sun blocks. • Use light pressure on face. • Use cool water for washing face and body. • Avoid hot baths, sauna/steam–use showers instead. • Avoid extreme temperatures. • Use proper products to decongest and soothe. • Use heavier moisturizers in winter. • Learn stress management. • Have relaxation massage regularly to reduce stress. • Carefully check product ingredients for allergies before purchase.

Nutritional Support for Skin Conditions *(cont.)*

Skin	*Appearance*	*Possible Causes*
Broken Capillaries	• Associated with blotchiness. • Fine thread-like blood vessels on skin's surface. • More visible on thin areas of skin such as the eyelids and temples.	• Constant dilation of capillary walls leads to weakened elasticity resulting in broken capillaries. • *Vasodilation*– diameter of capillary walls widened due to increased blood flow. • *Vasoconstriction*– diameter of capillary walls constricted. • Blood flows away from skin's surface. • Pores close to retain body heat.
Rosacea	• Chronic disorder affecting nose and cheeks. • Abnormally red, moderate to severe seborrhea, possibly pustular lesions. • Found in age groups 30–50. • More common in females than males, but worse in males.	• Possible etiology: aging, hormonal imbalance, menopausal symptoms, excessive alcohol intake, vitamin B deficiency. • Stress-related gastrointestinal disorders.

Treatment Recommended	*Nutritional Advice*	*Home Care Advice*
• Decongest. • Stregthen. • Use of cautery devices.	• Increase vitamins C and P to strengthen capillary walls. • Increase flavonoids intake. • Take antioxidants. • Drink eight 8-oz. glasses of pure water daily. • Consume omega-3 fatty acids. • Minimize inflammatory food consumption.	• Same as blotchy skin. • Avoid temperature changes–place hands on cheeks when coming in from cold. • Use heavier moisturizers in winter. • Use gentle pressure on face. • Use cool to lukewarm water. • Avoid hot water, baths
• Non-stimulating treatments. • Reduce redness with anti-inflammatory products/treatment ingredients. • Mild progressive exfoliation treatments. • Manual lymph drainage massage.	• Minimize stimulating foods. • Eat anti-inflammatory foods. • Try alternative proteins such as soy and legumes. • Avoid salt. • Eat more fresh foods • Eat antioxidant-rich foods. • Use dietary supplements such as vitamins A, E and C, selenium and vitamin B complex, but avoid niacin.	• Use cool water to clean face and body. • Use gentle pressure on skin. • Use high SPF products. • Avoid direct sun exposure. • Have regular stress therapy treatments. • Practice stress management. • Participate in mind-body exercise such as yoga, Pilates and meditation to reduce stress.

Nutritional Support for Skin Conditions *(cont.)*

Skin	*Appearance*	*Possible Causes*
Oily, acne prone	• Shiny seborrhea-like skin. • Greasy to the touch. • Asphyxiated pores. • Comedones, milias. • Enlarged pores. • Occasional pimples, pustules and cysts. • Usually medium to thick skin. • Sallow, devitalized complexion. • PMS–mild to severe breakouts occur 7–14 days before menstration. • Cravings for carbohydrates, reduced energy, moody, depression, bloating and edema.	• Main cause–over-production of sebum. • Hormonal imbalance due to puberty, PMS or pregnancy. • Heredity. • Improper cleansing. • High humidity environment. • Stress or nerves. • Drugs or medication.

Treatment Recommended	*Nutritional Advice*	*Home Care Advice*
• Deep cleansing. • Desincrustation using galvanic current therapy. • Tighten pores. • Regenerate. • Regular skin peelings.	• During PMS, minimize consumption of foods that promote inflammation. • Try soy milk. • Detoxify by increasing fiber-rich foods. • Reduce iodine-rich foods. • Avoid fried foods, eat more steamed or grilled foods. • Eat fiber-rich foods. • Drink eight 8-oz. glasses of pure water daily. • Increase antioxidant-rich foods. • Take dietary supplements–vitamin A and E for healing, vitamin B for stress. • Minimize caffeine intake during PMS.	• Deep cleanse pores more often during PMS to avoid breakouts. • Reduce/avoid smoking • Do some form of exercise. • Avoid touching the face. • Do not squeeze pimples. • Keep hair off face and wash often. • Change pillowcases regularly. • Shower immediately after exercise. • Learn to relax. • Avoid dairy products. • Minimize salt and caffeine intake.

Nutritional Support for Skin Conditions *(cont.)*

Skin	*Appearance*	*Possible Causes*
Acne	• Caused by *p. acnes bacteria.* • Inflammation, cysts, scarring. • Andogen related. • Four grades: 1 and 2: mild–face and neck 3 and 4: severe–spreads to chest and back. • *Acne vulgaris*–adolescent acne from hormonal imbalance. • *Acne cosmetica*–comedegenic cosmetics. • *Acne rosacea*–adults over 35 years old. Includes reddish, sore lesions–butterfly shape on nose and cheecks. More common in women but worse in men. • *Acne mechanica*–caused by poor habits such as touching the face with dirty hands.	• Same as oily skin

Treatment Recommended	*Nutritional Advice*	*Home Care Advice*
• Deep cleanse. • Healing. • Scar treatment. • Manual lymph drainage massage. • Peelings with AHAs and chemical peels. • Skin resurfacing procedures such as microdermabrasion and cautery devices. • Cryotherapy.	• Eat a more vegetarian diet, and increase fiber-rich foods. • Eat more steamed or grilled foods. • Avoid foods that promote inflammation. • Eat more anti-inflammatory foods. • Reduce or avoid stimulating foods. • Avoid salt. • Try alternative protein such as soy and legumes. • Increase zinc to boost immunity and improve protein metabolism. • Avoid refined carbohydrates and consume wholesome foods instead of convenience foods. • Increase consumption of antioxidant-rich foods. • Drink green and black tea • Use dietary supplements such as vitamin A 100,000 IU/d for three months, vitamin B-6 to reduce stress, vitamin E, zinc, selenium, black cohosh to reduce PMS symptoms and chromium to increase energy levels.	• Deep cleanse face more often before PMS to avoid breakouts. • Avoid using comedogenic products and use camouflage makeup instead. • Wash face and shower immediately after exercise. • Have regular deep cleansing facial treatments by an experienced skin care professional. • Have regular body massage. • Exercise regularly to improve mood and reduce depression. • Incorporate mind/ body fitness such as yoga, Pilates and meditation.

Nutritional Support for Skin Conditions *(cont.)*

Skin	*Appearance*	*Possible Causes*
Back acne	• Pimples, cysts and scars. • Perhaps keloids–raised, irregularly shaped scars. • Asphyxiated pores.	• Hormonal imbalance. • Environment–dirt, high heat/humidity. • Excessive sweating from exercise and not showering afterward. • Improper hygiene. • Exacerbated by certain types of clothing such as nylon and some wools. • Heredity.
Enlarged pores	• Found around T-zone–forehead, nose, chin and cheeks. • Common on thick, oily skin. • Also can be found on mature, dry skin that used to be oily in youth.	• Excessive secretion of sebum in sebaceous ducts leading to enlarged pores.

Treatment Recommended	*Nutritional Advice*	*Home Care Advice*
• Deep cleansing. • Exfoliating treatments. • Back acne treatments. • Skin resurfacing–microdermabrasion.	• Same as acne.	• Shower/clean skin immediately after exercise. • Use body products such as shower gels with a loofah mitt, but avoid open lesions. • Indirect sun exposure is beneficial in small doses to dry sebum. • Change clothing and linens regularly. • Check clothing if causing skin irritation. • Practice stress management to prevent breakouts. • Try 100% cotton clothing instead of nylon or plastic.
• Deep cleanse to minimize pores. • Have peelings such as AHAs, chemicals peels with salicylic acid.	• Consume a healthy balanced diet. • Use antioxidant therapy with vitamins A, C and E.	• Use deep cleansers with facial brush to keep pores clean. • Use astringent masks.

Nutritional Support for Skin Conditions *(cont.)*

Skin	*Appearance*	*Possible Causes*
Scar tissue	• Damaged epidermal or dermal tissues. • Includes keloids–inflammatory scars. irregularly-shaped scars caused from trauma resulting in excessive collagen formation.	• Scars from acne, falls, burns, insect bites or accidents. • Post-inflammatory hyperpigmentation. • Surgical procedures.
Dry	• Lines, wrinkles, leathery feel and crepiness. • Dry patches. • Feels tight without creams. • Usually thin skin that ages early. • Feels sensitve due to lack of sebum. • Dry, mature skin can have enlarged pores, but is dry from aging. • Body also can feel tight, dry and itchy. • *Alipoid*–young skin shows absence of visible pores and early signs of aging such as crow's-feet. • Skin feels dry and itchy.	• Aging process. • Heredity. • Improper cleansing. • Hormonal imbalance. • Endocrine disorders such as hypothyroidism. • Illness. • Negative lifestyle behaviors such as smoking and alcohol. • Environmental factors such as extreme cold, air conditioning and excessive sun exposure.

Treatment Recommended	*Nutritional Advice*	*Home Care Advice*
• Regenerate. • Skin resurfacing with microdermabrasion, chemical peels or cryotherapy. • Medical collagen injections.	• Use antioxidants such as vitamins A, C and E, and selenium. • Increase dietary intake of phytochemicals before surgical procedures to enhance healing. • Consume omega-3 fatty acids. • Consume first class proteins for tissue repair such as lean meat.	• Avoid direct sun exposure on post- • Use regenerating creams.
• Moisture. • Tone and firm. • Skin resurfacing treatments such as microdermabrasion, enzyme peels, AHAs and chemical peels. • Alipoids should use preventative treatments such as anti-aging therapies.	• Balanced diet. • Increase omega-3 fatty acids. • Increase intake of calcium, iron and zinc as well as vitamins C and P for collagen synthesis and to strengthen capillary walls. • Eat antioxidant-rich foods. • Consume phytochemicals. • Increase phytoestrogen intake. • Reduce diuretics such as caffeine and alcohol. • Drink green tea instead of coffee. • Take anti-aging dietary supplements to prevent premature aging of skin and body.	• Avoid soap and harsh products. • Use proper products for moisturizing, protective creams and sun blocks. • Avoid direct sun exposure, but enjoy early morning or late evening sun. • Use cool to lukewarm water. • Avoid hot baths/ sauna–use showers. • Avoid smoking. • Participate in active physical exercise.

Nutritional Support for Skin Conditions *(cont.)*

Skin	*Appearance*	*Possible Causes*
Wrinkles, lines	• Lines between eyebrows, eyes, forehead and labial lobe. • Lines and folds in neck.	• Same as dry skin. • Worry and stress. • Lack of sleep. • Poor posture. • Excessive facial expression. • Pressing on skin tissues.
Sagging	• Loose slackness on cheeks, jaw line and neck.	• Aging process. • Quick weight loss in a short time period. • Active person suddenly becomes inactive. • Poor posture. • High pillows.

Treatment Recommended	*Nutritional Advice*	*Home Care Advice*
• Moisturize. • Firm and tone. • Regenerating. • Peelings such as AHAs. • Skin resurfacing treatments such as microdermabrasion and chemical peels. • Anti-aging therapy. • Medical treatments such as injectable fillers, laser skin resurfacing and collagen injections/fat transter.	• Consume a healthy balanced diet. • Increase calcium and zinc. • Consume first class proteins such as vitamins C and P for collagen formation. • Consume omega-3 fatty acids. • Eat antioxidants such as beta-carotene, and vitamins C and E to decrease free radicals. • Drink eight 8-oz. glasses of pure water daily.	• Avoid soaps–use cleansing milks. • Be aware of facial expressions. • Use rich moisturizing creams. • Always use protective creams such as sun protection. • Avoid direct sun's rays. • Use lukewarm to cool water to wash face. • Avoid steam/sauna. • Correct posture–keep neck high and long. • Avoid high pillows. • Sleep on back. • Learn to relax.
• Firm and tone. • Regenerate. • Anti-aging treatments such as collagen and cell therapy. • Muscle toning therapy with interferential current or microcurrent therapy.	• Take vitamins C and P for collagen synthesis. • Eat antioxidants and phytochemicals for anti-aging.	• Correct posture–keep neck high and long. • Avoid pushing on jaw line with hands. • Avoid high pillows. • Use firming creams with collagen and elastin.

Nutritional Support for Skin Conditions *(cont.)*

Skin	*Appearance*	*Possible Causes*
Dehydrated	• *Superfical*–fine lines, flakiness and tightness. • *Deep dehydration*–usually found with extremely dry skin, lines are deeper. such as soap. • Occurs when causes of superficial dehydration have not been corrected.	• Lacking moisture on skin's surface. • Lack of protective creams. • Improper products. • Change in temperature. • Illness. • Climatic conditions. • Environment such as air conditioning and central heating.
Pigmentation	• Any color other than the normal skin color. • *Hyperpigmentation*–moles, freckles, age spots, strawberry marks or port wine stains. • *Hypopigmentation*–vitiligo, or partial loss of pigments, albinism, or total absence of pigment, or stretch marks.	• Heredity. • Hormonal disorder. • Post-inflammatory reactions such as trauma from burns, acne, chemical peels and squeezing pimples too hard. • Excessive sun exposure after waxing or electrolysis. • Reaction to UV rays while on drugs such as insulin, tetracycline and birth control pills. • Certain plants and metals. • UV exposure while wearing certain perfumes. • Photosensitive skin.

Treatment Recommended	*Nutritional Advice*	*Home Care Advice*
• Moisture. • Regenerate. • Exfoliation such as AHAs, enzyme peels and microdermabrasion.	• Drink eight 8-oz. glasses of pure water daily. • Consume more fruits vegetables and juices. • Consume omega-3 fatty acids. • Eat antioxidant-rich foods.	• Use a humidifier. • Avoid hot water, use cool to lukewarm water. • Avoid steam/sauna. • Avoid harsh products • Use protective creams for face and body.
• Regenerate. • Depigmentation treatments using various peeling modalities such as enzyme, chemical, microdermabrasion and cauterizing devices. • Nitrous oxide therapy. • Use preventive measures to avoid post-inflammatory hyperpigmentation with invasive skin peelings.	• Eat antioxidant-rich foods such as vitamin C and E to protect against free radicals formed from skin trauma. • Drink eight 8-oz. glasses of pure water daily. • Consume first class proteins for collagen formation. • Take dietary supplements.	• Wear sun blocks particularly after skin care and exfoliation procedures. • Use regenerating creams. • Avoid direct sun's rays.

- The presence of telangiestacia, or broken capillaries on the face, also can be a sign of weakened elasticity of blood vessels caused by constant vasodilation. Check if the client suffers from allergies regularly and recommend daily intake of vitamin C, citrus bioflavonoids and proanthocyanadins found in colorful purple/red fruits and green tea. Reduced intake of inflammatory foods also should be recommended.
- Dry, wrinkled skin infers an inadequate intake of water and essential fatty acids. Recommend drinking at least eight 8-oz. glasses of pure water daily and eating fish at least two times a week. Older people have reduced sensations of thirst and must be reminded to drink water throughout the day.
- Photodamaged skin, particularly on the décolleté, is a definite sign of inadequate use of sunscreens. Recommend using an SPF of 15 or more and avoid direct sun exposure. Remind clients to reapply sun block every half hour in the sun.
- Gray, devitalized skin accompanied by lines around the mouth indicate poor circulation induced by heavy smoking.
- Deepened lines between the brows, forehead, and a down-turned mouth can mark the presence of fatigue or stress. Recommend wearing sunglasses and make the client aware of excessive squinting and facial expressions. Various forms of stress therapy are highly recommended for these clients.

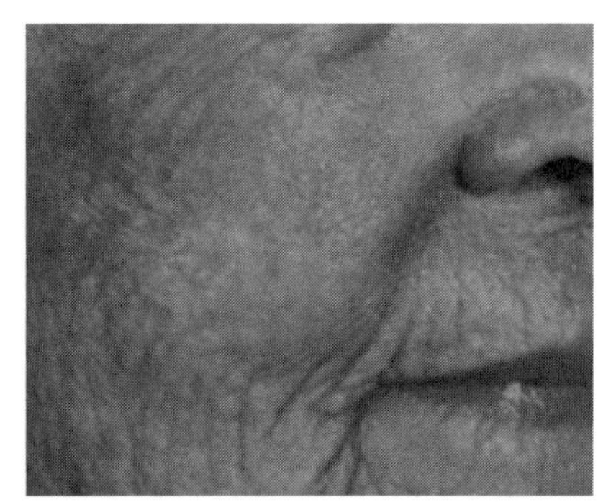

Dry, wrinkled skin infers an inadequate intake of water and essential fatty acids.

Vitamins and the skin

Vitamin A is essential to produce mucous secretions that soften, heal and protect the skin from infection. Synthetic forms of vitamin A are used to treat many skin conditions and certain forms of cancer. They include *Retin A*, a chemical derivative of vitamin A used to treat wrinkles, mild to moderate acne and other skin disorders by stimulating skin exfoliation. Also, *isotretinoin* is a topical form of retinoic acid used to treat cystic acne and any disorders of keratinization. Although isotretinoin is manufactured from vitamin A, it has a different chemical structure. It is beneficial for cystic acne but can cause birth defects in infants if taken during pregnancy. It only is given under a physician's care.

Toxicity. Excessive amounts of vitamin A, over 10,000 IU, do not help acne. Beta carotene does not cause toxicity but is stored in the fat just under the skin. Excessive intake from natural foods may turn the skin yellow and is not harmful, but toxicity can occur if taken in supplement form, particularly when smoking and drinking alcohol. Vitamin A supplementation in doses of 25,000–50,000 IU are recommended for use in pre- and post-surgery on a short-term basis for quick healing and recovery.

Deficiency. This results in skin infections. Reduced mucous secretions limit the absorption of nutrients leading to infections of the mucous membranes of the digestive, respiratory and urinary tracts. The skin's surface becomes dry, rough and scaly with keratinized cells forming hardened plugs in pores and hair follicles known as sebaceous hyperplasia, some appearing in the shape of doughnuts. Deficiency also leads to dry eyes and reduced night vision.

Recommended doses. As a preventive care for skin disorders, try to consume at least five servings of phytochemicals, brightly colored fruits and vegetables, to ensure an adequate supply of beta carotene, or take vitamin A dietary supplements because food processing removes it. Anti-aging experts advise no more than 15,000 IU (300% RDA) with no more than 5,000 IU in vitamin palmitate and the rest in mixed beta carotene foods.

Protein and skin

Collagen is the most abundant protein in the body and is the main constituent in connective tissue. It was discovered in the 1960s to be one of the greatest breakthroughs in skin care formulations. A skin care professional should possess a broader understanding of collagen formation and how it relates to the maintenance of the skin and body.

The main function of protein in skin care products is to form an occlusive film on the skin's surface minimizing moisture loss to the surrounding dry air. These proteins are known as Natural Moisturizing Factors (NMF). Under controlled environments, enzymes and acids are used to break down the animal proteins into lighter molecular weight to produce the desired chain lengths required for their cosmetic formulations. The level of processing, as well as the type of protein source, produce different effects in skin care products.

Collagen

Collagen gives support and rigidity to tissues. The collagen found in the dermis is composed of chains of both essential and non-essential amino acids which form the collagen and elastin fibers that are grounded in a fluid-like matrix called the ground substance. Three polypeptide chains formed of collagen fibers are wrapped around one another to form a triple helix rope-like formation anchored together at right angles and held together by cross linkage of fibers between these chains. The main amino acids in collagen are glycine and proline. The fibroblast cells in the dermis secretes *procollagen,* the precursor for **tropocollagen**, the basic unit of collagen. Tropocollagen cross-links with two polypeptide chains, **hydroxyproline** and **hydroxlysine**, each chain comprising of approximately 1,000 amino acids, to form a stable molecule of collagen. During collagen formation, an OH group is added to form a compound called hydroxyproline that is essential in forming the triple helix. Vitamin C and iron are needed for this conversion. For example, the disease scurvy in which vitamin C was deficient. was found to be responsible for many signs of connective tissue abnormalities. Collagen fibers are tough and hold a great deal of moisture, but do not stretch easily, while elastin fibers are highly resilient. The matrix holds a large amount of water and proteoglycans that are composed of a polysaccharide called glycoaminoglycans (GAGs), and a protein. One of these GAGs is called hyaluronic acid, and maintains water balance in the dermis. In aging, the cross-linking of the collagen fibers causing reduced solubility in the salt and acid solutions that circulates in body fluids. This leads to dry skin with lines, wrinkles and poor elasticity.

Collagen in skin care products. As the best NMF, collagen forms a natural film on the skin's surface to minimize transepidermal water loss (TEWL). Its low cost, availability and effective results make it one of the most popular and common ingredients used in cosmetic preparations today. When applied topically, it leaves the skin soft and smooth, with a high gloss and viscosity, and does not cause any allergic reactions. Being the main structural component in all body proteins—skin, nails, hair, bones, teeth, tendons, blood, enzymes and hormones—the skin care specialist must have a thorough understanding of its formation. Collagen appears in either soluble or hydrolyzed form. Soluble collagen has a higher molecular weight and is more effective and preferred because it has greater water-binding properties. However, the hydrolyzed form is the most common form used in cosmetics because of its lower molecular weight. Protein sources are derived from animal, vegetable or silk. Although animal-derived collagen is considered the best protein for excellent results, availability and cost, today's research is being done with plants because of the animal rights movement.

Collagen and cartilage health. Cartilage is soft bone containing more elastin than collagen fibers. During aging, the cartilage at the joints becomes dry and brittle leading to stiffness and inflammation ultimately resulting to arthritis. Glucosamine, a compound composed of glucose and amino acids, helps to form proteglycans and chondroitin, a chain of sugars, plays a vital role in cartilage health. Together with sulfate they form a compound called glucosamine sulfate that attracts liquids to the joints to aid in lubrication and reduce stiffness and inflammation. These substances are available as dietary supplements and are used as preventive care for arthritis and osteoporosis.

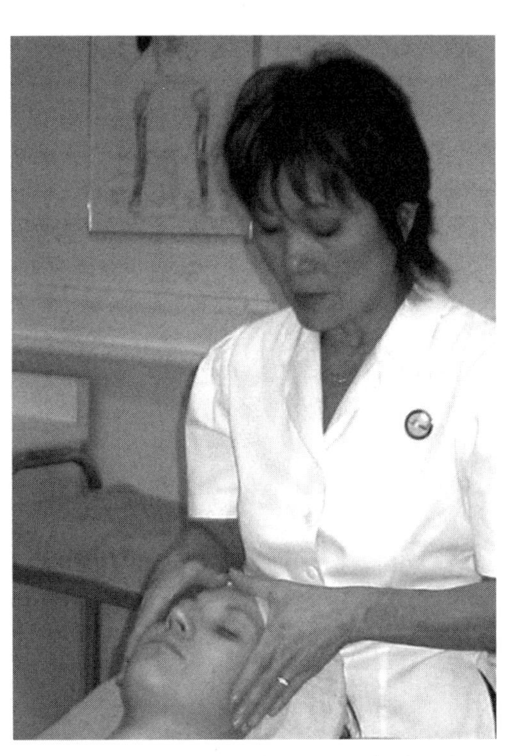

In addition to regular facial treatments, healthy skin needs a diet with adequate supples of both macronutrients and micronutrients in the correct proportions.

Vitamin C and the skin

During collagen synthesis, the amino acids **proline** and **lysine** must be present, and when an OH group is added, the compound **hydroxyproline**, which forms the collagen helix, is created. This conversion requires the bioavailability of both vitamin C and iron. Improper collagen metabolism may occur if an eating disorder exists, particularly in younger individuals because nutrients such as zinc and copper that are found in protein would lead to impaired tissue formation.

Antioxidants

Free radicals are generated naturally during oxidative processes within living tissues. The body typically produces natural antioxidants to neutralize free radical damage.

In the course of aging, this ability is diminished lowering the body's immunity and increasing vulnerability to disease. That is why teenagers can abuse their bodies by going without sleep, drinking excessive alcohol and eating junk food with few signs of premature aging. Think of the oxidative process that occurs when a car shows rust, or when fruit such as an apple turns brown when left exposed for a short period. However, if you pour an antioxidant substance such as vitamin C over the cut apple, it does not turn brown but maintains its freshness. During inflammatory conditions, one should avoid sugary foods and saturated fats, and choose foods that have anti-inflammatory effects such as monounsaturated fats including olive, canola and vegetable oils. Increase fish oils and flaxseed, which are excellent sources of omega-3 fatty acids. Unfortunately, the North American diet includes an excessive intake of saturated fats high in PG2, trans fatty acids and high sugary foods that promote inflammatory conditions such as acne, eczema and arthritis. Natural antioxidants found in foods are beta carotene, vitamins C and E, the minerals zinc and selenium, phytochemicals and certain amino acids.

CHAPTER 8

Free Radicals and Stress Management

Plants have been used for medicinal purposes for centuries, but it is only recently that Western society has begun to use plants as a source of preventive care. Researchers are conducting more studies on the health benefits of plants. A new health paradigm of "wellness" outlines ways in which preventive care can be integrated in many health care professions, including skin care. This involves not only new technologies that help prevent the aging of the skin and body, but also incorporates strategies such as nutrition and fitness. The protective values of nutrients must include knowledge of free radicals.

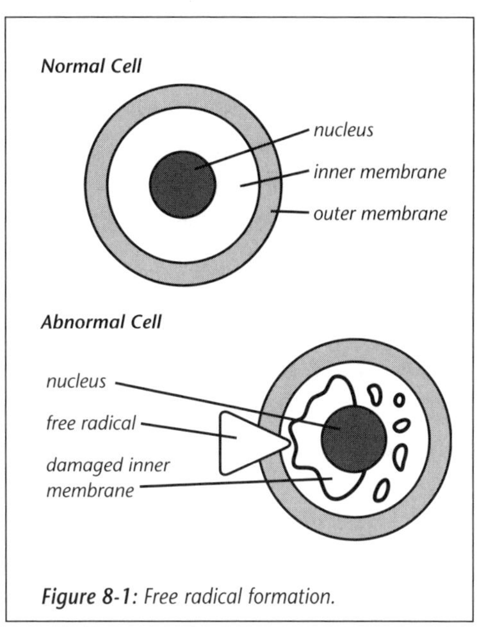

Figure 8-1: *Free radical formation.*

Free radicals

Free radicals damage cells, body tissues and promote the development of cancer. They are as deadly as a parasite but in a different way. Many people already have heard of free radicals and are somewhat aware that they are harmful to the body. However, most do not really understand how the chemical reactions occur. Health care professionals should possess some knowledge of the formation of free radicals to help their clients counteract their harmful effects on the body. Excess free radicals can trigger chronic disease such as cancer, heart diseases and autoimmune diseases such as diabetes and arthritis. But what are they? The following is an explanation of how free radicals are formed in each living cell of the body.

Chemical formation. Oxygen is essential to life, and during cellular metabolism, it is used to burn or metabolize food for energy. However, during this chemical process, some molecules are damaged. These damaged molecules are called free radicals, or **oxidants**, and they can create havoc by causing damage to the cells of the skin, brain, lungs, digestive tract and arteries as well as to DNA, the genetic code that controls cellular behavior. A free radical can be defined as a very powerful chemical that is capable of independent existence carrying one or more unpaired electrons in its outer orbit. Free radicals, therefore, are byproducts of your body's metabolism and can be described as the body's own "exhaust fumes."

Physics dictate that electrons circle around the nucleus in pairs for molecules to be balanced. If an electron is knocked out, the atom becomes unbalanced, and the remaining electron becomes a free radical that will try to stabilize itself by attaching to a nearby molecule that will then become unstable and biochemically inactive. This action turns the normal atom into a free radical. In its quest to achieve stability, it then tries to pass the extra electron to yet another stable molecule, or tries to grab an electron from a neighbor to make up a pair of electrons to revolve around its own nucleus. This sets off a chain reaction within the tissues forming more free radicals which continues down the line creating a cascading effect that first affects the cell membrane and then enters the cell hitting on the mitochondria, eventually leading to the damage of the DNA. (See **Figure 8-1**, page 121.)

But it is not only the human body that produces free radicals. They also penetrate the human body from the outside, mostly through the skin, lungs or intestinal tract. Free radicals also are produced during the detoxification process when the body neutralizes foreign substances such as medication, toxins, chemicals and alcohol.

Free radicals and the immune system. The immune system jumps into action to eliminate foreign substances such as viruses, bacteria or abnormal cells, or cancer cells, and white blood cells produce free radicals to attack these invaders. However, the excess free radicals remain in the body and can launch attack on the body's tissues. When immunity is low such as during illness and stress-related diseases, the body is more vulnerable to an attack from free radicals.

Free radicals and the brain. Since the brain uses so much of the body's available oxygen from the blood, brain cells, more than any other organ, especially are vulnerable to attack from free radicals. There is a positive correlation between free radical damage and brain diseases such as Parkinson's and Alzheimer's diseases, and even clinical depression. Free radicals can accumulate in the cell membranes causing them to break, affecting the mitochondria and eventually attacking the DNA. When this occurs, the impaired or denatured DNA will then form new unhealthy cells that will have an unhealthy, shorter lifespan. This accelerated mutation leads to cellular aging, and these reactions become a major contributing factor for a variety of stress-related diseases, cancer and cardiovascular conditions.

Free radicals are produced from two sources. External sources include toxic elements produced by skin and body trauma, pollution, ultraviolet (UV) rays, poor diet, smoking, alcohol, excessive exercise and other negative lifestyle behaviors. Internal contributors include emotional stress, infection and chronic disease.

Free radicals and health. When excessive amounts of free radicals are formed, they cause great damage to cellular tissue. The most common free radicals formed in the human body are the **superoxide radicals**, and scientists have developed many mechanisms to control their production. Other common free radicals include nitrogen dioxide, or nitric oxide, that reacts with blood vessels to cause vasodilation. The most dangerous free radical is the **hydroxyl radical** capable of reacting with almost any compound in the body including proteins, carbohydrates, lipids and enzymes. Fortunately, they are not produced in humans as often, but when they are, they cause severe cellular damage. **Hydrogen peroxide** is relatively non-toxic to cells but in large amounts, can accelerate free radical production. The hydrogen atom contains only one electron in its orbit and is therefore a free radical. Often, it bonds itself to carbon backbones, such as lipids, to form saturated fats. Unsaturated fats, particularly polyunsaturated fats, are more unstable than saturated fats and therefore are more easily attacked by free radicals. Fatty deposits such as LDL cholesterol also are highly susceptible to oxidation, or lipid peroxidation, leading to plaque formation in blood vessels, a major factor in arteriosclerosis, or hardening of the arteries. The resulting inflammation produces highly oxidative free radicals. When proteins such as collagen are attacked, its fibers become cross-linked, and the cell membrane becomes damaged or hardened. Nutrients cannot enter the cell, leading to premature cellular aging, evident as wrinkles and lines on the skin's surface.

Antioxidants and health

Antioxidants, literally meaning against oxidation, are vitamins and minerals that neutralize free radicals by donating electrons, limiting the damage they cause. They stop the oxidative process by removing the catalyst, the free radical. By giving electrons to free radicals, they stabilize the unpaired molecules stopping chain reactions in the tissues. Some vitamins are described as free radical scavengers because they "scoop up" the free radicals preventing the chain reaction of peroxidation in lipids inhibiting the formation of unwanted LDL cholesterol in the body.

Natural antioxidants. Luckily, the body possesses natural antioxidant enzymes that keep free radicals under control and minimize cellular damage. These are **superoxide dismutase** (SOD), **catalase** and **glutathione peroxidase**. They deactivate the free radicals, minimizing cellular damage. Other antioxidants manufactured inside the body include co-enzyme Q10 (CoQ10) used in treating heart diseases.

However, when the body is bombarded with excess free radicals produced from both internal and external sources, the body's immunity is weakened and becomes more susceptible to tissue inflammation. This leads to various skin disorders including pimples, as well as cellulite, or cellular inflammation, inflammatory conditions such as arthritis, bursitis and tendonitis, and many other diseases.

Reduced antioxidant defenses. The body's ability to respond to oxidative stress is reduced due to aging, illness and environmental stressors such as heavy exercise, improper diet, inflammation and obesity. The key to combating excess free radicals is to use preventive measures and strategies that reduce free radical formation. One of the most acceptable theories of anti-aging is the Theory of Calorie Restriction. (See **Chapter 6**.) It states that in aging, a decreased consumption of calories will decrease oxidative processes, reducing free radical production. Nutrition experts highly recommend the dietary intake of foods that are rich in antioxidants to stem free radicals that are produced in many inflamed skin conditions such as sunburn, contact dermatitis, wrinkles and premature aging, and even before undergoing stressful events such as surgery. For post-care surgery, select foods that are low in fat and high in antioxidants to accelerate the healing process and fortify the immune system. Check food labels to see if these antioxidants appear at the beginning of the list—this would indicate higher concentrations.

Dietary sources of natural antioxidants. Many natural foods contain substances that act as antioxidants. For preventive care, simply increase antioxidant intake through dietary intake or supplements. One of the largest groups of antioxidant foods is the flavonoids, found mainly in fruits, leaves, stems and roots of vegetables, legumes and tea. (See **Figure 8-2**.)

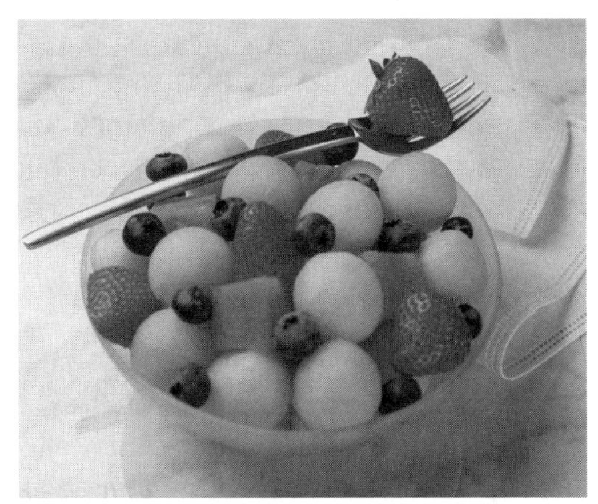

Figure 8-2: One of the largest groups of antioxidant foods is the flavonoids, found mainly in fruits, leaves, stems and roots of vegetables, legumes and tea.

Proanthocyanidins refers to a family of flavonoids from plants that popularly are known as antioxidants, such as those found in red wine and grapeseed extracts. They finally become **anthocyanins**—the pigments that give the rich red colors to berries such as cranberries and grapes.

The "French Paradox" is an excellent example of how proanthocyanidins in red wine contribute to a lower mortality of heart disease among the French who are notoriously known to eat a high fat diet yet drink large amounts of red wine.

A diet high in antioxidants such as beta carotene, vitamins C and E, bioflavonoids, and the minerals zinc and selenium, can play a major role in delaying the aging process and preventing degenerative diseases such as cancer and diabetes. Other natural plant compounds called phytochemicals also aid in the body's defense. Botanicals such as **catechins** in tea are believed to quench free radicals. Reduce coffee consumption and try green or black teas because they are very rich sources of polyphenols.

Preventing free radical formation with nutrients

Many plants contain protective nutrients that can help to prevent the formation of these toxic substances. Although they appear to be similar, they can be classified as either antioxidants and free radical scavengers or phytochemicals. The stresses of the modern lifestyle lead to increased free radical production, while modern diets provide inadequate antioxidant nutrients to support the body's defense systems creating an imbalance. Some health experts believe that the balance between your antioxidant intake and exposure to free radicals could become the balance between life and death. Therefore, tip the scales in your favor by making simple changes to diet and antioxidant supplementation.

Free radical overload. The production of free radicals increases substantially due to prolonged and uncontrolled stress, competition, chronic diseases and infections, environmental exposure to smoke, UV rays and heavy metals, and an unhealthy diet composed of high fat, fried foods and eating foods cooked at high temperatures where they turn black—burnt meats. Protect yourself and prevent diseases by making changes to your diet to avoid free radical overload.

Nutrition and stress management

Stress is one of the five pillars of anti-aging, and one of the main attractions of the spa is stress therapy or anti-stress treatments. It is essential to life because body tissues need to be stimulated to stay alive. Most people can tolerate normal stress if it is minor. However in modern society, people live in an over-stressed world where countless stressors have an impact both physically and psychologically often leading to maladaptive or abnormal behaviors.

What is stress? **Stress** is a catch-all word that describes a reaction in response to a stressor. It encompasses abnormally high levels of emotional and physiological arousal in the body and is associated with some degree of personal unhappiness. Stressors can be defined as physical or psychological demands placed on the body in various situations and can be viewed as either negative or positive, depending on how they are perceived. Most are viewed negatively and thus produce high levels of free radicals leading to premature skin and body aging, and even violence or death. Because of this, an individual who is suffering from high stress appears haggard and old with deep wrinkles in the labial lobes, between brows and around the eyes. While most normal stressors can be tolerated by most people, if they are severe or if an individual is confronted with an excessive amount of stressors all at one time, the coping ability diminishes and an abnormal response occurs. These could include becoming irritated or angry very quickly or sinking into depression. Stress is recognized as playing a significant part in the causes of many physical and psychological illnesses. See **Symptoms of Stress**, page 127.

Stressors can be induced by various sources, from the outside world or from within our bodies. **Biological stressors** manifest due to malnutrition, illness and trauma; **psychological stressors** manifest due to low self-esteem, fears and guilt; and **social stressors** manifest due to relationships, finance, war, as well as other causes.

Indications of stress. If you observe closely, several physical and psychological symptoms of high stress easily can be recognized. There are two key transmitters affecting stress: serotonin and noradrenaline. Adequate sleep is absolutely essential for long-term health and regeneration. Insomnia, or sleep deprivation, is a common behavioral disorder when suffering from high stress and appears to accelerate premature aging. **Serotonin** is a neurotransmitter important in the regulation of sleep, appetite and body temperature. The presence of the essential amino acid tryptophan together with vitamins B-6, niacin and magnesium are important co-factors needed to convert tryptophan into serotonin. If stress destroys sleep, serotonin levels are reduced resulting in insomnia, depression, mood swings during PMS and menopause, and fatigue. Therefore, it is important to ensure adequate levels of protein are taken under stress.

Noradrenaline, released by the adrenal glands, gives feelings of pleasure and motivation. The body uses high levels of energy under duress and noradrenaline helps to release immediate energy at this critical time. Lack of this hormone results in reduced energy and fatigue.

Common stress-related diseases include cardiovascular diseases such as angina and hypertension, asthma, autoimmune diseases, cancer, type II diabetes, depression, headaches, PMS and ulcers.

Symptoms of Stress

Overt Symptoms	*Covert Symptoms*	*Emotional Symptoms*
• Fatigue • Lack of energy • Shallow breathing • Allergies, frequent colds • Emptiness • Tightness in jaw, neck • Hunched shoulders, curled toes • Talking quickly • Open darting eyes • Constantly moving in a nervous manner • Heavy smoking • Biting nails constantly	• Insomnia • Lack of concentration • Lack of decision-making • Tight unnatural smile • Avoids eye contact • Obsessiveness	• Anxiety, fear, irritability • Negative self-talk • Low self-esteem, anger • Feeling of pressure • Depression, despair

Stressors: Highest to Lowest

Highest	High	Moderate	Low
• Death of spouse/ child • Divorce • Death of a close family member	• Retirement • Illness/ injury • New marriage • Job loss • Change of finances • Pregnancy • Death of close friend	• Borrowing/ lending money • Change in living status • Marital difficulties • Work problems • Chronic allergies • Change in job • Spouse begins/stops work	• Change in residence • Change in sleep habits • Change in eating habits • Minor law violation • Vacation/ holidays

Modified Major Stress Evaluators of Han Seyles, PhD.

The stress scale

According to psychologist Hans Seyles, PhD, different life experiences carry varying stress potential. For example, the death of a close relative rates the highest on the stress scale while a change of eating habits ranks the lowest. See **Stressors: Highest to Lowest** for these rankings.

If you suffer from several low stressors, they can accumulate over time to become high stressors. The following hypothesis developed by Seyles shows the systematic development of a stressor. These three phases are controlled largely and regulated by the adrenal glands. If it is understood what happens in the body during each phase, perhaps the skin care professional can learn how to help clients deal with their stressors. When a stressor impinges on the body, three phases of development occur.

1. *The Alarm Phase.* This is the initial and normal response to a stressor and also is referred to as the "fight or flight" response. Physiologically, this response is triggered by reactions in the brain that ultimately cause the pituitary gland to release adrenocorticotropic hormones (ACTH). This leads to the release of adrenaline and other cortisols from the adrenal glands.

The fight or flight response mobilizes the body's resources for physical action causing the heart and respiratory rate to rise in order to increase blood and oxygen to the muscles and brain for immediate response to the stimulus. Nutrients for the skin are diverted to the organs that respond to the stressors—muscles, heart and lungs. As a result, the skin receives less nutrients leading to reduced skin immunity and breakouts. The errector pili muscle contracts causing the hair shaft to close pores to maintain heat in the tissues. They stand erect, creating "goose bumps" on the skin's surface. The liver converts glycogen to glucose and releases the extra energy into the blood stream to meet the needs of the body in combating the stressor. Vasoconstriction occurs and blood drains away from the skin's surface giving a pale appearance. Sweat production is increased, and the body's temperature is reduced; digestive secretions are inhibited so it is difficult to eat. The heart beats faster, blood pressure increases, and the body breathes faster. This response is an involuntary action governed by the autonomic nervous system.

If the stressor occurred unexpectedly, the alarm reaction will be greater than normal and higher anxiety levels will result. If stress is triggered but there is no outlet for the extra energy produced, there will be negative effects on the body. Some of the symptoms to be noted during this phase include pangs of anxiety, lack of concentration, sleeplessness, easily irritated reactions and lack of appetite. For some individuals, the opposite reaction may occur such as gaining psychological comfort in eating excessively, resulting in weight gain. The alarm phase usually is short-lived.

2. *The Resistance or Adaptation Phase.* The cortisol hormones largely are responsible for the resistance phase where the individual must either learn to adapt to stressors, or learn strategies to handle them by developing a positive attitude toward them. This phase allows the body to continue fighting the stressor long after the effects of the Alarm Phase have worn out. The individual must either learn to handle the stressor or have a stress therapist intervene to give support. This is a voluntary action controlled by the central nervous system. If the stressors are overcome during this phase, the individual has learned to control the stress. If this period of resistance action is prolonged, the risk of diseases such as high blood pressure, diabetes or deteriorating mental health occurs.

3. *The Exhaustive or Fatigue Phase.* The individual is overwhelmed with the stressors and no longer can adapt to them. Various organs including

heart and blood vessels began to weaken leading to a weakened immune system and eventually ending in stress-related diseases.

The stress of life

What causes the response is the individual's reaction to the stressor. Each person is likely to respond differently to the same stressor as a result of their individual perception or life experiences. Anticipation and imagination also can trigger the stress response. For example, getting married usually is viewed as a happy event, but also can be very stressful, or some people may find waxing painful, while others practically can sleep throughout the procedure. Type A individuals, characterized by their quick tempers, intense drive for success and aggressive, competitive nature, are highly susceptible to stress. They need to take the time to analyze their behavior because constant strains to stressors may lead to high blood pressure and other cardiovascular diseases.

Stress management

Psychological stress management. The key to stress management is teaching the client how to recognize stress symptoms that occur in the Alarm Phase and how to use effective strategies to improve the client's psychological ability to cope with her stressors. In doing so, the maladaptive stress response is reduced or eliminated. The goal is to accept the stressors or use positive thinking in dealing with them. Turn the negative viewpoint to a positive one, and the problem will not appear as threatening.

Physiological stress management. The chronic stress that occurs in the Fatigue Phase releases high levels of the steroid hormones cortisol, adrenaline and norandrenaline to meet the energy demands stimulated by the stressors. If the high levels of hormones are not checked eventually, the individual eventually may suffer from high blood pressure, a prelude to heart disease. Constant high cortisol levels result in high oxidative stress because more energy is burned and there is an excess production of free radicals. By teaching the client how to recognize the occurrence of intense levels of muscular tension resulting from stress, and using mind/body relaxation techniques, a person can learn to control the physiological action of the body to the stressor. An example is deep breathing, which helps to slow down the heartbeat and promotes relaxation.

If these hormones levels, released by the adrenal glands, can be reduced with nutritional strategies, they will not have such a strong effect on the body. Remember that high oxidative stress produces excessive production of free radicals that attack the cell membrane, mitochondria and eventually the DNA. Oxidative stress decreases DNA repair and may increase the likelihood of the development of pathological tissues, leading to premature aging of the skin and body.

Diet and stress management

In addition to stress therapy, massage and mind/body exercise, dietary modifications can be used to counteract the effects of free radicals and help in stress management.

According to the anti-aging Theory of Calorie Restriction, reduced calorie intake will result in lower free radical production. Studies also have shown that the size, composition and when meals are eaten can affect cognitive behavior. Experimental evidence suggests that in particular, those who skip breakfast do not perform well in memory and problem-solving skills when compared to those who eat breakfast. Remember that the brain utilizes at least 90% of the body's energy. Furthermore, those who ate a large lunch made more errors than those who ate a normal sized lunch. Therefore, eating lighter and smaller meals can reduce production of free radicals and increase memory and retention skills.

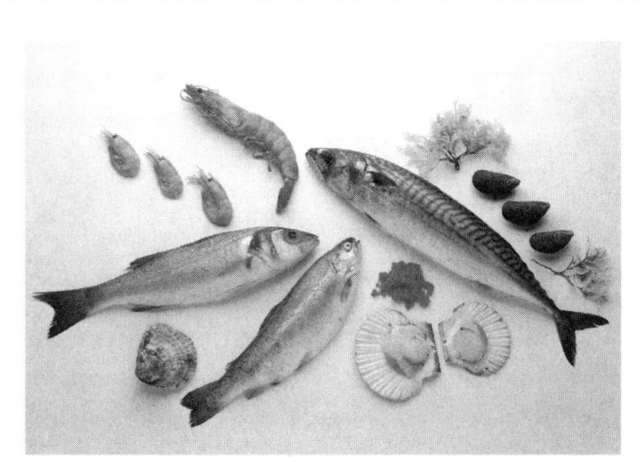

Increase intake of anti-inflammatory foods such as omega-3 and flaxseed by eating more fish and soy foods.

A high carbohydrate, low protein diet is associated with reduced levels of cortisol and is preferable for highly stressed individuals. Other studies suggested that monounsaturated and polyunsaturated fats did not increase cortisol levels as saturated fats.

High alcohol intake in healthy subjects had a negative impact on the endocrine system by stimulating high steroid production.

To summarize, smaller meals, unsaturated fats and eating breakfast are essential for mental alertness. Scientists also recommend that several small meals throughout the day instead of three large ones may be preferable to maintain normal amounts of blood glucose levels for the body's use to reduce hunger pangs.

The stress response and skin

The skin is a mirror that reflects the emotional health of the skin. Stress triggers and aggravates skin conditions such as eczema, psoriasis, warts, cold sores, and aggravates PMS and rosacea. It stimulates the sebaceous glands to produce more sebum. As a result, skin breaks out in pimples, clogged pores and hives. If a client shows some of these conditions, she is exhibiting signs of stress, and nutritional counseling can help to reduce these symptoms. Ongoing stress reduces the immune system, and the body is more susceptible to free radical attacks. A diet rich in vitamins, particularly antioxidants, beta carotene, vitamins C and E, the B Complex, and minerals such as zinc and selenium, strengthens the immune system, decreases anxiety, nervousness and depression, improves concentration and mood and results in a healthier, smoother complexion.

Beta carotene—Beta carotene is essential for the growth and repair of all epithelial cells and for the production of secretions that keep the skin soft and moist. Deficiency would cause the water-insoluble protein keratin in the epidermis to harden, resulting in thick, dry skin that may be prone to disorders such as milias and keratoses. In addition, skin infections such as seborrhea and acne vulgaris may form. Beta carotene is non-toxic since it is derived from plants and not from animals. Adequate levels of this pro-vitamin would prevent the formation of unwanted skin lesions that cause embarrassment and stress among those who suffer from them. Beta carotene also has been found to inhibit the stimulation of adrenaline and noradrenaline hormones indirectly. Certain conditions such as stress from wound healing may require higher doses of vitamin A for short periods of time, but long term supplementation at high doses can result in toxicity.

Tryptophan—As mentioned earlier, this essential amino acid is a precursor of serotonin, a hormone that initiates sleep and must taken in the diet during stress. Tryptophan is used by brain cells to manufacture serotonin which improves mood, anxiety and insomnia.

Deficiency in vitamin B complex—This results in skin inflammation and disorders such as dry cracked lips (B-2), dermatitis (B-3), hyperpigmentation (B-3), acne vulgaris and anemia (B-6). Certain B vitamins such as B-2 and B-6 act as co-factors to synthesis of prostaglandin hormones that affect the skin's complexion. Vitamin B-6 may function as a physiological regulator of the action of steroid hormones and conversion of tryptophan to serotonin.

Vitamin C, or ascorbic acid—Vitamin C is essential for synthesis of collagen, the main protein of the skin. It acts as a co-factor for several enzymes and affects the regulation of circulating thyroid and cortisol hormones. Studies have found that vitamin C supplementation led to decreased nervousness, depression and improved mood. This water-soluble vitamin is not stored in the body and needs to be taken daily.

Vitamin E—This lipid-soluble antioxidant has been established for maintaining the structural and healthy functioning of the nervous system.

Essential fatty acids—Increase intake of anti-inflammatory foods such as omega-3 and flaxseed by eating more fish and soy foods. Avoid or reduce eating inflammatory foods, including animal-derived foods such as meat and dairy products.

Stimulating beverages/foods—Reduce or avoid stimulating foods and drinks such as alcohol, caffeine and spicy foods. Try drinking herbal teas such as green tea, as well as juices such as black currant and cranberry juices to calm the nervous system.

Potassium to sodium ratio—One of the key dietary recommendations to support healthy adrenal glands is to ensure sufficient levels of potassium within the body. A dietary potassium-to-sodium ratio of 5:1 is best, but most Americans have a ratio of less than 1:2. Fruits and vegetables contain the highest levels of potassium, and a diet rich in these foods will contribute to reduced steroids levels.

Refined carbohydrates—Minimize consumption of sugar and white flour from the diet to reduce irritability and depression.

Other nutrients—Zinc, magnesium and pantothenic acid also play a critical role in the functioning of healthy adrenal glands.

Dietary supplementation—Diets rich in phytochemicals have been shown to induce a lower incidence of stress than those with lower phytochemical consumption. Nutrition experts, in particular anti-aging health practitioners, preach the hazards of insufficient amounts of vitamins and minerals to fight high stress levels in preventing skin and body aging. In today's world where drugs and processed foods reign, it is important to eat not only a more natural wholesome diet, but also to take dietary supplements to augment the daily

Stress Management Strategies

After stress reduction treatments, the client should feel relaxed and usually is in a positive mental frame of mind. Following is advice on coping strategies or stress management.

1. Adopt a more positive attitude toward the stressors or learn to adapt to them.
2. Practice healthy nutrition and participate in regular exercise.
3. Get adequate sleep.
4. Get regular face and body massages.
5. Eat, talk and move more slowly.
6. Don't be so competitive, but have fun.
7. Practice mind/body awareness activities such as deep breathing, yoga, meditation, Pilates and tai chi.
8. Take some time to do things that you like—stop and smell the roses.

nutrient intake. Many people do not realize that medications, even oral contraceptives, may impair absorption of nutrients, so it is wise to take supplements separately from medications. Note that dietary supplements must be taken with food and water.

Supportive stress reduction techniques

Learning to control life's stressors is of key importance to maintain health and well-being and truly is anti-aging. A number of stress reduction techniques have been proven effective in treating stress-related syndromes. See **Stress Management Strategies**. Therapies are based on altering or controlling one's response to stressors, whether internally or externally induced. An experienced therapist can detect areas of tension in the upper arms, shoulders and facial muscles, and skillfully manipulate using specific massage techniques to alleviate the tension knots. All stress reduction methods include some elements of suggestion, and the therapist must focus on developing voice modulation to induce relaxation for the client. Psychologists who specialize in stress reduction stipulate that in order to calm the mind and body, it is necessary to relax all the complex interacting systems of the body. It is important that the therapist possesses good communicative skills and be an active listener to the client.

Progressive relaxation. Progressive relaxation methods first were introduced in psychology to reduce fear in patients by using techniques of "counter-conditioning." This strategy was modified later by other psychologists to teach patients to attain deep muscle relaxation in a progressive way. The goal of progressive relaxation is to help the client to learn to reduce muscle tension in the body by first tensing and then relaxing each large muscle group to create awareness of muscular tension. As muscle tension diminishes, the effects of various components of the autonomic nervous system are reduced such as heart rate and blood pressure.

As the client becomes deeply relaxed, she learns how to become more "conditioned" against the stressors. Voluntary skills then can be developed to counter-condition the body against the arousal of stressors. The key goal in stress management is to create an awareness of the response to stressors and through this, the client can learn to control the stress responses.

CHAPTER 9

Glycemic Index and Health

The term **glycemic index** has been cropping up regularly in health news in recent years. What is it, and how does it impact health? How does it affect skin and body care professionals? Since many skin care professionals now work within the realm of wellness, this chapter attempts to explain the correlation between the glycemic index and health. In the past, the glycemic index has been associated with the treatment of diabetes, but in recent years, health care professionals have begun to use it in other areas of health such as weight control and exercise. It was developed by Canadian researchers working on diabetes who wanted to measure how quickly foods, particularly carbohydrates, were digested into the bloodstream.

The glycemic index

Blood glucose levels are maintained by several hormones. Insulin from the pancreas converts excess blood glucose to glycogen and is stored in the muscles and liver. When the body needs more energy, the hormone glucagon that is secreted by the liver converts the stored glycogen back into glucose and puts it back into the blood for immediate use. Ephinephrine hormone released by the adrenal gland increases glucose production when the body is under stress and requires more energy. The glycemic index is a guide that indicates how quickly blood glucose and insulin levels show up in the blood immediately after digesting carbohydrate-laden foods. Different carbohydrates result in varying glycemic index responses. When blood glucose levels rise quickly, the food is given a higher glycemic index value than those that take longer to digest. High blood sugar levels inevitably increase the hormone insulin that converts excessive glucose to glycogen to be stored in the liver and muscles for later use. Excessive blood insulin levels are detrimental to those who suffer from low blood sugar. The glycemic index of a food is measured to a standard food or "control" food. An arbitrary glycemic index value of 100 is given to glucose or white bread, and other foods are classified in comparison. For example, glucose carries a glycemic index value of 100 while a peach carries a low glycemic index value of 28.

Glycemic index and diabetes. High blood sugar levels inevitably lead to increased insulin levels that convert any excessive glucose to glycogen. Excessive insulin levels in the blood are detrimental to individuals who suffer from type II diabetes and **hypoglycemia**, or low blood sugar. That is why physicians always insist that diabetic patients limit or avoid certain carbohydrates that raise blood sugar too quickly. Several observational studies have shown that high glycemic index foods were associated not only with increased risk of developing type II diabetes, but also with cardiovascular diseases and certain cancers. In the past few years, type II diabetes, usually found in mature individuals, has been discovered among children at alarming rates and is positively correlated to obesity, a phenomena that is threatening to be one of the fastest growing epidemics in Europe, North America and even developing countries such as China. The foods eaten in Western society typically are high in fat and carbohydrates, and produce a high glycemic index response ultimately promoting weight gain. In contrast, low glycemic index foods help control weight gain and ultimately lead to better health. Diabetes is the fourth leading cause of death in the world, and both obesity and diabetes now are emerging as major causes of morbidity in the United States. Some surveys have shown that some parents are outliving their children who die from the ramifications of obesity and diabetes.

Glycemic index and carbohydrates. Carbohydrates provide the main source of energy in foods and are the quickest form of getting the energy. Health care professionals recommend a daily intake 55% or more of carbohydrates, 15–20% protein and less than 30% fat out of which no more than 10% should be saturated fats. The quality of the carbohydrates that constitute the majority of the daily diet should be checked carefully. Carbohydrates are categorized as simple—sugars, and complex—starches. All carbohydrates must be broken down into monosaccharides before they can be absorbed by the cells. There are three types of monosaccharides: glucose, fructose and galactose, each having different physical and chemical properties. This accounts for their varying amount of sweetness, fructose being the sweetest. Glucose constitutes 80% of all monosaccharides. With the onset of hunger, many crave sugars because they help curb hunger immediately. This is because sugars are digested quickly appearing immediately in the blood stream in the form of glucose. However, complex carbohydrates such as vegetables, rice and pasta take longer to digest because they have to be broken down by enzymes in the gastrointestinal tract before they can be available to the cells.

Understanding the glycemic index

The research in glycemic index indicates that food that is digested and absorbed slowly has the least impact on blood sugar levels. At the moment, not all carbohydrates have been assessed, and the process still is ongoing. Many Western diets produce a high glycemic response that promotes weight gain in contrast to low glycemic index foods that may enhance weight control. With this mind, a glycemic index table has been devised to inform health practitioners and patients of the glycemic index value of foods. The more refined the food, the quicker the absorption and higher the glycemic index value. Natural, unprocessed foods such as non-starchy vegetables and fruits are digested slowly and are assigned a lower glycemic index value. High sugar foods are absorbed quickly, placing a strain on blood sugar levels that are harmful for diabetics. Learning to read and interpret food labels gives clues to sugar content. Contrary to popular belief, many high glycemic index foods include starches such as bread, cereals and potatoes regardless of high or low fiber. This is due to the starch becoming fully gelatinized so that it is easily digested and absorbed. Glycemic index values are influenced by the following factors.

Type of sugar. Fructose has a lower glycemic index than sucrose or glucose and is found in about 15% of all simple carbohydrates. Foods high in fructose have little effect in raising high levels of blood sugar and insulin, so check the amount of fructose in comparison to sucrose or glucose in food.

Type of starch. The more glucose, the higher the glycemic index. More refined carbohydrates carry a higher glycemic index value than wholesome, coarse grains.

Fiber content. The more fiber, the lower the glycemic index response. Fruits and vegetables contain large amounts of fiber.

Size of portion eaten. The less food eaten, the lower the glycemic index response.

Degree of food processing. In general, the more processed the food, the higher the glycemic index. However, some processed foods such as potato chips have a lower glycemic index than boiled potatoes.

Amount of protein and fat in food. The more complex the protein, the higher the glycemic index. Higher amounts of proteins and fats in food slow down digestion.

Method of food preparation. Soft, overcooked foods are digested more quickly than firm, raw foods and intact grains.

Low glycemic index foods include oatmeal, legumes, pasta, apples, pears, oranges, peaches, plums, dried apricots, grapefruit, yogurt, low fat milk and carrots.

Moderate to high glycemic index foods include processed foods such as bread, muffins, crackers, cereals, rice, potatoes, popcorn, honey, raisins, bananas and grapes. Many other carbohydrates still are being assessed for their glycemic index values.

Glycemic index and diabetes. Since the quick rise of insulin and blood sugar levels are detrimental to diabetic and hyperglycemic individuals, they are advised to eat foods that reflect low glycemic index values.

Glycemic index and weight loss. In recent years, health care professionals have become aware that the glycemic index can be used as a tool to help in weight reduction. Low glycemic index foods may enhance weight loss by promoting satisfaction and reducing the secretion of insulin and blood sugar levels. For weight management, the consumption of low to medium glycemic index foods can prove to be quite useful. A high fiber diet incorporating low glycemic index foods will slow food digestion because it enhances satiety by maintaining constant blood sugar levels for a longer period of time thus helping to curb excessive food intake.

Glycemic index and exercise. Studies by Kirwan et al suggest that consumption of lower glycemic index foods before exercise would be beneficial to sustain blood glucose levels, leading to improved exercise performance and duration. Since a person should not exercise on an empty stomach, simple sugars such as fructose are very beneficial before a workout. Several studies suggest that high fiber foods have low glycemic index because they enter the bloodstream slowly, such as sweet potatoes and whole wheat, instead of regular potatoes and white rice.

Glycemic index and growth hormone. If taking growth hormone supplements, high glycemic index foods should be avoided before taking them because high insulin levels are produced that will prevent the hormones from being released.

New insights

Some researchers believe that the glycemic index permits new insights into the relationship between the physiological effects of carbohydrate-rich foods and health. They see the glycemic index as a more useful concept in nutrition rather than the traditional classification of carbohydrates as sugars or sugars as simple or complex. Furthermore, the glycemic index often is used to help people eat healthy, reduce the risk of diabetes, control weight and improve exercise performance.

CHAPTER 10

Nutritional Counseling in Pre- and Post-care Surgery

New research in nutritional science may provide fresh insights in optimizing not only the body's health, but also the physical appearance of the skin and body. While most studies are focused on preventing skin conditions such as cancer and skin disorders, more studies are being conducted on how to combat the aging of the skin. Due to the pursuit of youth and beauty, the number of individuals undergoing cosmetic surgery and skin resurfacing treatments has escalated in the past few years. These treatments can result in much pain, discomfort, inflammation and bruising. However, many health professionals believe that the healing process can be accelerated with proper dietary intake before, during and after surgical procedures. Many estheticians now are working with dermatologists and plastic surgeons who perform cosmetic procedures, most of which cause wound injury. These skin care professionals should learn as much as possible about certain nutrients and their effects in enhancing the healing of tissues.

The importance of nutritional status in wound healing

Good nutritional status is essential for wound healing, and although this has been studied for centuries, sufficient knowledge in this area still is lacking. During surgical procedures, body tissues experience extreme trauma and oxidative stress. Wound healing is dependent on healthy nutritional status for speeding recovery after surgical procedures. Deficiencies in carbohydrates, proteins, fatty acids and certain micronutrients can put a damper on the healing process and prolong the stages of wound healing.

Pre-operative care

The esthetician who is working with physicians should know not only how to physically prepare the skin for surgery, but also be able to give the patient advice on nutrition before, during and after surgery. This will lead to increased credibility in the "wellness" component of the health care team and give the patient a sense of comfort that she is in good hands. A thorough personal history of the patient should be done to review nutritional status and lifestyle behaviors.

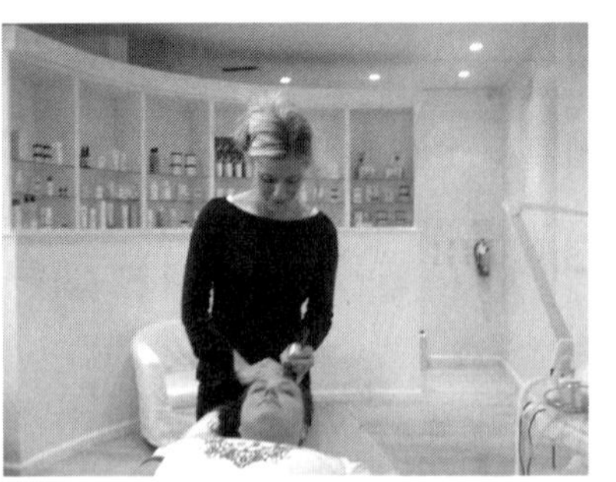

The esthetician who is working with physicians should know not only how to physically prepare the skin for surgery, but also be able to give the patient advice on nutrition before, during and after surgery.

To prepare for surgery, the body should be nourished with optimal amounts of nutrients such as proteins, essential fatty acids and antioxidants to arm the immune system and minimize inflammatory reactions. Adequate amounts of glucose provide energy to tissues and deposition of new tissue. Protein, particularly the amino acid arginine, is essential for tissue renewal. Protein, particularly the amino acid arginine, is essential for tissue renewal, and increased intake of zinc will enhance the immune system and prepare for the expected trauma on body tissues. Adequate water intake is also necessary to replenish dehydration of tissues. Antioxidants such as vitamins A, C and E quench the excess free radicals formed from oxidative stress due to surgery. Avoiding inflammatory foods and drinks such as fatty meats, caffeine, alcohol and spicy foods are part of preventative care preparing the body for the impending tissue damage.

Before surgery, advise the patient to avoid smoking but exercise regularly to strengthen the muscles that would help maintain the body's strength and stamina during the "downtime" period when no physical activity can be performed. The esthetician's role in pre-op is to prepare the skin for surgery using deep cleansing, light exfoliating and moisturizing facial treatments as well as recommending appropriate skin care products for home care use. Mental support provided by the skin care specialist can help the patient prepare for surgery with a positive mind.

Post-operative care

Immediately after surgical procedures, the skin appears inflamed or bruised, and it is during this critical time that infection is most likely to set in. Dietary intake can play a significant role as a therapeutic agent in skin healing. Proteins, certain types of fats and vitamin supplementation are necessary to enhance wound healing and promote recovery for clear, healthy, smooth skin.

Protein. First and foremost, a high protein diet is essential for wound recovery. Amino acids are necessary in nutrition for collagen renewal and repair. After surgery, the patient must follow the physician's orders, but when signs of recovery are seen, first class proteins should form an integral part of the daily diet to promote strength and quick healing. Nutritional supplements should include the amino acid arginine to promote wound healing.

Glucose. The patient will be weak and lacking energy after surgery, therefore adequate amounts of glucose will provide the body with extra energy for healing and deposition of new tissue.

Essential fatty acids. Omega-3 and omega-6 are necessary for their anti-inflammatory effects and their role in cell structure. Supplementation with fish and flaxseed oils would be of benefit since the patient will not have a good appetite. Eating and drinking flavonoids such as soy products, green tea, black currant, borage oil and evening primrose oil will have protective benefits.

Water. Plenty of fluids replenish the dehydration that occurs during surgery.

Antioxidants. Beta carotene, vitamins A, C and E, and minerals selenium and zinc are of vital importance to maintain an efficient immune system and prevent excess free radical formation that occurs from wounds.

Vitamin A—Vitamin A has been shown to be beneficial in wound healing since it stimulates collagen synthesis. Vitamin A is needed by epithelial cells for production of protective secretions such as mucus on the skin's surface for lubrication and resistance to infection. Any openings in the skin are susceptible to infection and some physicians recommend high doses of some dietary supplements on a short-term basis to enhance wound healing. For example, 25,000–50,000 IU vitamin A are recommended as pre-op and post care supplementation to promote healing of the traumatized connective tissue.

Vitamin C—Vitamin C is an extremely important nutrient involved in the synthesis of collagen and connective tissue, and is vital for the healing process. Collagen is a component of the intracellular matrix, the glue that holds all cells together in the dermis and strengthens the walls of the capillaries. When the skin is injured during surgical procedures, capillaries need to be strong and healthy to prevent hemorrhaging, bruising and edema. Vitamin C also has anti-inflammatory effects on the skin by reducing the release of histamine and other inflammatory substances into the tissue, reducing symptoms of allergies. Deficiency of vitamin C contributes to fragile tissue.

Bioflavonoids, or vitamin P—These have been used as nutritional support to reduce bleeding and enhance wound healing. They help to reduce pain, inflammation, bleeding, bruising and edema that occur during injury. They are found together with vitamin C in plants with yellow, red and blue hues, and are known to improve capillary strength and help reduce the symptoms of allergic reactions.

Vitamin E, or alpha-tocopherol—High levels of free radicals produced in any skin injury can be counteracted with vitamin E. This fat-soluble antioxidant protects the cell membranes from destruction. It has a protective action on lipids, particularly polyunsaturated fats (PUFA). Therefore those who consume large amounts of PUFA will need to take more vitamin E. Luckily, both vitamin E and PUFA usually are found in the same foods. Significant sources of vitamin E are nuts and most vegetable oils, especially wheat germ oil. It is readily destroyed by heat, so avoid frying of vitamin E-rich foods. Toxicity is rare, and in post-care surgery, taking vitamin E supplements at the upper levels of 1,000 mg/d would accelerate the healing process. There are different forms of vitamin E, so look for the term **alpha-tocopherol** on the label because it is the only tocopherol that is active in the human body. Vitamin E or tocopherols consist of four different compounds—alpha, beta, gamma and delta—that are distinguished by the positions of their chemical side chains. The alpha tocopherol is the only one that is biologically active in the human body—it acts as an antioxidant. The other tocopherols are not converted readily to alpha tocopherol in the body, nor do they perform the same roles.

Vitamin K—Vitamin K is known for its clotting properties and deficiency is rare. After surgery, effective blood clotting is vital for healing. Vitamin K is produced endogenously in the GI tract by bacteria flora. Once synthesized, it is absorbed and stored in the liver. Dietary sources of this vitamin include liver, green vegetables and cabbage.

Aloe vera—Aloe vera reduces the edema that occurs in wounds and has an anti-inflammatory effect on traumatized tissues. It is believed that the *topical* application of this well-known cactus-like plant contains a number of compounds that accelerate healing, including vitamins C and E, and zinc. The glycoproteins found in the plant break down certain substances that cause pain and inflammation and have been shown to stimulate fibroblasts, connective tissue formation and epidermal growth, thereby promoting wound repair.

Flavonoids—Flavonoids give plants their colorful pigments. They sometimes are considered "nature's biological response modifiers" due to their anti-inflammatory actions against allergens, viruses and carcinogens. There are many different types of flavonoids such as the citrus bioflavonoids, rutin and bromelain. Quercetin shows the greatest activity among flavonoids and as supplements, it is available in powder and capsule. In general, flavonoids prevent the release and synthesis of compounds such as histamine and prostaglandins that promote inflammation and allergies.

Camouflage makeup

The skin is inflamed and bruised after surgical procedures, and the client normally stays away from work and avoids social contact during this period of recovery. Skin care professionals can introduce complementary therapies such as camouflage makeup, a specialized form of makeup that gives excellent coverage for the inflammation, scars or bruising and makes the skin appear clear and flawless. This type of makeup does not harm the skin and originally was created for burn victims. Although the application is simple, it usually requires specialized training and is an excellent adjunct service to help the client feel more confident about her appearance during downtime.

Promoting recovery

The days when you were confined to bed after surgery are gone and in fact, recent studies have shown that those who were physically active, regardless of age, recovered quite quickly. Wounds place increased metabolic demands on the body and physicians must consider the nutritional support for their patients, particularly older individuals, through adequate dietary intake and supplementation to help promote a safe and rapid recovery.

CHAPTER 11

Skin Sensitivities or Allergies

Modern mankind has come a long way from early times when eating patterns consisted of relatively non-toxic foods such as whole grains, fruits and vegetables. Today, in order to feed and please everyone on the planet, modern technology has developed a plethora of refined foods containing chemicals such as food additives, artificial colorings and flavorings, preservatives, pesticides and hormones. In fact, some additives are not even required to be listed on the food label. These hidden ingredients in many commercialized foods have given rise to an increase in food and environmental allergies during past decades.

The genetic manipulation involved in the cross-breeding of various plants has led to a loss of control in defining food antigens entering the circulatory system so rapidly, they often can result in fatal situations. The manifestation of these practices has resulted in a high number of food allergies, skin sensitivities and disorders, and oxidative stress as well as various body metabolic disorders.

The body's immune function is known to decline with age. Research into mechanisms for enhancing the immune system with vitamins such as antioxidants, and polyunsaturated fats such as omega-3 fatty acids, to reduce inflammatory skin disorders are proving fruitful.

Skin care professionals sometimes are challenged to recognize skin reactions triggered by the use of certain cosmetics, food intake or environmental allergens. With a higher incidence of hypersensitive skin, more education in determining whether the allergy may be due to cosmetic applications or food allergens can prove very beneficial to a professional's practice. Asking more questions about known food allergies and having knowledge of cosmetics and their origins also may prove to be very helpful to the skin care professional. This chapter deals with the protective effects of nutrients on skin sensitivity and sun exposure, and their relationship to the immune response and food toxins.

The immune response

The skin is the largest organ in the body and continuously is exposed to internal and external influences that affect its condition and function. It is supplied richly with free nerve endings that transmit sensations of temperature, pain and touch to the central nervous system to be interpreted. When the skin comes in contact with a foreign substance that is intolerant to the body, certain cells called **Langerhans cells** in the upper layers of the skin migrate to the lymphatic vessels and then to the lymphatic nodes. This leads to the immune response where the mast cells in the dermis release a substance called **histamine** that causes inflammatory responses such as swelling, pain, itching or hives, erythema and even fever. Since Langerhans cells are susceptible to UV rays, excessive sun exposure can suppress the body's immunity by reducing their actions.

Although many substances may cause an allergic reactions, certain ones are more likely than others to stimulate a response. If a substance is applied topically on the skin for a prolonged period of time, a physiological reaction will occur. Although many people can be exposed to a foreign substance, only a few may have an allergic reaction to it. For example, when poison ivy comes in contact with the skin, it may have varying effects on different individuals, but it can be quite severe in some cases. The skin may become very red, itching and swollen but these symptoms can disappear quickly.

An **antigen** is a foreign substance that enters the body and includes any microorganism, some drugs such as penicillin, toxins, animal and vegetable proteins, and foreign tissues such as transplanted organs. An **allergy** is the inflammatory response to an antigen, resulting in vasodilation. Antigens or allergens stimulate the production of proteins called **antibodies** released by the lymphatic system rendering the antigens harmless.

The immune system consists of the lymphatic system and certain protein molecules that defend the body from infection and disease. Immunity is body's ability to resist infections. Some individuals are very lucky to possess **natural immunity**—a natural protective ability to easily resist certain allergens. An example would be the individual who receives chicken pox injections with no resulting allergic response. **Acquired immunity** refers to the body's ability to develop powerful immunity against foreign agents such as viruses and toxins, a result of receiving flu or vaccine shots. There are two basic types of acquired immunity.

Humoral or B-cell immunity. In this immune response, the B cells transform into plasma cells and secrete antibodies that circulate in the bloodstream to neutralize antigens.

Cell-mediated or T-cell immunity. When encountering antigens, T-cells attach to them quickly forming a large number of lymphocytes to engulf and digest the antigen.

Toxins in food

A toxin is any compound that has a detrimental effect on living tissue. A compound is a molecule formed from several other elements and has new properties from that of the individual elements. The body's immunity can be reduced by the presence of toxins taken into the body through dietary intake. Toxins may be heavy metals such as lead, mercury and aluminum; chemicals such as solvents, drugs, alcohol, pesticides and food additives; and various microbes. Some plants contain lethal toxins in high concentrations and are unfit for human consumption while others contain mild toxins and are benign.

Food allergies. Ironically, although food is essential for human survival, nature has endowed plants with the ability to manufacture toxins for protection from predators. Therefore, many plants contain naturally occurring toxins and may cause allergic reactions in some people. True food allergies are abnormal responses of the immune system to specific nutrients in foods usually with serious symptoms. Reactions to food intake are far broader than the common symptoms of hives, erythema, swelling and itchiness that show up on the skin. They manifest themselves in either immediate or delayed hypersensitive reactions. Severe reactions usually show up within a few minutes to about an hour after ingesting the offending food, while delayed reactions begin to appear after 24 hours or more. A wide variety of symptoms are mild to life threatening, and are associated with a class of antibodies known as immunoglobulin E (IgE) that affects only 1–2% of the total population.

Some symptoms include: erythema, hives, dermatitis, skin inflammation, eczema and swelling of the skin; nausea, vomiting, diarrhea, cramping and flatus in the GI system; asthma and rhinitis—inflammation of mucous membranes of nasal cavities, in the respiratory system; or migraine, anal itching, flushing, laryngeal edema, or swelling in larynx, asthma, and anaphylactic shock, the most dangerous reaction that involves many body systems, usually is fatal.

Several metabolic disorders also can be reflected by the pH of urine, but this abnormality can be corrected through proper nutrition and dietary supplementation. Similar dietary interventions also can be used to control or eliminate food allergies and skin sensitivity.

Common food allergens. Surprisingly, the foods that have been found to cause the most allergies usually are those eaten on a daily basis, not necessarily those eaten occasionally. Most often, naturally occurring proteins have been found to be the culprit of food allergies. The most common food allergens known as the Big Eight are cows' milk, eggs, fish, shellfish, peanuts, soybeans, tree nuts and wheat. Tree nuts refer to almonds, walnuts, pecans, cashews, Brazil nuts, pistachios, hazelnuts, pine nuts, macademia nuts, chestnuts and hickory nuts.

Hidden sources of allergens. Knowing the hidden sources of these food allergens will help prevent attacks. Some ingredients in foods that have been reported to be common triggers of migraine attacks include amino acids, tyramine and histamine. These are found in higher levels in a range of foods such as cheese, alcohol, sausage and tinned fish. Mackerel and tuna contain high amounts of histamine. Caffeine, which has a diuretic effect, has been found to stimulate gastric secretion and can cause heartburn, nausea, vomiting and diarrhea, as well as irregular heartbeat, sweating, anxiety and sleeplessness. In general, any excess dietary intake of known toxic foods may be harmful so if intolerance to these common food allergens is suspected, it is prudent to limit their intake. If a milk allergy is present, check for casein, a milk derivative, in some meats and in foods such as canned tuna fish. Many restaurants cook their steaks with butter. According to the Mayo Clinic Food and Nutrition Center, ingredients such as calcium lactate, cocoa butter, cream of tartar, sodium lactate and most forms of lactic acid do not contain milk, although lactic acid starter culture may contain milk.

Many people are severely allergic to peanuts and must be aware that arachis oil is peanut oil, and that many foods sold in bakeries and ice cream shops contain peanuts. Wine and beer contain significant amounts of sulfites which have been linked to food allergies. Gluten is the ingredient that causes the wheat allergy called **celiac disease**, a permanent adverse reaction. The major grains that contain gluten are wheat, rye, oats and barley. Many bakeries now have developed gluten-free grains for these individuals.

Indigestion. In some cases, the acid base balance of the body needs to be checked. Has the person eaten too many acidic foods such as tomatoes, citrus fruits and coffee? Do they regularly suffer from heartburn or gas and resort to taking antacids or acid controllers? These indigestion problems have been associated with eating too quickly or overeating.

Tracking allergens in cosmetics

In the clinic or spa, if the client experiences a breakout following a facial treatment, the tendency is to point the finger to the skin care product used during the treatment, particularly if the reaction occurred within 24 hours. However, sometimes it may be caused by skin sensitivity to a particular food allergen instead. Many cosmetics use aracidis oil, a peanut oil used for its softening, healing properties, and lactic acid in their formulations. Lactic acid is a preservative, moisturizer or exfoliant, and is derived from sour milk and foods such as beer and pickles. Certain food coloring used in cosmetics may be a possible source of the skin irritation. The goal is to locate the allergen using a two-fold process to narrow down the offending substance. Check the personal history of the client, particularly the Big Eight allergens.

The most common cosmetics that cause contact dermatitis are lipstick and nail polish due to the eosin dye they contain. Detergents, strong alkalis and petroleum products are potential allergens in cosmetics as well as plant and plant products such as essential oils, animal products such as lanolin and collagen or the influence of various medications such as antibiotics, antihistamines and steroids.

The elimination strategy for skin care. Stop using the potentially offending products for a few days and wash the face with only water. Begin using the products one by one and wait for any sign of reactions. If you get a reaction, the next step is to scrutinize the ingredients on the product label.

Derivatives of known allergens. It is very helpful to have some knowledge of hidden allergens in the product labels since many of them are derivatives of other substances. For example, milk derivates are found in cheese, lactose, whey, casein, yogurt and ice cream, while certain ethnic foods such as Thai use specific ingredients in cooking, such as peanuts. Other hidden allergens include petroleum jelly, a common cosmetic ingredient obtained from petroleum; royal jelly comes from the queen bee; lactic acid is a product of milk; paraffin wax is derived from petroleum; potassium hydroxide and sodium hydroxide are strong alkalis; spermaceti is the fatty acid from the sperm whale; and thioglycolic acid found in chemical depilatories are highly irritating to the skin.

Nutrition and sun protection

Epidemiological and experimental studies have established firmly that premature skin aging and a wide range of skin disorders are the result of excessive sun exposure. The effects of UV rays are very damaging to the skin and cause biological effects such as erythema, inflammation, hyperpigmentation, burnt skin and, over time, skin cancer. Anyone who was a sun lover in their youth often has skin that looks old, dry, wrinkled and crepe-like with many sunspots, or hyperpigmentation, all over the face and body. Although there are many treatments both surgical and non-surgical for photo-damaged skin, topical applications and oral consumption of certain nutrients can play a beneficial role in reducing the incidence of changes in the skin associated with UV radiation.

Ultraviolet radiation. UV rays consist of UVA, UVB and UVC. The ozone layer absorbs UVC leaving UVA and UVB rays. The continuing breakdown of the protective ozone layer has led to the increasing incidence of skin diseases during the past few decades. The subsequent formation of free radicals destroys not only the structural cell components of the skin, but also the genetic component, or DNA. UVB, or burning rays, penetrate the epidermis causing erythema, peeling and burning while UVA rays penetrate deeper into the dermis and contribute to malignant cancers and benign conditions including wrinkles and premature skin aging. The epidermis is the first line of protection against free radicals and carries several natural antioxidants, however, recent studies show that after a certain amount of sun exposure, they are destroyed.

Antioxidants and skin protection

Studies have shown that skin damage from UV rays can be reduced or prevented with the use of antioxidants. Vitamins C, E, beta carotene and flavonoids, all found in fruits and vegetables, have significant antioxidant effects in the treatment against photodamaged skin.

Vitamin C. High levels of vitamin C usually are present in the epidermis, and topical applications of vitamin E have been shown to be effective in protecting the skin from UVB, or photodamaged skin. Wound healing is dependent on vitamin C because it is essential for the production of collagen.

Vitamin E. Considered the main antioxidant in skin and body tissues, vitamin E offers significant protective photoaging effects. However, it is most susceptible to be depleted by UV light and needs vitamin C to prevent its degradation in the skin. Vitamin E is listed in many sunscreen products as either tocopheryl acetate, an oil derived from peanuts and used for moisturizing and soothing, or other derivates of vitamin E, including tocopherol nicotinate, tocopheryl sorbate or vitamin E acetate.

Beta carotene. The carotenoids, beta carotene and lycopene, were found to have photo protective effects in several studies which showed that erythema in sun-exposed skin was reduced when using beta supplementation. The data suggested that the slight skin hyperpigmentation from the beta carotene supplementation might have given extra skin protection against the sun. Beta carotene supplementation before and during sun exposure provided protection against sunburn on the *whole* body as compared to sunscreens that protect only the application points of the skin. Researchers concluded that using both carotenoids and topical sunscreens together gave the most protection against sunburn.

Omega-3 fatty acids. Several studies indicated that long term dietary intake of omega-3 fatty acids, most commonly found in marine animals with a high level of fats such as salmon, mackerel and cod liver oil, was shown to protect the skin at the macroscopic and cellular levels despite the increased oxidative stress from sun exposed skin.

Flavonoids. These polyphenols from fruits and vegetables help to strengthen an immune system weakened by UV rays. They are believed to have anti-inflammatory effects, and studies have reported that flavonoids may act as a sunscreen in preventing DNA damage in epidermal cells. Significant dietary sources of flavonoids include soy products, green and black tea, citrus fruits with a red or wine color, cruceriferous vegetables and red wine.

A combination of habitual dietary intake and supplementation of vitamins, carotenoids and polyunsaturated fats may protect the whole body against photodamaged skin. In contrast, topical sunscreens have to be applied regularly and work only on the areas to which they were applied. Therefore, using both approaches is best for skin protection.

Detoxification

Any substance that can disturb the body's natural metabolic functioning can be termed toxic or harmful. Normally, the body can regulate homeostasis of toxic levels through its natural elimination system—the liver, kidneys and sweat glands. If a person is both physically and mentally healthy, the imbalance can be controlled to keep toxic levels low in the body. However, if more toxins are taken in than can be eliminated, then several symptoms can occur to indicate the presence of toxic buildup. Fasting, detoxification and cleansing are the oldest treatments known to man and are natural processes to eliminate toxins from the body. Toxicity occurs in the body on both external and internal levels. People are exposed to external toxins daily from the environment by breathing pollutants and ingesting food, drink and drugs. The body produces internal toxins from oxidative processes. These include biochemical, cellular and free radicals. If they are not eliminated, they can cause a buildup leading to the body malfunctioning and eventually cause damage to its systems.

What is detoxification? Detoxification is the process of removing, neutralizing or transforming toxins and clearing congestion. Almost everyone needs to detoxify their body at some point. In fact, there are many signs that may indicate that your body needs some form of cleansing. They include bad breath, constipation, diarrhea, foul odor in urine or feces, headaches, frequent colds, sore throat, sinus congestion, anxiety, indigestion, hives, fatigue, insomnia, diabetes and cancer. The complexion also can serve as an indicator for internal health. Skin congestion, acne, pustules, cysts, eczema and psoriasis are signs that an internal cleansing is needed, no matter how good the topical skin care regimen. Fats, especially oxidized fats, also act as toxins in the body. Body conditions such as cellulite, menstrual problems, varicosity and obesity also infer that the body needs to detoxify.

Why detoxify? The world is fraught with toxins. Externally, people are confronted with toxins from the environment such as industrial pollution, chemicals on crops and heavy metals such as lead or mercury in the water. The common use of pesticides, particularly DDT, one of the most common environmental contaminants, in the soil and water contaminate foods, and the excessive use of drugs in today's society contribute toward a high build up of toxins internally. Although DDT has been banned from the United States since 1972, it is believed that it comes from produce imported from countries where it still is used. Free radicals are produced inside the body during metabolic activities adding to the toxic buildup. Natural toxins also are present in certain types of seafood, particularly shellfish.

Many nutritional experts recommend that some form of cleansing or detoxification should be practiced occasionally, particularly when there are signs of toxicity. Some extreme detoxification programs using laxatives, enemas, colonics and diuretics can be detrimental to health. Fasting among some individuals, such as those who suffer from allergies, may be beneficial and should be done under the guidance and advice of a dietician or nutritionist. Detoxification helps reduce toxic buildup, relieve congestion, improve elimination and rejuvenate the body's systems. Experts in this field give many reasons for detoxification. (See **Reasons for Detoxification**, page 157.)

Natural detoxification system. If you are healthy and proper food preparation techniques are used to remove these toxins, the body will not suffer any ill

Reasons for Detoxification

Detoxification helps reduce toxic buildup, relieve congestion, improve elimination and rejuvenate the body's systems. Experts in this field give many reasons for detoxification.

1. Considered an anti-aging program for slowing the aging process by treating or preventing disease.
2. A form of cleansing and purification.
3. Helps in weight loss.
4. Decongests the skin for a clearer complexion.
5. Rejuvenates the body.
6. Can contribute to spirituality.
7. Improves fertility.
8. Enhances the senses.
9. Increases environmental awareness.

effects of toxins from consumed foods or liquids. The immune system, liver and kidneys are responsible for producing antitoxins and antibodies to remove toxic substances absorbed from the gut. The liver filters passing blood every minute while the kidneys eliminate urine, and sweat is removed from the skin and sweat glands. This natural detoxification process helps to clear wastes and revitalize the body's natural functions.

Voluntary detoxification. Lifestyle measures can be taken to detoxify the body by voluntarily reducing intake of known toxic foods and increasing elimination. Raw foods, particularly fruits and vegetables, are wholesome, healthier to eat and carry higher levels of nutrients than cooked versions. The trade-off is that the potential for toxicity is greater for uncooked foods, but the nutrient values are higher. Although the body has an amazing internal mechanism for removal of toxins, sometimes these systems break down for various reasons such as illness, resulting in toxicity. Some people can sense an oncoming cold or congestion and know that it is time to go on a natural cleansing program to clean out the body from the inside. Some claim that they experience spiritual wellness after a light detoxifying program, and this feeling reinforces their commitment to reduce the abuse on their bodies.

How often to detoxify? Almost everyone needs an internal cleansing of the body occasionally. This is analogous to having your car overhauled or cleaned regularly for overall improved function. Detoxification is highly recommended for those who tend to live an abusive lifestyle such as consuming a diet high in fats, meat, rich dairy products, deep fried or refined foods, inadequate sleep, excessive alcohol or smoking. Or, it may be better simply to cut back on those foods that contain high levels of toxins instead. (See **Recommendations to Prevent Skin Sensitivity or Food Allergies**.)

If you feel that you have overindulged in rich foods or excessive portions one day, cut back the next day and eat a lighter fare such as fruits, vegetables and herbal foods to reduce the toxic levels in the body. Coupled with regular

Recommendations to Prevent Skin Sensitivity or Food Allergies

1. Reduce or limit intake of common known allergic foods—the Big Eight.
2. Avoid or minimize cured meats, refined or canned foods, sugar, salt, saturated fats, fried foods, coffee, alcohol and nicotine.
3. Eat a more vegetarian diet by consuming more fruits, vegetables, whole grains, legumes, nuts and seeds, and avoid or limit animal-derived foods. The high fiber content helps detoxify the colon. Anti-aging health practitioners recommend 20–40 grams of fiber daily. The average American diet contains only 11–15 grams.
4. Eat natural foods that are in season, focusing on organic choices whenever possible.
5. Drink at least eight 8-oz. glasses of pure, filtered water to help dilute and eliminate toxins. It cleans skin and kidneys, and helps in electrolyte balance. It is suggested that 2–3 glasses of water be taken before meals to help in digestion and elimination.
6. Avoid taking drugs and instead substitute with natural herbs, which have fewer side effects.
7. Try natural therapies such as acupuncture, chiropractic and homeopathic therapy.
8. Indulge in treatments to promote sweating such as steam and sauna with massage, body peelings to remove dead cells and promote new cell formation, and skin and body wrap treatments in spas to promote rejuvenation.
9. Get attuned with your body both physically and mentally by building up sweat during physical exercise—practice yoga, Pilates and meditation.

exercise and stress management skills, detoxification achieves and maintains both mental and physical health. Many people visit spas to detoxify, lose weight or rejuvenate their bodies. While this is good for business, it should be part of normal life and not just for specific occasions. If a skin care professional observes any signs of toxicity, advice on cutting back or improving the client's diet can be given to optimize the results of the skin and body treatments. A good time to detoxify is in the spring and fall. In fact, it is recommended that women follow a cleansing program the week before their menstruation to reduce some premenstrual symptoms. When feeling congested or suspect that a cold is coming, try a more nontoxic diet by eating lighter foods, drinking lots of fluids and getting a good night's sleep. Furthermore, avoid those foods that are most congesting to the body. These include fats, fried foods, organ meats, refined foods, coffee and alcohol. Least congesting foods include fruits, vegetables, purified water, roots and herbs.

In general, balancing both acid and alkaline foods is the key to a detoxifying diet. Colon cleansing is one of the most important components of detoxification. Acidic-forming foods such as milk products, meats and refined foods such as sugar will lead to increased production of mucus that will cause congestion while the more alkaline-forming foods of fresh fruits, vegetables and whole grains will help to balance the acid-alkaline base of the body's chemistry. Green vegetables, especially high-nutrient leafy greens, carry good cleansing actions since their high fiber content helps to clear the GI tract. A more stringent level of detoxification involves fasting or going on a liquid diet by intake of juices, vegetable broths and teas to purify the body. Some experts recommend taking **miso**, a paste of fermented soybean, during fasting or adding spirulina, an algae powder, to juices. However, do not try rigid detoxification diets unless under a naturopathic doctor's care. If the body is deficient in nutrients or low in energy, it is wiser to go on a higher nutrient, higher protein building diet to energize and improve health instead of a cleansing diet. Each individual's needs change over time. A regular healthy diet with no excess will not require any intensive detoxifying program.

Dietary supplements. Herbs such as echinacea, garlic, goldenseal, licorice and parsley are commonly taken by many individuals as supplements in their detoxifying diets while others take wheatgrass and sprouts. Some nutritional experts believe in using supplements to restore a healthy balance of flora to the large intestine. They recommend taking **probiotics** such as lactobacillus and bifidobacteria, a particular kind of fiber that encourages the growth of friendly gut bacteria. They balance the flora in the GI tract, build up the immune system by producing vitamin K and some B vitamins as well as improve the motility of the colon. There are many types of lactobacillus, each having a specific therapeutic role in the colon. This especially is beneficial to women who tend to produce reduced amounts of pancreatic and intestinal digestive enzymes leaving them prone to the absorption of partially digested proteins and other substances that can trigger inflammatory reactions leading to skin lesions and poor complexion. If going on a lighter diet, take dietary supplements such as antioxidants, vitamin B—particularly niacin, and minerals such as zinc, selenium, calcium, magnesium and potassium.

Broader perspective

The modern world places oxidative stress on the body by creating numerous forms of skin sensitivities and allergies. Therefore, it is very beneficial for skin and health care practitioners to have a broader perspective in tracing possible causes of skin reactions. In addition, nutritional approaches in skin care should be used as a natural and holistic approach to treatment.

CHAPTER 12

Weight Management

With the growing prevalence of obesity around the world, particularly North America, this chapter is devoted to the theories and investigation of this ubiquitous problem in society. Skin care professionals can play an active role in weight management for their clients. If health care professionals practice healthy nutrition themselves, they most likely will counsel their clients about nutrition and weight management. In recent years, the number of clients visiting esthetic establishments for body treatments has increased significantly. They come for relaxation and for cellulite, detoxification and toning treatments, therefore the skin care therapist who is trained in body therapy is in a prime position to offer services to attain and control a healthy body weight.

Obesity

The terms *overweight* and *obesity* are not to be used interchangeably because they actually carry individual meanings. **Overweight** refers to an excess amount of body weight, including all body tissues such as muscle, bone and water, while **obesity** is defined as an excessive amount of body fat relative to height. The ideal amount of fat varies for each individual. For example, the body fat for a normal man should be 12–20% of total body weight while that of women should be 20–30%.

Obesity exists when the percentage of body fat exceeds 30% for women and 20% for men. Athletes need less fat, while an Alaskan fisherman requires more fat for insulation from the cold. However, too little fat among individuals who smoke, suffer from an illness or have an eating disorder can lead to infertility, depression and reduced body metabolism. Whether a person needs to lose weight depends on several factors such as the amount of excess weight, age, genetic makeup and health. Not all obesity will cause death or shorten the lifespan. Some healthy, obese people can exist just like individuals carrying normal weight but leading unhealthy lifestyles.

In the early part of this century, obesity became a world epidemic, prevalent everywhere among all ages, ethnic groups and educational levels. The percentage of obesity during the past decade has risen significantly in industrialized countries including France, the United Kingdom and Germany. Recent surveys indicate that obesity even has stricken some developing countries such as Latin America and even China. Scientists studying this phenomenon believe that contributing factors are related to the movement of people from rural to urban areas where there is reduced physical activity and more access to fats and oils thanks to the prevalence of fast food chains.

Social discrimination. Modern society places such emphasis on being thin that in many instances, obese individuals may be discriminated against. Almost 30–40% of women and 20–25% of men in North America always are trying to lose weight, and they spend millions of dollars to do so, mostly without success. Many people are judged by their physical appearance instead of their character. Obese people are perceived as being lazy and stupid, with lack of control over their bodies. This discrimination may lead to deep psychological problems and reduced self-esteem. As a result, many seek refuge in eating more to feel good about themselves.

On the other hand, beauty is in the eye of the beholder, and some cultures do not carry the same prejudices, but tend to view obesity as a sign of robustness and beauty. Various ethnic groups also possess striking differences in body composition. For example, Asians are of small stature and small-boned while certain Europeans such as Germans possess large body stature and heavier body mass. For some obese people who have tried countless diets, it almost is impossible to lose weight. They should be treated for what they are worth in their character, and not for their physical appearance. The main goal of losing weight should be to prevent the potential health hazards associated with being overweight or obese, particularly if the cause is genetic.

Who is obese? As many as 80% of people among American-Indian and Australian Aborigine descent have been recorded as obese. A survey conducted by the Centers for Disease Control and Prevention from 1991 to 1998 showed that almost one in five American adults now is considered obese compared to earlier records, and a report by the Rand Corporation found that in the year 2000, the number of severely obese people increased from one in 200 in 1986 to one in 50. The North American Association for the Study of Obesity claims that more lives are being lost to obesity than to any war or terrorist attack, and studies at the Behavioral Medicine Research Center in Houston, Texas, estimate that almost every American will be overweight or obese by 2040. Obesity is more prevalent among women, blacks, Hispanics and low socio-economic populations. Being overweight or obese places a high risk for developing serious health problems such as heart disease and stroke, diabetes, cancer and gallbladder disease.

Obesity among children is a grave concern in modern society; the latest research estimates more than 30% are obese. Studies have shown that if both parents are obese, there is 80% chance that their children will be obese, so controlling obesity during the growing years is critical in weight management during the adult years. The obesity problem can place a huge economic burden on health care systems in all countries. It is given low priority in health care because it is not viewed as a disease, but as a self-inflicted condition that can be self-controlled and easy to correct. Health authorities now are funding more research to investigate this growing problem in society. The Health Mandate for 2010 is to reduce the prevalence of obesity to less than 15% of the population and to increase the number of adults who are a healthy weight to 60%. This refers to authorities that are concerned with the healthy and wellness of the population. The Health Mandate promotes health within the region and works to prevent diseases and injury saving the government huge future health costs. It can be federal or state organized.

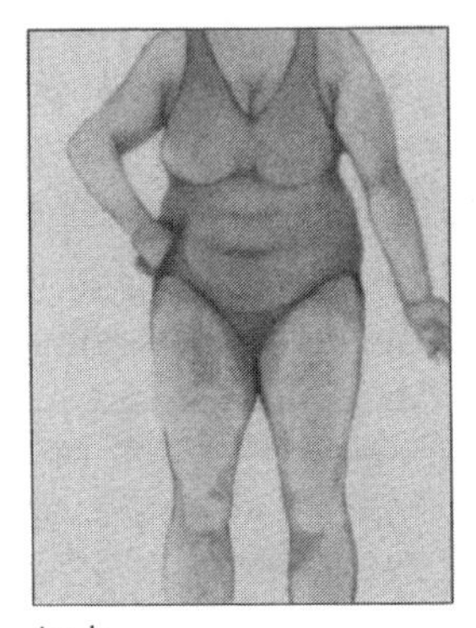

Apple

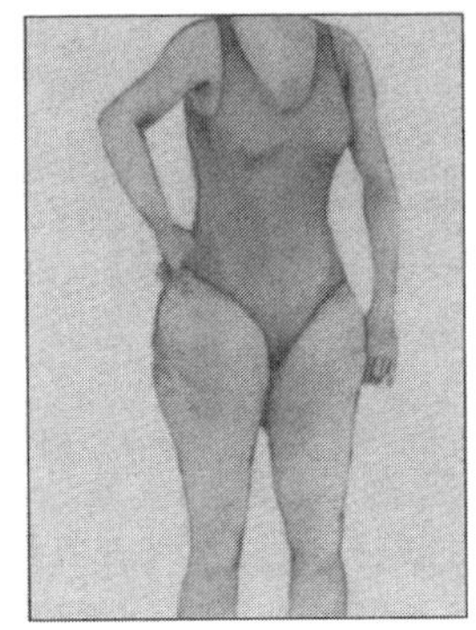

Pear

Figure 12-1: *Apple-shaped and pear-shaped bodies.*

Fat distribution. Distribution of body fat rather than the amount of fat carried is a more critical factor to consider in health. Individuals who store excess fat in the chest and abdomen—**apple-shaped**—are at a higher risk for cardiovascular diseases such as hypertension, diabetes and high blood cholesterol than those with excess fat in the hips, thighs and buttocks—**pear-shaped**. Apple-shaped is associated with deficiency of testosterone and poor lifestyle factors such as alcohol and smoking, most commonly associated with men. **Syndrome X** is a term used to describe a set of cardiovascular risk factors associated with apple-shaped individuals.

Pear-shaped body types mainly are found among post-menopausal women who tend to lead a sedentary life, but are considered a lower risk for heart disease than men. (See **Figure 12-1**.)

Body weight is not an accurate index of obesity because it does not show the location of fat in the body. For example, a muscular person such as a body builder may be overweight relative to height, but has a low body fat percentage while a slender man may be not be visually fat except in the abdomen.

Causes of obesity

Obesity is a disorder of energy balance and is associated with cardiovascular disease, insulin resistance and an overproduction of lipids that leads to high concentrations of fatty acids, triglycerides and very low density lipoproteins (VLDL). Diabetes is a disease associated with obesity and involves abnormalities in insulin secretion and insulin action. Insulin resistance is a common feature of obesity and diabetes and is affected by the type of dietary fat intake.

Theories of obesity range from internal factors such as genetics, psychological and metabolic to environmental factors such as cultural, socioeconomic and external cues, or a combination of several of these factors. Although some people are predisposed to obesity, environmental factors play a significant role in weight gain. While the causes of obesity are multifaceted, the underlying theory is based on energy consumption being greater than energy expenditure. This leads to excess energy stored in fat cells of adipose tissue.

Energy expenditure. A simple mathematical component can be used to explain weight loss or gain.

More energy intake (kcals) than energy output = weight gain
Less energy intake than energy output = weight loss
Energy intake is equal to energy output = weight maintenance

The best strategy to lose weight and maintain an appropriate body weight is not only to reduce daily food intake, but also increase regular physical activity.

Genetic theories of obesity

Fat Cell Theory. This theory states that the number and size of fat cells of adipose tissue formed during childhood determines obesity in adulthood. During the growing years, the number of fat cells increases rapidly. Because of this, monitoring the eating behaviors of children is critical. With excess food intake, fat cells increase in number—**hyperplasia**, and maximize in size—**hypertrophy**. During weight loss, the number of fat cells remains the same, but the size atrophies. If excess food is consumed, they multiply again. This hypothesis states that

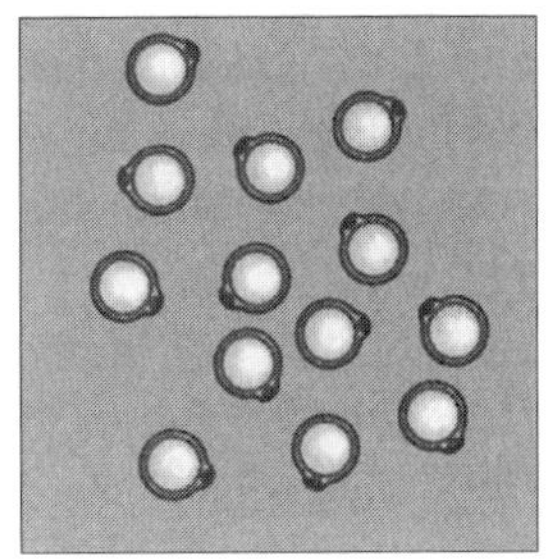
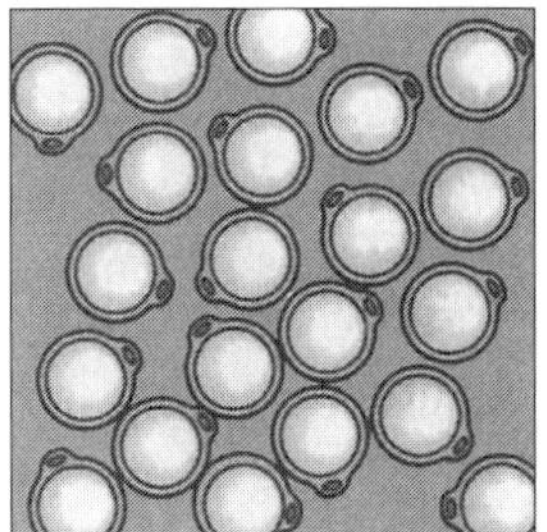
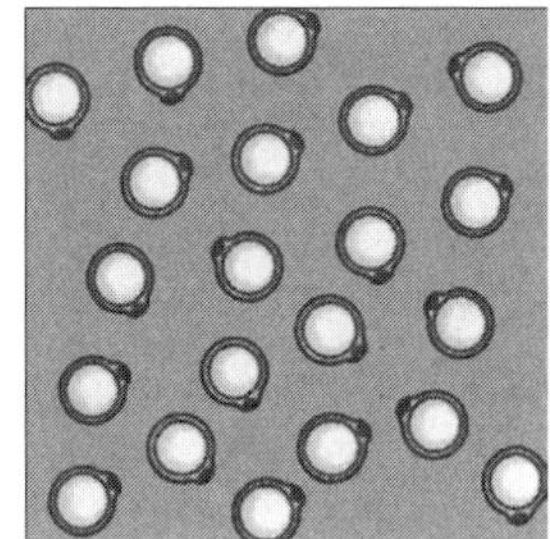

Fig 12-2: Fat cells atrophy in weight loss.

the fat cells always will become stimulated through psychological or environmental cues making it very difficult for the obese to lose weight. (See **Figure 12-2**.)

Set Point Theory. This controversial theory proposes that the body has an internal clock that automatically reverts to its original body weight in order to maintain homeostasis, regardless of any effort to reduce it. When one is full, satiety signals the brain to stop eating. The size of the individual determines the set point or satiety, so that a larger person will have a higher set point and require more food intake to reach satiety than a smaller person. During weight loss, the natural set point will be reduced, but there always is that tendency to return to it in order to feel satisfied. This theory seems to be tied in with the Fat Cell Theory where the fat cells become stimulated to get refilled due to other factors. In other words, the body will fight attempts to lose weight. This may help to explain why most diets do not work. The obese can fight off impulses to eat for a time, but eventually the signal becomes too strong to ignore, making it very difficult to lose weight. Research indicates that a strong determination to achieve a lower set point for gradual weight loss can be practiced and a new set point can become internalized over time. In other words, the set point is not as set as it is defined.

Lipoprotein Lipase (LPL) Theory. This is an enzyme found in the fat cells of obese people that determines the rate at which fat is stored. The obese have more LPL to store fat, and during weight loss, LPL increases, enhancing the body's ability to regain the lost weight. More LPL is produced in fat cells of the hips, thighs and breasts of women and in the abdomen of men. Upper body fat is easier to lose than lower body fat. Therefore, men tend to lose their abdominal fat quicker than women can lose fat in the lower body. Some studies have shown that weight loss activates the LPL genes making it easier to regain weight.

Leptin Gene Theory. Researchers have located an obesity gene called **leptin** that is produced by fat cells. It acts as a hormone that binds to receptors in the hypothalamus gland in the brain that, in turn, affects appetite and energy expenditure. Increased body fat is associated with high levels of leptin. Individuals lacking this gene show poor control of appetite and always are hungry with a tendency to overeat. Research shows that although obese people generally show high leptin levels, their receptors may be defective or insensitive—because of this, obese people are unable to suppress their appetite.

Thermogenesis. There are two types of fat in the body, white and brown fat. White adipose tissue stores fat, and brown fat burns white fat. **Thermogenesis** is the process by which fat is burned to release heat. This theory poses that impaired thermogenesis can contribute to weight gain. If not oxidized, fat is stored as white adipose fat leading to weight gain. Brown fat constitutes only 1% of total body fat and is found primarily around the shoulder blades, under the arms, along the spine, on the top of the kidneys and in other discrete locations. Brown fat plays a key role in thermogenesis by burning up excess calories. Some theories suggest that lean people have a higher ratio of brown fat than overweight people. **Uncoupling Protein** (UCP) is another important component of brown fat that helps to burn the stored white fat for energy. One way to stimulate brown fat metabolism is to expose your body to colder temperatures daily so that your body must burn additional energy to stay warm. Walking or jogging outdoors would be an example of stimulating your brown fat.

Psychological factors of obesity

The eating behaviors of many people are affected by psychological factors. Stress, anxiety or any arousal can lead some individuals to eat for comfort or to relieve boredom. This response to stress can become internalized resulting in frequent overeating. Parents often respond to a child's crying by offering food as a soothing agent, but this reward may become habitual, leading to conditioned stimuli in later years.

Environmental factors of obesity

External Cue Theory. Some people eat in response to external stimuli such as smell and sight of food, or to the time of day instead of internal pangs of hunger. Overweight people tend to overeat, especially when exposed to environments where food looks and smells good, and particularly when the food is cheap and in large portions with a wide variety. The high fat convenience foods that are ubiquitous in western society are hard to resist, sometimes even for disciplined and health conscious individuals. Fast food, with its large portions, promotes obesity because it not only tastes delicious, but the high fat content stimulates people to eat more, even if they are not hungry, so it is very difficult for those predisposed to weight gain.

Physical inactivity. The easy lifestyle of industrialized society promotes little exertion. People have become dependent on the use of escalators, cars, remote controls, televisions and computers all which contribute toward a sedentary lifestyle. Recent studies suggest that a lack of physical activity is one of the main proponents in the development of the current childhood obesity phenomena. With this in mind, health authorities are conducting many changes to increase physical activity in schools by developing fitness programs and building gyms for students to exercise regularly.

Assessing body composition

Body composition is one of the main variables considered in assessing health status. According to researchers involved in anti-aging, 30% of the body's composition can be attributed to genetics and 70% to environmental factors. This hypothesis infers that the responsibility of a person's health status lies primarily on lifestyle factors and, therefore largely can be controlled. Body weight alone is a poor reflection of body fat composition.

Basal Metabolism

Food is taken into the body and, in the presence of oxygen, is burned or oxidized to produce energy. **Basic metabolism** refers to basic internal life processes within the body that tend to go unnoticed, such as breathing, digestion, excretion and even resting, while **cellular metabolism** refers to processes that take place within the cell.

Basal Metabolic Rate (BMR) refers to the rate of energy used by the body under basic, non-active conditions. An appropriate value can be estimated approximately 12 hours after a meal when digestion is finished, for example, when you first wake in the morning, resting at a comfortable room temperature when no energy is used to maintain constant body homeostasis. For the average adult, the BMR is calculated approximately at 1 kcal per kilogram (kg) of body weight per hour.

$$\text{BMR} = 1 \text{ kcal} \times \text{kg (body weight)} \times 24 \text{ hours}$$

Factors that increase the BMR include fever; growth—higher among children and pregnant women; height—higher in tall, thin people than the overweight or obese; gender—males have about 10% higher BMR than females due to greater body mass; muscle tissue is highly active even during rest while fatty tissue has low BMR. The larger and leaner the tissue, the higher the BMR; stress—high stress levels release more cortisol hormones for "flight/fight" effect; systemic disorders such as hyperthyroidism; and temperature—BMR is higher in a cold environment.

Factors that decrease BMR include age—after age 30, BMR drops 5% every decade; nutritional status—starvation diets, fasting and very low calorie diets slow the BMR; and endocrine systemic disorders such as hypothyroidism and Cushings Disease.

Every person uses some form of energy expenditure in daily life, some more than others. The daily energy requirements or basic energy needs (BEN) of an individual is calculated from the BMR, plus the degree of daily physical activity.

BEN = BMR + % daily activity levels

Measuring body fat

Anthropometric measurements are the most common methods used to measure the physical characteristics of the body and compare against a similar individual specific for that age and gender. Although measuring body weight is easy, inexpensive and quite accurate in assessing body composition, it does not indicate necessarily the location or the amount of body fat present. Therefore, several methods are used by health care professionals to assess body composition, each with their advantages and disadvantages.

Ideal Body Weight (IBW). Measuring height against weight is the most commonly used benchmark for determining obesity. This chart, know as the Ideal Body Weight (IBW), was formulated in 1957 by the Metropolitan Life Insurance Company for insurance purposes to determine the relationship between weight and life expectancy. (See **Appendix IV**, page 291.)

If an individual was obese, life insurance was considered a high risk for the insurance company. Ultimately, it encouraged people to try to keep their weight down. However, it has been criticized for several shortcomings such as it doesn't necessarily reflect optimal healthy weight, and it failed to recognize that weight alone is a poor reflector of body fat composition.

Waist circumference and waist-to-hip ratio. This is the most valuable and simple indicator for abdominal obesity. If using waist circumference only, a measurement of greater than 35 inches for women and 40 inches for men indicates higher health risks. In the waist-to-hip ratio, the circumference of the waist is divided by the hip measurement. A ratio of 0.8 and higher for women, and 0.9 and higher for men is indicative of health hazards.

Body Mass Index (BMI). The BMI is the most current method used to indicate probability of health risks and is obtained by dividing the body's weight by the square of its height.

$$\text{BMI} = \text{weight (kg)} / \text{height}^2 \text{ (m) OR weight (lbs)} / \text{height (inches)} \times 705$$

Scientific evidence indicates that a body weight above or under an estimated range is positively correlated with risks of disease or high mortality. A BMI of 30 or higher indicates obesity with very high health risks leading to cardiovascular related diseases such as stroke, hypertension and diabetes, while a BMI under 18 may reflect a propensity for health problems such as anemia, chronic fatigue and eating disorders. The least overall risk is a BMI between 20 and 25. However, the BMI does not reflect body composition or location of excess body fat.

Skin fold thickness. This is the easiest and least expensive method to measure body fat. Using skin fold calipers to measure the thickness of subcutaneous fat on certain sites of the body such as the triceps and biceps, a rough percentage of body fat can be estimated. For example, skin fold measurements in the triceps greater than 18–19 mm in men or 25 mm in women suggests excessive body fat. The skin fold increases proportionately as body fat is gained or lost. However, this method has low accuracy, particularly on obese people. (See **Figure 12-3**.)

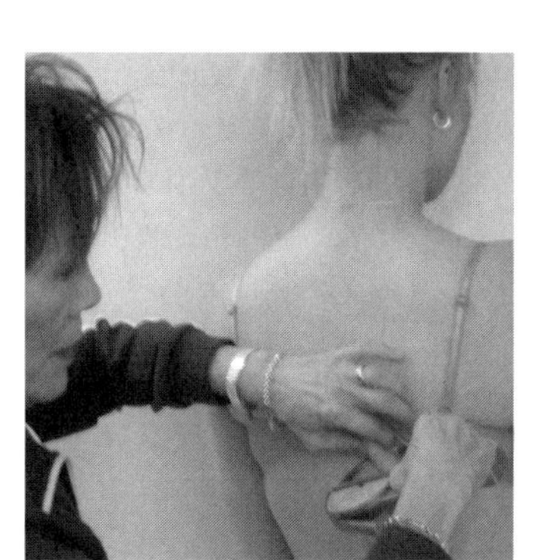

Figure 12-3: *Taking skin fold measurements.*

Bioelectric impedance. This is a quick, safe and non-invasive procedure that gives a measurement of body fat composition. Using a low-frequency alternating current, electrodes are attached to the hands and feet. The amount of body fat is measured by checking the speed at which the current passes through the body. Since fat is a poor conductor of electricity, the current is impeded by the presence of body fat. Lean body mass can conduct more electricity than fat mass—the more fat present, the more resistance to the current.

Underwater weighing. This method is used mainly in research labs. The body is immersed in a tank of water and weighed. Although very accurate, it is very expensive, impractical, bulky and inconvenient for the ill, very young, very old and those fearful of water.

Body types and their characteristics

According to American anthropologist William Sheldon, PhD, people come in different shapes and sizes. Although most people can be placed in one of the following three categories according to human physique, some individuals may exhibit characteristics of more than one type. The three main body types briefly are described here but a fuller description can be found in **Chapter 15**.

Endomorph. This body type is rounded, often plump, with a heavy body and small, short limbs. The body type usually is hereditary and has trouble losing weight.

Mesomorph. This body type is characterized by muscular, well-developed shoulders and slim boyish hips. Mesomorphs usually are athletic.

Ectomorph. This body type has a long, thin frame and small muscles with a bent-over posture. Ectomorphs have a tendency to be underweight and are associated with low energy levels.

Underweight

Although most people are concerned about being overweight, there are some individuals who are underweight by anthropometric measurement standards, and are subject to health hazards as well. It is just as hard to gain weight as it is to lose it. Underweight people tend to have high metabolic rates that burn energy very quickly, even without exercise.

Strategies for weight gain. Underweight people should eat larger portions of high caloric foods, such as whole milk instead of non fat milk, salmon instead of snapper, avocados instead of cucumbers and select whole wheat muffins, nuts and cheeses. Nutritious foods that not only are high caloric, but also nutrient-dense, are favorable. It is recommended to eat 700–1,000 kcals daily above normal energy needs to support regular exercise, and increase strength training exercises to build up more lean muscle.

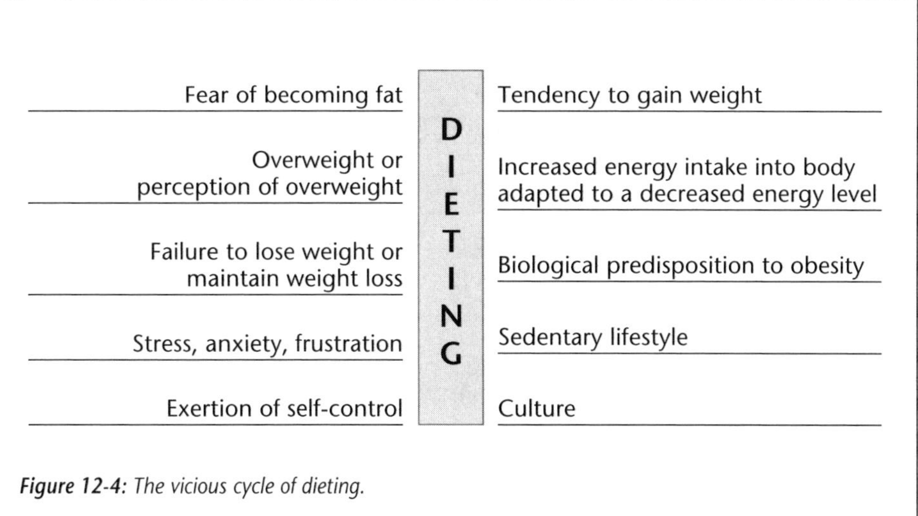

Figure 12-4: *The vicious cycle of dieting.*

The dynamics of dieting

In a society where there is a large amount of pressure to be thin, and both males and females constantly are on a diet, both social and psychological dynamics of dieting must be addressed. **Figure 12.4** indicates how dieting behavior can evolve from an array of various psychological and environmental factors. See **Psychological Profile of Dieters** on page 172.

Changes of weight gain and loss. Gaining or losing one pound on the scales does not necessarily mean that body fat is reduced—it only reflects changes in the different body materials, such as water, bone tissue or lean muscle. It is important to maintain the lean tissue that is vital for health and life. For the underweight individuals who wish to gain weight, the priority is to gain weight—not just fat, but *both* lean and fatty tissue.

What happens to the body when dieting? In order to understand why fad diets don't work, it is necessary to understand what occurs when excess food intake, or overeating, occurs and when dieting, or inadequate food intake, takes place. Proteins, carbohydrates and fats are metabolized into amino acids, glucose and fatty acids, respectively. Carbohydrates are the main fuel for energy and are used by the body before it turns to its fat storage. Reserves of carbohydrates and fats normally are stored in the body for later use—carbohydrates as glycogen in the liver and fatty acids in adipose tissue. Protein is used to replace body proteins such as muscles, skin, hair, nails, blood and other substances. Any excess is converted to fat and cannot be converted back to protein.

Psychological Profile of Dieters

- Dieters have both psychological and emotional attachments to food.
- Dieters show numerous adaptations such as constant preoccupations with thoughts of food and reduced control of eating making dieting very difficult.
- Many obese people use different excuses to rationalize their eating.
- Stress levels are high during dieting and this restraint sometimes can lead to eating binges making dieting counterproductive.
- Dieters use appearance as a measure of self-worth to gain approval for love or affection.
- Perpetual dieters always are trying different diets, particularly extreme ones.
- The therapist has to constantly motivate clients to try to change lifestyle behaviors.

During severe dieting or fasting, the body has to use any food reserve to maintain life. Glycogen is first taken from the liver and converted to blood glucose when depleted, fat stores are used. It is estimated that the brain alone uses approximately 2/3 of a day's energy, so that with little or no food intake, one will experience dizziness, weakness and irritability with loss of concentration. The nervous system cannot use fats as a secondary fuel source, but muscles and other organs can. With continued dieting, the body eventually turns to its last source of energy—the lean protein tissues such as muscles and skin. In the extreme last resort, the body eventually begins to devour its own tissues to maintain life by converting fat stores into a form called **ketone bodies** to feed the nervous system.

Ketosis, or the formation of acidic ketone molecules, is an adaptation to prolonged food deprivation and is very harmful because it upsets the acid-base balance of the blood. The body's lean tissues continue to be lost rapidly to supply glucose to the brain and the body's metabolism also slows down to conserve as much as energy as it can. That may explain why some people who are on a fad diet show dramatic weight loss within a few days—they are using their own protein tissues as fuel. Protein contains half the amount of kcals as fat, so dramatic weight loss is apparent. During the first few days of a low carbohydrate diet, a great amount of water is lost, but it is only temporary. With continued starvation, the liver, heart, skeletal muscles, lungs and blood are being burned as fuel to maintain life. The dieter then begins to look emaciated with atrophied muscles and unhealthy looking skin. This is most commonly seen among those suffering from eating disorders such as anorexia nervosa. Eventual death will occur with loss of all vital tissues such as the liver, blood and heart.

The Yo-Yo Syndrome. The tremendous pressure to lose weight in society can lead to desperation in the overweight or obese. This results in trying different diets that claim to work miracles. New fad diets with different names are cropping up regularly to entice dieters. The initial rapid weight loss makes them credible at first, but after that, the weight returns, greater than before. Most people cannot live forever on fad diets, and when the dieter eventually resumes normal eating habits, the metabolism remains low to preserve its energy so even if little food is eaten, it is burned very slowly and weight recurs, hence the name. (See **Figure 12-5.**)

Most weight loss programs are ineffective and pose some health risks by losing large amounts of fluids quickly. Long-term studies have indicated that most diets will lead to 95% regain of weight within two years. When undergoing a low-calorie diet, the body experiences semi-starvation states, and the metabolism is lowered in order to survive.

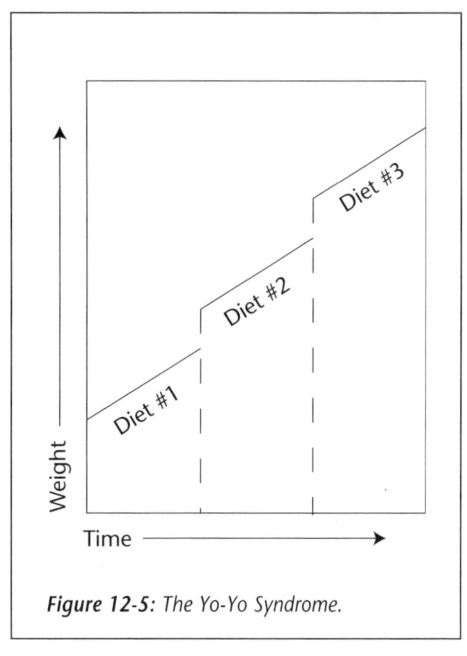

Figure 12-5: *The Yo-Yo Syndrome.*

Weight loss diets

The best weight loss results come from a long-term relationship between a nutritious, low fat diet supported by a regular exercise program and other positive lifestyle changes. Since one pound of fat is equivalent to 3,500 kcals and to lose this pound, it is necessary to reduce the daily kcal intake by 500, weight loss is very difficult to accomplish through diet alone. The most sensible approach would be losing 0.5–1 pound per week gradually through healthy lifestyle habits that incorporate less food intake combined with physical exercise. Weight loss can be achieved with a kcal intake of no less than 1,200 kcal/d or 1,500 kcal/d respectively for normal-sized females and males combined with physical exercise three or four times a week for a minimum of 20 minutes. Besides increasing the BMR, physical exercise will increase lean body mass and reduce body fat as well as improve mood and self-esteem. The key to successful long-term weight loss is to make healthy substitutions for non-nutritious foods. The diet must be modified for each individual. The following is an attempt to explain how some popular diets affect the body. *Text continued on page 176.*

Strategies for Behavior Modification

The main goal is to have a healthy body weight by consuming fewer kcals and simultaneously performing physical exercise. Other behavioral changes include the following:

- Emphasize nutrient-dense with minimal kcals.
- Always check fat content, especially saturated fat, when selecting foods.
- Consume more legumes, whole grains, fresh fruits and vegetables, and fewer meat products.
- Eat more fish and lean poultry. If you must eat red meat, consume small portions of very lean red meat for iron and B-12.
- Evidence is emerging that dietary phytoestrogens play a beneficial role in obesity and diabetes due to the ingestion of isoflavones and lignans found abundantly in soy protein and flaxseed. These have been found to improve glucose control and insulin resistance conditions as well as cardiovascular disease and cholesterol levels. A diet rich in soy protein will be greatly beneficial in weight management.
- Choose foods with low glycemic index values to maintain normal blood sugar levels to appease hunger pangs.
- Trim all visible fats and remove skin from meat.
- Use smaller portions and smaller plates.
- Use low-fat versions of fatty foods and limit empty calorie foods such as alcohol and sugary foods.
- Eat a healthy breakfast and lunch, and less for dinner, or alternatively, eat several small meals throughout the day.
- Eat more steamed, grilled and broiled foods, and avoid or limit fried foods.
- Exercise moderate consumption or avoid alcohol—no more than two drinks per day for men or one drink per day for women.
- Drink adequate water, a minimum of eight 8-oz. glasses a day, especially before and during meals to aid digestion, absorption and excretion.
- Chew foods slowly for proper digestion.

- Avoid salty foods and use more spices.
- Eat fresh, whole, unprocessed foods with high fiber as much as possible and avoid or cut down on processed convenience foods.
- Avoid trans fatty acids found in processed foods. They are just as harmful as saturated fats.
- Don't grocery shop when hungry.
- When eating out, share an entrée with someone or take a portion of the food home for the next day.
- Eat your own meals at home and arrive at parties after food has been served.
- Identify your rationale for eating excessively, making incorrect food choices and avoiding exercise.
- If you don't eat a healthy diet or are on a weight loss program, take dietary supplements to support your diet.
- Lose weight slowly, 1/2–1 pound a week.
- Increase your BMR through regular physical exercise.
- Exercising in the morning is best because it activates your metabolism and you burn more energy easily throughout the day. Exercising outdoors instead of indoors also will improve the body's metabolism.
- Use both aerobic and strength training to build up lean muscle mass that is more metabolically active even during rest.
- Get physically active. Join a club, hire a personal trainer and meet people.
- Minimize the association between food and celebration—organize a popular physical activity instead of a dinner party.
- Adopt a positive mental attitude toward your body image by working on improving your personality.
- Good posture helps to increase the oxygen supply to the body to burn kcals quickly.
- Set a goal for a healthy but realistic weight. If you are overweight, aim first to prevent further weight gain rather than trying to lose a huge amount of weight immediately.

High protein, low carbohydrate diet. With this diet, the loss of appetite is the same as in any low-calorie diet, and the body will go into the ketosis state as previously described. The body responds to a low carbohydrate diet in the same way as fasting. It has used up the small amounts of glucose and then turns to protein for energy. But the excess protein is stored in the form of fat. Why not give the body the carbohydrates it wanted in the first place? Why give it the excess protein when it will convert it to fat? Furthermore, there are several side effects such as constipation, nausea, headaches and fatigue. The Atkins Diet is an example of this diet.

Very Low-calorie Diets (VLCD). This is an extreme diet of less than 800 kcals/d and usually is under medical supervision. The protein intake is very high but the very low carbohydrates supplemented by vitamins and minerals are in the form of powdered formulas. They usually are prescribed for the morbidly obese who have had no success with most traditional diets. High health risks are associated with these diets, and they sometimes can be fatal.

Medical treatments

Many medical treatments are given by physicians to help the obese.

Drugs. These aggressive treatments for severe cases of obesity are reserved for medical professionals and pose health risks. Drugs have been used unsuccessfully in the past. They are appetite suppressants that work on brain chemicals to control appetite and make people feel full. Some work by blocking the absorption of fatty acids in the intestine so fewer kcals are absorbed by the body. At the present, 50–100 new products are in the early stages of development, some to burn kcals and others to tinker with body chemistry. Once the drugs are discontinued, the weight returns. Two prescription drugs, **sibutramine** and **orlistat**, currently are on the market and must be taken in conjunction with a reduced kcal, low-fat diet and increased physical activity. Several side effects such as hypertension, constipation, insomnia, gas and headaches may occur and must closely be monitored by a physician. The FDA has approved some over-the-counter drugs for weight loss such as benzocaine, in a candy or gum form, which anesthetizes the tongue.

Surgery. Liposuction is a popular surgical procedure to suction undesirable pocket of fat from the body. It is considered comparatively safe at the present time if performed by a knowledgeable and experienced physician, but some serious complications can occur for some individuals. However, this does not help the patient to manage body weight. Another extreme operation to make the stomach smaller is called **gastroplasty**, or stomach stapling, which forces the person to eat less. In very serious, life-threatening cases, medical costs may be covered by the government, depending on the country's medical policies. Overall, cosmetic surgery can help improve self-confidence, but behavioral changes in eating must be learned for long-term results.

Non-medical strategies

Herbs. Consumers use several herbal products as "natural" sources to lose weight. For example, **St. John's Wort** is believed to suppress the appetite by enhancing the release of the serotonin hormone. Weight-loss supplements containing **ephedrine** from the Chinese plant **Ma Huang** are combined with caffeine and/or aspirin, and have been linked to heart attacks and seizures. Use of ephedrine has been banned where the jurisdiction of the FDA is withheld throughout the United States. Other herbal laxatives containing castor oil, aloe, senna and buckthorn are sold as "dieters' tea" and also may have side effects.

Spa treatments. Beauty treatments in spas have limited results. These include cellulite reduction, spot reduction using a variety of electrical equipment, and massage—they must be supported with lifestyle behavior changes that include a healthy diet, regular vigorous exercise and stress management tactics. Strategies for dieting and physical exercises for different body types are discussed in **Chapter 15**.

CHAPTER 13

Anti-aging and Nutrition

Gerontology is the scientific study of aging. Many theories explain aging, but it can be defined as the progressive changes that occur in the body with the passage of time associated with degenerative diseases and culminating in death. Aging can be viewed as chronological or biological. **Chronological age** is age by date of birth—40 or 50 years, while **biological age** refers to the functional ability—the physical and mental state of the individual rather than the age in years. Both chronological and biological aging are affected by two factors.

Intrinsic factors are genetic factors associated with chronological age. They are inherited DNA programs in the individual who suffers from diseases such as cardiovascular diseases, cancer, diabetes or osteoporosis, or skin conditions such as thin skin, wrinkles or dyschromias—abnormal skin discolorations.

Extrinsic factors are factors associated with aging caused by environmental influences including solar radiation, pollution and negative lifestyle behaviors such as unhealthy diet, food toxins, alcohol, smoking and stress.

While chronological age cannot be controlled, individuals have some control over biological age. For example, a 70-year-old man sometimes can look, feel and have the physical strength and vigor of a 30-year-old man *if* he practiced preventive measures early in life. In fact, anti-aging experts estimate that 30% of aging effects are attributed to intrinsic factors while 70% are caused by extrinsic factors such as lifestyle behaviors. In other words, you have major control in extending your lifespan and preserving the health of your body, but it depends on the amount of effort you used early in life.

How long can humans live?

Humans are living much longer than they did in prehistoric times since human life has more than doubled in the 21st century. According to a study reported in *Nature 2003* and supported by the National Institute on Aging, the average life expectancy in G-7 Industrialized Nations, or Greater Seven industrialized nations that show the highest income per capita, is 85 years. These countries include Canada, France, Germany, Italy, Japan, the United Kingdom and the United States. It is predicted that by the end of this century, the advanced technologies in medicine, sanitation and nutrition will enable humans to live an average lifespan of 100 years. However, the question is not only if humans can live longer, but also would quality of life exist as well? No one wants to live an extended lifespan suffering from disabilities and diseases. Humans want to live an active, healthy and productive life in their later years.

Changing perception of aging

In today's society, the word *aging* tends to infer negative intonations. Thoughts go to frail, weak individuals suffering from degenerative diseases such as heart problems, cancer, osteoporosis and Alzheimer's disease. In other words, older people are thought of as being helpless or dependent on others.

This notion is beginning to change, and the focus is now on biological aging. The 78 million baby boomers expected to converge on society during this decade are changing the perception of aging. Before discussing anti-aging, a short synopsis of the various theories of why and how the body ages will be discussed. Many theories have been proposed by famous scientists and some of them overlap, but the anti-aging therapist should possess a basic knowledge of the most acceptable ones. Following is a brief description of each.

Theories of aging

Free radical theory of aging. This is the most well-known theory developed by Denham Harman, MD, PhD, in 1955 and accepted by most health care professionals. More details of this theory are covered in **Chapter 8**.

The Wear and Tear Theory. This hypothesis by August Weismann, PhD, a German biologist, stipulates that over a long period of time, the body's organs suffer wear and tear from toxins in the environment. In youth, even with heavy drinking and inadequate sleep, the body can maintain and repair its systems, but with aging, the body loses the ability to repair and heal itself.

Calorie Restriction Theory. Proposed by gerontologist Roy Walford, MD, of California, this theory has proven to be viable and is accepted by all scientists. It holds that with reduced calorie intake, less oxidative processes occur resulting in minimal free radical activity. However, vitamin and mineral supplementation must be taken with regular exercise to offset the reduced nutrient intake.

The Telomere Theory. Studies in genetics and genetic engineering spurred this latest hypothesis. In the DNA of the cell, sequences of amino acids called **telom-**

eres are found at the ends of chromosomes. Every time the cell divides, a telomere is lost, and the Hayflick Hypothesis proposes that the cell dies after the 50th cell division. Scientists have come to accept that the length of the telomere is shortened in aging. They also have discovered that the enzyme **telomerase** is responsible for repairing and replacing telomeres in germ and cancer cells, and is the cause of cell proliferation. Anti-aging scientists speculate that if a telomerase enzyme was used to continue the cell division, cellular life can be extended.

Conversely, research work is being continued on enforcing telomere shortening to kill germ and cancer cells. Therefore, the tip length of your chromosome may be a gauge of your cancer risk.

The Neuroendocrine Theory. The nervous and endocrine systems are the basis of the aging system. The body's hormones work together with the nervous system to regulate many functions for maintaining a healthy body. Reduced body functions and age-associated diseases are linked closely to reduced levels of hormones in the body. Hormonal replacement therapy therefore is considered an important component in anti-aging therapy.

The leading causes of death

In Western society, particularly North America, the leading causes of death are all age-related. They are in order below.

1. Cardiovascular diseases
2. Cancer
3. Diabetes
4. Drug-related diseases
5. Alzheimer's disease
6. Arthritis
7. Osteoporosis
8. Obesity

Note that apart from genetics, all these diseases are related to nutritional deficiencies. It should be clear that a person's destiny could be controlled simply by correcting or modifying dietary intake to reduce the risks of debilitating age-related diseases. Why wait for them to occur when you can take measures to prevent them from occurring?

The aging of the skin

It seems inherent in human nature to be attracted to beautiful things. From the earliest times, people always have been seeking ways to achieve physical beauty. Cleopatra was considered one of the most beautiful women in history, and people still think favorably of her today simply because of her attractiveness. Many psychological studies have shown that attractive people are more favored in life than unattractive individuals. Furthermore, when a person looks beautiful, she acts and feels more confident. As the body's physical appearance deteriorates in aging, many people show discriminating behaviors toward older people, not only because of their age, but also because they are not as attractive as before. This fact drives most people to seek treatments to improve not only their physical beauty, but also their health and functional ability.

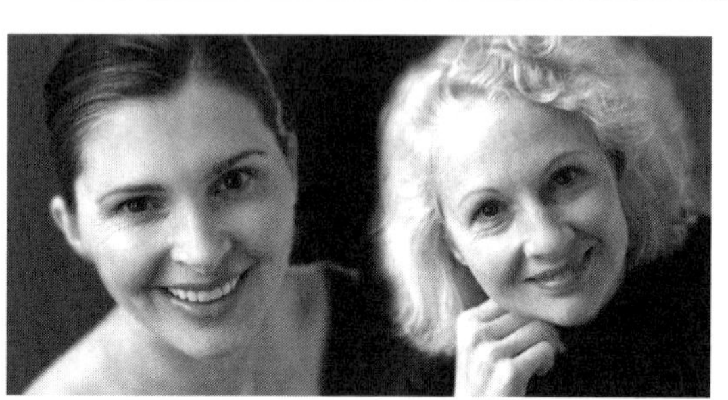

Figure 13-1: *The skin begins to show signs of aging beginning in the mid-20s and appears crepey, wrinkled and sagging with a dull complexion by menopausal age.*

Causes of skin aging

The aging of the skin concerns everyone. The skin begins to shown signs of aging beginning in the mid-20s and often appears crepey, wrinkled and sagging with a dull complexion by menopausal age. (See **Figure 13-1**.)

What are some of the mechanisms that cause the skin to age and can they be prevented or delayed? Causal factors can be both internal and external.

Intrinsic, or internal factors of skin aging

- A thinner epidermis.
- Reduced vascularization—the epidermal-dermal junction flattens out resulting in reduced nutrient exchange and slower cellular metabolism. This results in a dull and devitalized complexion.
- Increased transepidermal water loss (TEWL).
- Changes in the structure of connective tissue. Collagen and elastic fibers

begin to degenerate and the soluble collagen becomes insoluble leading to reduced moisture content and resulting in dry, wrinkled skin.

- Atrophy of sebaceous glands causes less sebum production resulting in dry, crepey, wrinkled skin.
- Weakened capillary walls atrophy resulting in broken capillaries, spider naevi or hemangiomas—small blood spots, on the face, décolleté and body.

Extrinsic, or external factors in skin aging

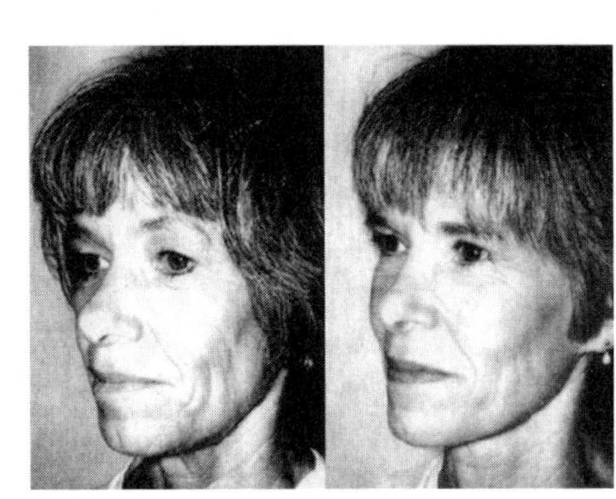

Figure 13.2: *The ravages of external factors on the skin.*

- Excessive sun exposure, especially during youth, has been found to be the single most devastating factor that leads to premature skin aging. Wrinkles are caused from epidermal tissue damage from UVB exposure whereas skin sagging is due to the UVA rays penetrating deeper into the dermis. Fine lines around the mouth and eyes appear as early as in the late-20s or early-30s, and the skin begins to sag around the jaw line, neck and other parts of the body. Twin studies show how an unhealthy lifestyle incorporating excessive sun exposure and smoking can accelerate skin aging. (See **Figure 13.2**.)

- Pigmentary disorders such as **lentigine**, or age spots, **solar keratoses**, or sun spots that appear profusely on sun-exposed areas, and **melasma,** or larger patches of hyperpigmentation from reduced hormonal levels, begin to appear on the cheeks. In addition, epidermal protrusions such as **fibromas** and skin tags, or smaller fibromas, appear on the neck, breast and face. **Sebaceous keratoses** such as milias and **xanthalasmas,** or cholesterol deposits under the eyes, become more visible on the face from poor skin exfoliation. Many people find these minor skin lesions unsightly and unwelcome, particularly the aging baby boomers, many of whom already are unhappy with their deteriorating physical appearance.

- Using incorrect skin care regimens and products can dry the skin's surface and makes it look wrinkled and devitalized with rough skin texture.

- Unhealthy lifestyle behaviors such as poor nutrition, excessive smoking and alcohol intake, inadequate sleep and high stress levels accelerate the aging process making a person appear older than their chronological age. **Rosacea** is a middle-age syndrome that appears in the late-30s or early-40s where the skin becomes red and blotchy, and is aggravated by any stimulating food or drink such as spicy foods, alcohol, stress and hormonal problems.

- Lack of physical activity and poor posture contributes toward sagging tissues on the face and body. **Kyphosis**, or convex curvature of the back, is a visible sign of an aging body. Regular physical exercises and strength training exercises in earlier years can prevent, reverse or delay these visible signs of aging.

Anti-aging

In the past ten years, the term anti-aging has been cropping up in health-related literature. Many therapists and skin care manufacturers utilize the word anti-aging to describe benefits or services. Even spas have included anti-aging therapies in their menus to describe their face and body treatments. What does this really mean? This chapter will help inform health care professionals, including estheticians, how anti-aging can work within the scope of their profession.

History of anti-aging. The term **anti-aging** infers "against aging" and applies to any form of preventive care for slowing down the aging process. The notion of anti-aging first was explored in 1993 by a small group of physicians and scientists dedicated to developing strategies for extending the human lifespan. They were concerned about the economic and social impact of the impending aging population and how the quality of an extended lifespan can be maximized. This is how The American Academy of Anti-Aging Medicine (A4M) was born. Seen as a new paradigm of medicine, these scientists viewed aging not as an inevitable process, but as a disease that can be treated, and perhaps prevented or slowed down. Since then, anti-aging therapies have been popularized by the news media and have spread to the beauty industry.

This interest in anti-aging also was driven by a dynamic baby boomer generation actively seeking strategies for maximizing good health and longevity. They lost some confidence in Westernized drug therapy and were seeking alternative health care. This led to the rebirth of natural therapies which accelerated a massive boom in healthy living and sales of vitamins. This proactive group viewed themselves as still youthful and were the driving force behind the fitness boom in the '80s. They are more educated, possess more disposable income than their predecessors and want to stay attractive and healthy as long as possible. They continue to ski, jog or work out to maintain their physical energy and youthfulness. They do not intend to sit in a wheelchair in a retirement community like their parents, but are strongly motivated to lead quality lifestyles in their later years. In seeking optimal health, this cohort initiated the development of the wellness ethic in the spa ndustry to enhance their physical and mental development. They are willing to spend their financial assets to fight aging symptoms such as wrinkles, lines, graying hair, age spots and fatty deposits on their body. Best of all, they are open to new therapies that promise to make them feel and look good. This has led to a greater demand for qualified therapists to work in wellness and medical spas. The political and social impact of the baby boomers in modern society is shaping the nature of the health and beauty professions as they gain momentum and more respect in society.

The science of anti-aging

Anti-aging is a science that has been documented over time by some of the world's top researchers. Anti-aging medicine is a medical specialty that incorporates three components: detection, prevention and intervention.

The aims of anti-aging medicine are to extend the length and quality of the human lifespan and to prevent, delay or, in some cases, even reverse the deleterious or damaging effects of diseases that commonly occur with age.

Advanced technologies. Anti-aging therapies include the use of advanced technologies to detect medical problems and then use appropriate measures to prevent, intervene or reverse the condition. Prescreening devices now are available for early detection of many medical conditions. For instance, mammograms are used for early detection of breast cancer, cancer screening equipment is used to detect early formation of melanoma skin cancer, PSI level testing is used for prostate cancer, bone density screening is available for osteoporosis and sophisticated equipment such as MRI and CAT scans are available for other medical problems. Regular blood tests show the onset of high cholesterol levels, hypertension, homocysteine and blood sugar levels. Upon detection, various interventive strategies such as surgery, medication and adopting positive lifestyle behaviors such as healthier nutrition and regular exercise can be implemented to reverse conditions.

Anti-aging program. Following are the cornerstones of an anti-aging program.

- *Nutrition.* This is the top priority in health and anti-aging. Optimizing nutritional needs with a healthy diet supported by dietary supplementation has been recognized as one of the main pillars of anti-aging. Proper dietary intake maximizes the immune system and strengthens the body's defense mechanisms to disease. Antioxidant-rich foods and dietary supplements play a very important role in keeping the body healthy and free of toxins, able to combat free radicals.

- *Physical exercise.* Participate in regular exercise at least three times a week for a minimum of one hour to increase bone and muscle mass and reduce fatty tissues. Exercise also helps to increase growth hormone levels, reduce stress and improve mood. Since physical exercise is one of the most important components of an anti-aging program, **Chapter 15** in this book has been devoted to exercise and its benefits.

- *Hormonal Replacement Therapy.* The etiology of aging includes hormone deficiency. This leads to the popularity of Hormone Replacement Therapy (HRT) in the past. It has been established that the body's levels of hormones decrease significantly with age, and that the levels of most hormones such as sex hormones and growth hormones are reduced significantly by age 60. This is believed to contribute toward decreased muscle mass and increased fat mass in older people. For decades, HRT for females was believed to have significant anti-aging benefits by supplying the aging female body with an alternative form of estrogen therapy. However, in recent years, scientists have unearthed evidence that showed positive correlation of HRT with an increased risk of aging diseases such as cancer and cardiovascular diseases among those women who were on HRT for a long period of time.

  It now is recommended that a high intake of soy protein that contains phytoestrogens can be used to offset estrogen deficiency in women. Phytoestrogens have been found to have a similar chemical structure as estrogen and may act to block estrogen receptors in tissues reducing the risk of cancer. Growth hormone, produced abundantly during adolescence, is released from the pituitary gland and carried in the blood stream to the body tissues and organs to stimulate the growth of tissues in the body such as muscle and bone. Anti-aging scientists believe that hGH or growth hormone levels should be restored to ensure healthy functioning of the systems of the body because, with reduced levels of hGH, the body begins to age.

Anti-aging therapy includes growth hormone replacement therapy in the form of injections or dietary supplements. Synthetic growth hormones in various forms have appeared on the market in the form of dietary supplements or sprays. **Secretagogues** (pronounced se-cre-ta-gogs) are dietary supplements formulated from 191 natural amino acids, the same as growth hormones. They do not act as growth hormones but as precursors to growth hormones to stimulate the release of hGH from the pituitary gland. Although their potency is low, it is a safe alternative for those who do not wish to use growth hormone injections. Secretagogues can be sold by health care professionals including skin care practitioners. Studies have shown that resistance training, particularly on the lower part of the body can increase levels of hGH.

- *Lifestyle behavioral modification.* Stress plays a major factor in accelerating the aging process by producing excessive free radicals. Positive lifestyle behavioral modifications can reduce free radicals. Those who suffer high levels of stress show deep wrinkles and are more likely to eat more food for comfort leading to weight gain. Therapists should offer stress management therapies such as yoga, Pilates and meditation to relax both mind and body, and encourage clients to have various types of massage regularly as well as be taught stress management strategies to control stress levels. Sometimes having a simple facial treatment not only improves skin complexion, but also can help relieve stress.

The estheticians role in anti-aging

The holistic approach for anti-aging therapy in esthetics should include treatments for the total well-being of the individual. This includes preventive care and interventive measures that include treatments and products to smooth and rejuvenate the skin. Any products or treatments that promote anti-aging infer that they will prevent or remove some visible aging signs on the face and body. As a result, cosmetic manufacturers are developing more powerful active ingredients to combat aging skin.

Several interesting anti-aging products and devices have appeared in the market to fight free radicals and rejuvenate the skin. Treatments to soften the wrinkles, smooth the skin's surface, brighten the complexion, even out skin tone and remove minor skin protrusions are in high demand to make the skin

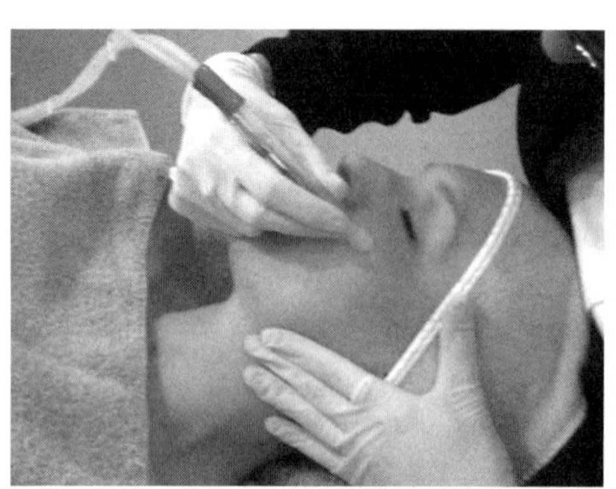

Figure 13-3: Facial skin treatment.

appear fresh and youthful. The function of the esthetician is to achieve or maintain a healthier, more youthful-looking skin and body for the client. The esthetician is strategically positioned in society to become an anti-aging therapist. In fact, clients who flock to spas are beginning to view estheticians as part of the wellness team. (See Figure **13.3**.)

The health model of esthetics

With the emergence of the medical spa, the role of the esthetician is changing to a more health-oriented one. The anti-aging field attracts those individuals who are more health than beauty oriented. Those who incorporate healthy aging into their work do so by performing anti-aging treatments or by referring their clients to anti-aging health practitioners. The following Health Model of Esthetics proposes the different levels of esthetics and how they relate to the healthy aging market.

The Cosmetics Model. This includes those who work in the beauty industry and perform a more superficial level of work such as makeup artistry, hair, nails, waxing and facials.

The Wellness and Health Sector. This includes those spas where therapeutic massages, stress therapy, more in-depth facial treatments, nutritional advice and exercise may be offered.

Clinical Estheticians. They are more results-oriented and specialize in a higher level of work, particularly in problem skin such as sensitive skin, acne, rosacea, and wrinkled, sagging skin by using deeper forms of peels such as microdermabrasion and light chemical peels combined with active ingredients in the form of serums and ampoules to nourish and regenerate the skin. They are more results-oriented and use a more holistic approach in their practice by including nutrition and offering stress therapy treatments.

Medical Esthetics. This practice occurs in a medical setting where the skin care professional assists the physician in pre- and post-operative surgery by performing deep cleansing skin treatments as well as giving nutritional guidance. The medical spa may offer anti-aging services through a certified anti-aging physician or health care practitioner. Medical spas also offer medical services such as cosmetic surgery or dermatological services including chemical peels and laser surgery for aging and problem skin.

Anti-aging and the skin

The skin care professional can work within the framework of the three components of anti-aging—detection, prevention and intervention.

Detection. Studies suggest that many clients visit their esthetician more frequently than they do their physicians. Because of this, a knowledgeable and skilled skin care professional may have initial access in detecting unhealthy conditions. Since the skin can reflect the results of many negative lifestyle behaviors, estheticians can be trained to detect underlying health problems by closely observing certain conditions of the skin and body. See **Skin and Body Anti-aging Observations**, pages 190-193.

Prevention. A more educated population will be more aware of preventive strategies that will help reduce and defer high medical costs in society, particularly among the aging.

Home care advice. Preventive advice for those individuals with a family history of skin cancer includes efficient use of broad-spectrum sunscreens and referrals to certified anti-aging health practitioners. Preventive care also involves teaching the client positive lifestyle behaviors to prevent the onset and control dry, blotchy skin, dilated capillaries and all the skin conditions described above.

Motivate and support. Motivating and supporting clients to participate in other positive lifestyle changes that impact skin and body conditions all are part of preventive skin care. Teach them the pitfalls of smoking and excess alcohol intake, inadequate sleep, a sedentary lifestyle and poor posture. Guiding clients to healthier eating can reduce a multitude of health problems including cardiovascular diseases, osteoporosis, diabetes and obesity.

Referral to medical care. Note and advise clients to check suspicious looking lesions with their dermatologist. The advanced technology of cancer detection systems for early detection of melanoma can save lives.

Skin and Body Anti-aging Observations

Symptoms	*Possible Indications/ Recommended Lifestyle Changes*
Photodamaged skin, including excessive actinic keratoses–sun spots and moles.	*Indicators:* • Excessive sun exposure. • Not using sunscreens or sun blocks. • May lead to skin cancer. *Recommendations:* • Eat a healthy diet including antioxidant-rich foods and drink more water. • Take preventive measures including wearing broad spectrum SPF, avoiding direct sunlight, and getting regular skin resurfacing treatments such as microdermabrasion and chemical peels. • If unusual pigmented lesions, refer to a dermatologist.
Skin congestion–blotchy, telangiectasia, mottled complexion, skin hot to touch.	*Indicators:* • Possibly gastrointestinal problems including bloating, gas, indigestion and diarrhea; excessive alcohol intake or menopausal hot flashes. *Recommendations:* • Limit or avoid stimulating foods and drinks such as alcohol and caffeine. • Reduce inflammatory foods such as meat, dairy and deep fried foods, and trans fatty acids. • Increase omega-3 foods, soy foods, high fiber and antioxidant-rich foods. • Use sun blocks and avoid direct sunlight. • Practice stress management such as yoga and meditation.

Symptoms	*Possible Indications/ Recommended Lifestyle Changes*
Dry, dehydrated skin.	*Indicators:* • Insufficient water intake can be indicated by bright yellow urine with arid odor. • Deficiency of omega-3 foods. • Improper use of skin care products. • Excessive sun exposure. *Recommendations:* • Drink a minimun eight 8-oz. glasses of water daily, one before and after meals. • Have regular skin peelings with nourishing products such as ampoules and serums. • Use quality skin care products.
Pale complexion, fatigue, poor cold tolerance and whiteness in eyes.	*Indicators:* • Anemic conditions. *Recommendations:* • Eat iron-rich foods such as lean red meats and soy, dark green vegetables and beans. Check food labels for high iron content. Cook foods in iron pots. • Eat iron-rich foods together with vitamin C-rich foods for better absorption of iron. • Extreme anemic individuals may require vitamin B injections by a health care practitioner.
Deep wrinkles around the mouth and a sallow, grayish complexion.	*Indicators:* • Expressive laugh lines. • Excessive smoking impairs oxygen intake. *Recommendations* • Reduce or avoid smoking. • Have regular skin resurfacing treatments. • Be aware of excessive facial expressions such as frowning and laughing.

Skin and Body Anti-aging Observations *(cont.)*

Symptoms	*Possible Indications/ Recommended Lifestyle Changes*
Regular breakouts on chin and jaw line.	*Indicators:* • Habit of touching the face with hands that may be contaminated with dirt or bacteria. • Stress-related. • Improper diet. *Recommendations:* • Check for improper diet during breakouts. Limit PG2 foods, fried foods, shell fish, smoking and alcohol consumption; eat soy foods, steam broiled foods and increase water intake. • Avoid stimulants such as alcohol, nicotine and caffeine. • Be aware of habits. • Check if using comedogenic cosmetics. • Use deep cleansing products and have regular deep cleansing treatments.
More lines on one side of face.	*Indicators:* • Habitual pressing hands on the face or sleeping with one side of the face consistently on the pillow. *Recommendations:* • Sleep on back instead. • Be aware of pressing hands on face.

Symptoms	*Possible Indications/ Recommended Lifestyle Changes*
Deep lines or wrinkles between brows, may be accompanied by small, flat, reddish macules with no fluids on skin.	*Indicators:* • High stress levels. • Excessive facial expression. *Recommendations:* • Check diet–eat more omega-3-rich foods, increase water and vitamin intake. • Take dietary supplements such as viatmin B for stress. • Correct and be aware of excessive facial expressions. • Go for relaxation therapies regularly such as stress therapy and management. • Do exercises for developing mind/body awareness such as yoga, Pilates, tai chi and meditation.
Lines on the neck, even in the young.	*Indicators:* • Poor posture or using high pillows. *Recommendations:* • Hold head high and tall. • Use low pillows. • Practice yoga and Pilates to stretch body and improve posture.

Intervention. The main area of intervention of the skin care professional is to provide treatments for aging, sun-damaged skin to produce a softer, smoother, toned and more youthful complexion. Interventive therapies offer a quick fix to offset the visible signs of aging.

Medical procedures. Medical interventive procedures include cosmetic surgery, injections, fillers, fat transfer and even gene intervention.

Non-medical treatments. Numerous topical therapies are available to reduce or remove hyperpigmentation and rejuvenate the skin. They include topical applications of embryoblasts, collagen and antioxidants.

Skin resurfacing technologies include applications of various chemical peels, microdermabrasion and specialized equipment to remove minor skin lesions by skin care professionals to improve the physical appearance and help boost self-esteem.

For the body therapist, helping the client to improve posture and achieve or maintain a healthy body weight and a stronger body is part of intervention therapy. Under close scrutiny of the client's lifestyle behaviors, the skin care professional can make possible inferences and give advice to prevent and correct many of the conditions in **Skin and Body Anti-aging Observations**, pages 190-193. Cross referrals to other health care professionals such as personal trainers, naturopaths, chiropractors and other physicians can prevent further damage to the individual's health and build positive rapport between professions.

Skin resurfacing

Skin resurfacing refers to any procedure or tool that can smooth or rejuvenate the skin resulting in a more youthful, glowing complexion. Essentially, all resurfacing treatments work in the same manner. They remove the rough outer layers of surface tissues, and the traumatic effect on the skin stimulates the collagen fibers to heal and regenerate resulting in smoother, tighter, more youthful looking skin. Besides minimizing the fine lines, they also are effective in reducing scars and treating uneven skin tone.

Physical treatments can be either cosmetic or medically oriented depending on the skill and knowledge of the skin care practitioner and whether she is working in a spa, clinic or medical spa environment. Advanced technological systems used in the area of intervention are viewed as anti-aging tools. Skin resurfacing modalities include laser skin resurfacing, microdermabrasion, chemical peels and impulse light therapy, or photo facials. However, many of the above procedures do not remove the minor skin irregularities that proliferate in aging including fibromas, skin tags, cholesterol deposits, telangiestasia, hemangiomas and the ubiquitous age spots, or liver spots. Unique devices utilizing heat for cauterizing and cold therapy are available to remove these unsightly skin lesions that psychologically affect the aging baby boomers. Following is a short description of each skin resurfacing modality and how it can be used as an anti-aging tool.

Laser skin resurfacing. This surgical procedure first was used by an American dermatologist in the 1960s. Various types of laser systems have been developed since then. The energy of a specific wavelength can be absorbed by the skin to stimulate cell regeneration. A *laser* is a device that produces a beam of intense light acting as the energy source. For example, a carbon dioxide (CO_2) laser is used to literally burn the skin's surface layers. This **dermal wound** initiates the healing process when collagen fibers in the dermis contract and tighten. **Collagen tightening** occurs as part of the repair process resulting in smoother, tighter and more youthful looking skin.

The ideal candidates for laser skin resurfacing are light-skinned individuals with fine wrinkles or Fitzpatrick Skin Type I. There is a certain amount of downtime and the patient must be mentally prepared for the procedure. With proper skin care preparation and nutritional advice from the medical esthetician, healing time can be accelerated. Low doses of soft lasers are non-medical and used by skin care professionals to increase healing time.

Microdermabrasion. This alternative procedure to traditional dermabrasion initially was developed to avoid the risk of AIDS. This safe, non-invasive system was introduced in 1997 to the esthetic industry by entrepreneurs who believed that this device was a safe tool that can be used by skin care professional for deeper skin peeling. Referred to as "closed" dermabrasion, this procedure involves the usage of inert crystals that are pushed at a high speed through a tubing system across the skin's surface to abrade the dead skin layers. The dead superficial epidermal cells and used crystals are collected in a sealed container reducing the risk of contamination.

This treatment became instantly popular with the public because immediate noticeable results can be seen, and there is no downtime. Wrinkles appear minimized, the skin is smoother and more youthful looking, and active ingredients to nourish the skin can be penetrated for maximum results. The esthetic industry has taken this modality to its utmost heights in a short time, and the market now is saturated with almost every spa or clinic offering this service to their clients as an anti-aging tool.

Chemical peels. European estheticians brought chemical peels to America, but they only became popular within the last 15 years when the media promoted Retin-A* for treating wrinkles instead of just acne conditions. There are various types of chemical peels, but essentially they are acids applied on the skin's surface to break down the glue-like cement called **ceramides** that hold the epidermal cells together. Stronger levels of acids produce a wound or injury to the dermis as well, and this leads to formation of new skin cells in recovery. The most popular chemical peels are alpha hydroxyl acids (AHAs), and they commonly are used by physicians and trained estheticians. Physicians use stronger formulations of chemical peels while estheticians use milder strengths.

There are several contraindications and darker-skinned individuals and those with Fitzpatrick Skin Type III–VI are not suitable candidates for chemical peels. Other products used to lighten hyperpigmented areas include natural skin lighteners such as ascorbic acid, or vitamin C and licorice, as well as chemicals such as hydroquinone and kojic acid. They work by acting as blockers to the enzyme **tyrosinase** that converts the amino acid tyrosine to melanin, the pigment produced by melanocytes in the epidermis.

Devices to remove minor skin abnormalties. Minor skin growths seem to proliferate in aging and include pigmentary disorders such as sun spots, liver spots, fibrous disorders such as skin tags and fibromas, as well as sebaceous disorders such as milias and cholesterol deposits. Physicians have been using cautery devices for ages, but the tools used were quite painful and often caused scarring. During the past ten years, devices have become available to treat these disorders.

The aging body

Visible signs of an aging body are defined by poor posture indicated by a round back or humped appearance, as well as excess adipose tissues. Males tend to carry excess abdominal fat while women suffer from heavy hips and thighs. Older people also tend to have poor flexibility and low metabolic rate, so they burn energy slowly resulting in weight gain. Syndrome X is the term given to excess abdominal fat that indicates a high risk for cardiovascular diseases, high blood pressure, an unfavorable cholesterol profile and diabetes, all leading causes of death in today's society. See **Identifying and Relieving Signs of the Aging Body**, page 197.

** Tradename of Ortho-McNeill Pharmaceutical, Raritan, NJ*

Identifying and Relieving Signs of the Aging Body

Aging Symptoms	*Possible Indications/ Recommended Anti-aging Strategies*
Bent over posture with forward head tilt, round back, sagging breasts, protruding abdomen, possibly *lordosis*, or concave lower back, and arthritis.	*Indicators:* • Poor posture constricts proper breathing leading to fatigue quickly. • Lordosis indicates overstretched abdomen and tight lower back muscles resulting in hyper-extended knees. Presence of lordosis indicates lower back problems. *Recommendations:* • Eat a healthy diet. • Take dietary supplements such as glucosamine sulfate for arthritis and calcium for osteoporosis. • Practice postural exercises and resistance training to strengthen upper body and core muscles such as abdomen and lower back. Practice stretching and toning exercises such as yoga and Pilates to improve flexibility, balance and coordination.
Slow moving individuals include endomorph body type and may have dry skin	*Indicators:* • Slow mobility indicates sedentary lifestyle and low BMR. • Overweight or obese individuals may have difficulty losing weight. • Possibly suffers from hypothyroidism. *Recommendations:* • Participate in a more active lifestyle including regular exercise. • Eat a healthier diet consisting of low kcals, low saturated fats and high fiber. • Reduce sugar and salt intake. • Increase omega-3 rich foods and antioxidant-rich foods.

Anti-aging body therapy

It is important to note that the anti-aging therapist should only treat overweight individuals with no serious medical problems and refer the obese to medical practitioners. Anti-aging body care treatments in the spa or clinic should focus on achieving or maintaining a healthy body weight. They should include weight management strategies by using physical exercise to increase lean body mass, decrease fat mass, improve body posture and strengthen or improve muscle tone, flexibility and mobility. Stress therapy and management also are part of an anti-aging program to reduce or prevent excess formation of free radicals. Toning and cellulite treatments are components of a healthy body program.

Utilizing a series of body treatments such as various fitness modalities, nutrition, dietary supplements and various stress therapies, the body therapist can help the client improve the body's health. As an anti-aging treatment, a more comprehensive questionnaire regarding health and lifestyle behaviors must be filled out by the client to identify the body's needs. Serious medical problems must be referred to medical specialists. A series of body treatments using a support team to incorporate electrical therapy, regular physical exercise, nutritional guidance and stress management should be offered in the spa or clinic to maximize results. Body therapies may include the use of specialized equipment such as vacuum suction, non-invasive mechanical body contouring machines, gyratory massage and other electrical therapy devices that help increase blood circulation, improve body metabolism or tone muscles. Massage treatments incorporating stress management techniques will help reduce the formation of excess free radicals in the body. Many spas and medical clinics now offer exercise modalities such as aerobic exercise, weight training, Pilates and yoga to complete the holistic approach to body therapies.

Series of body treatments

The client must fill out a comprehensive form detailing some personal and medical history including nutrition and exercise. Before the treatment, baseline measurements of the body including percentage of body fat should be taken, recorded and used to compare with post-treatment to record changes. This enables the client to become more comfortable with the therapist who also can monitor the client closely and give support. At the end of the series, the client can be measured, weighed and another series of treatment may be offered if necessary. The following is a series of treatments combining multiple uses of the following machines where the client must come in at least twice in order to see results. Each machine should be used three times in succession before changing to another piece of equipment.

Vacuum suction. This involves the usage of various types of special suction cups made of glass or plastic. They are contoured on the treatment area, and the body tissues are suctioned and released creating a vacuuming effect. This is a form of mechanical lymph drainage and the cups are moved in the direction of the nearest main lymph nodes. This treatment improves poor circulation and helps to remove toxins found in cellulite conditions.

Electrical therapy equipment. This is a form of passive exercise and may include the use of special electrical equipment that carries faradic-type current. Special pads are placed on motor points of the muscles to create muscle contraction. Various programs are set according to the client's body metabolism and body type, and treatment time varies from 15–45 minutes. Interferential current is an excellent electrical therapy that gives good results for increasing blood circulation and improving muscle tone. This current is created from the crossing over of two medium frequency currents to form a super-impositioned field of low frequency current very similar to the body's own oscillations making it more comfortable for the client.

Gyratory massage. This is a form of mechanical massage or an alternative form of stimulating massage. Especially good to use on heavy tissues such as the buttocks or thighs, it is very handy to use on males who possess thick, heavy muscles. Several massage heads simulate the five classical massage movements and the equipment gives a vibratory effect.

Non-invasive body contouring machine. This is a sophisticated and expensive form of gyratory massage. Used by many medical professionals, it claims to reduce cellulite conditions by increasing blood circulation and removing toxic buildup in cellulite conditions.

The anti-aging triangle

Nutritional guidance has proven to be a key component in anti-aging therapy since most of the leading causes of death in the developed countries of the world include heart disease, cancer and diabetes, which can be prevented or controlled by eating a healthy diet. Yet it continues to be one of the most difficult behavioral changes to make for most individuals.

As mentioned before, physical exercise including the mind/body fitness treatments of yoga and Pilates should be incorporated into body treatments. They are further discussed in **Chapter 15**. Clients expect skin and body care professionals to be knowledgeable about health issues because they rely on them to keep their skin and body looking younger and healthier. By educating your clients about lifestyle management skills, you can contribute not only toward improving the quality of a longer lifespan for yourself, but also for family and friends.

Anti-aging is a new area of expertise for all health care professionals including the skin care specialist and can prove to be both psychologically and financially rewarding. Anti-aging only can be achieved through a holistic approach—mind, body and spirit using the components of nutrition, physical exercise, growth hormone replacement therapy and stress management. If true wellness therapy is to be incorporated in spas, both nutrition and fitness must be considered. Although body wraps, massage and aromatherapy are beneficial treatments, results are temporary. Nutrition and physical exercise need to be included to maximize the wellness ethic of the profession. In fact, many resorts and destination spas already have integrated these treatments within their programs. But what about the individual skin care professional in the urban or rural area? They can become anti-aging therapists by taking courses and reading about it in the numerous resources available. There are on-line courses on anti-aging available as well. The future of health care can be placed in a triangle. Conventional medicine is overlapped by alternative health care, including esthetic care, but in the end, the ultimate responsibility for anti-aging rests on the client.

CHAPTER 14

Food Labels

The fast lifestyles found in modern society leave little time to prepare or cook healthy meals at home. The close family unit where the mother or caregiver prepares meals from scratch to feed the family has been reduced to a minimum, and convenience foods have become the norm for most people, including students who live away from home. Today, the shelves of modern supermarkets are full of a vast array of prepared foods for the busy family and food preservatives are used to keep them as fresh as possible.

Food labels appear on most packaged foods, but many of them lack sufficient information and have yet to comply with the guidelines of the federal government. To determine the nutritional status of the foods you select, a clearer understanding of food labels must be developed. In 1973, the United States Food and Drug Administration (FDA) issued a mandate that the nutritional values of foods must be stipulated on food labels. Consumer awareness of food labeling has increased over the years and consumers now are demanding that proper nutritional information be provided on all foods. Over the last two decades, it became mandatory to list standardized serving amounts of nutrients including macronutrients such as sodium and calcium.

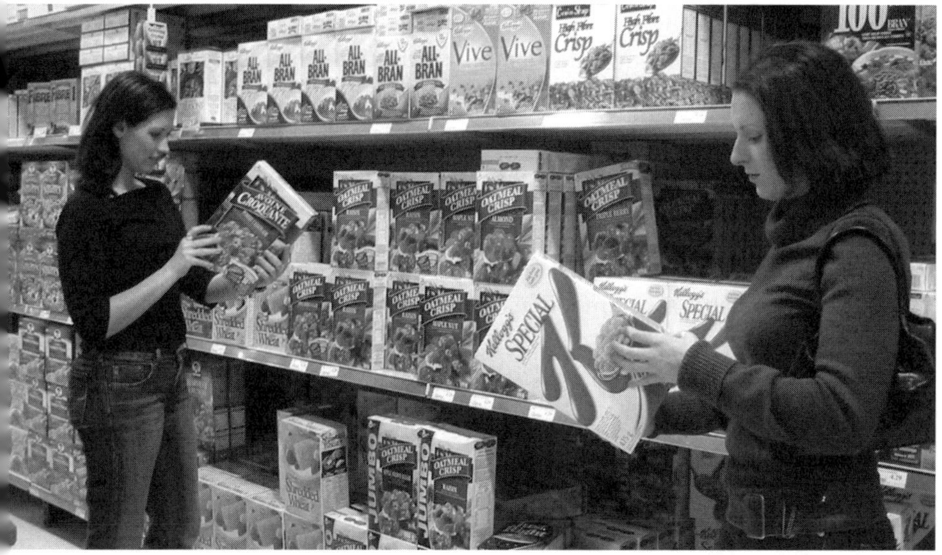

Food labels provide a wealth of nutrition information. Food label claims, calories per serving, serving size, percentage daily values (DV), minerals and vitamins, nutrients and percentage of fats give valuable information to the consumer who is interested in healthy food choices. The most recent mandatory guidelines released in July 2003 require food labels also to list the amount of trans fatty acids due to new scientific evidence showing that consumption of trans fatty acids raises low density lipoproteins (LDL), increasing the risk of coronary heart disease.

The requirement to list trans fat, saturated fats and cholesterol also applies to dietary supplements. Consumers need to learn the nutrition jargon on food labels to know what they are buying and eating, especially those who suffer from food allergies or skin sensitivities. The new labeling requirement evolves from the United States' Health Department's greater effort to inform consumers of the health consequences of their dietary choices. But how many people actually understand the meaning of the terms on food labels? Some may be nutrition savvy, but most do not really understand the meaning of these terms. The following information on deciphering food labels may shed some light on these terminologies and help consumers make quick, informed food choices for a balanced diet.

Food label claims

Although some manufacturers may make a claim on the front of the package, the FDA only allows those that are supported by scientific evidence. These include low-fat, cholesterol-, sodium- and fat-free foods. Even though these claims are regulated, caution must be taken about their validity because a low-fat food may not necessarily mean that it is nutritious or good for your health. For example, pretzels may be low in fat, but they are high in sodium and low in nutritional value. Low cholesterol does not necessarily mean that the food really is low in fat, but simply that it is not derived from animals. Certain information must be provided on the food label, including:

- Common name of all the product ingredients.
- Name and address of manufacturers or distributors.
- Net contents.
- Ingredient list.
- Serving size as well as number of servings per package.
- Quantity of specific ingredients.

Learning from food labels

A food label gives a quick snapshot of the nutritional values of a food, the ingredient listing, more detailed information per serving and nutrition claims by manufacturers. Note that the ingredient with the greatest weight is listed first, while the second one contains the most nutrients per kcal. For example, the first ingredient in a yogurt product is milk solids, followed by sugar, the most nutrient-dense ingredient. Ingredients that fall under the same category are placed under the collective term then listed by name in order of predominant weight. For example, sweeteners is the collective name for sugar, corn syrup, molasses, honey or jam. Different fats or oils also are listed such as coconut oil, hydrogenated fats or cholesterol because of their positive link to heart disease. Furthermore, specific well-known allergens such as peanuts and additives such as monosodium glutamate (MSG) are required to be listed. The nutrition panel lists the nutrients that concern public health such as fats, saturated fats, cholesterol and certain micronutrients such as sodium, vitamins and iron. **Figure 14-1** shows a good example of a nutrition panel food label and its nutritional facts.

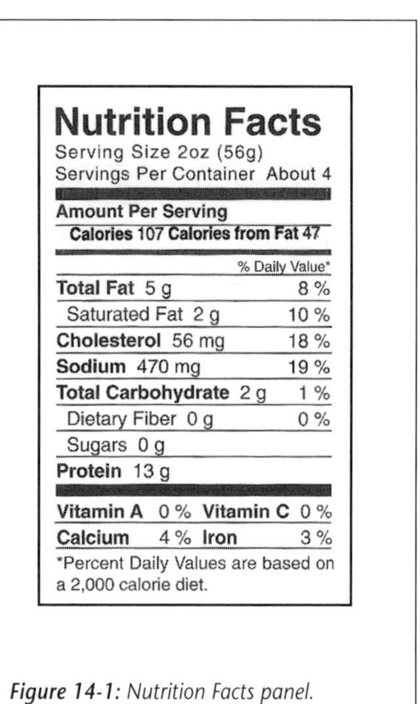

Nutrition Facts
Serving Size 2oz (56g)
Servings Per Container About 4

Amount Per Serving
Calories 107 **Calories from Fat** 47

	% Daily Value*
Total Fat 5 g	8 %
Saturated Fat 2 g	10 %
Cholesterol 56 mg	18 %
Sodium 470 mg	19 %
Total Carbohydrate 2 g	1 %
Dietary Fiber 0 g	0 %
Sugars 0 g	
Protein 13 g	

Vitamin A	0 %	**Vitamin C**	0 %
Calcium	4 %	**Iron**	3 %

*Percent Daily Values are based on a 2,000 calorie diet.

Figure 14-1: *Nutrition Facts panel.*

Top panel of food label. On the top left hand side of the Nutrition Facts label, specific information on the product is given. This includes serving size, calories and different nutrient information for each product. The bottom part contains a footnote that is standardized dietary advice based on the normal male and female individual and not relevant to that particular food. This only is found on larger packages. See **The Nutrition Facts Panel and the Consumer**, pages 204-205, for a better understanding of the meanings behind the terminology.

Footnote of the Nutrition Facts panel. In larger packages, this footnote appears on the lower part of the Nutrition Facts panel, and the information listed is not relevant to the particular food, but is standardized dietary advice for everyone

The Nutrition Facts Panel and the Consumer

General Terms	Meaning
Serving size	This is indicated by cups or pieces followed by the metric measures and must be a standard serving size for consumers to evaluate the amount consumed more accurately. Serving sizes are based on an amount of food a person normally eats, so that one serving size is the amount of that food containing the amount of listed ingredients. The new standard serving size of beverages is 8-oz. (240 ml) or 12-oz. (360 ml). The label tells you how many servings are in the total package, so that if there were five servings in the package and you ate all of it, you would have eaten five servings or five times the amount of the listed ingredients of one serving.
Calories and fat calories	Calorie requirements vary for each individual depending on age, weight, gender and activity level. The amount of calories indicates how many calories are in one serving of the food. The label also tells how many calories in one serving are from fat. For example, if there are 250 calories in one serving of potato chips and the amount of fat calories is 150, then one serving of this food contains more than half of the total calories from fat. If you ate the whole box, then you would have eaten the number of fat calories multiplied by the number of servings stated. This may be too much fat if you want to lose weight. Cookies with high fiber may not be the best choice if you don't know how much fat they contain while lightly salted chips can still be quite high in sodium and fat.
Percent DVs	The DVs on food labels help consumers become aware of which nutrients contribute a lot, or too little, of the daily recommended intakes. Like calories, the FDA uses 2,000 kcal/d as the reference amount for calculating the percentage of DVs. This is listed as a percentage of

General Terms	Meaning
Percent DVs (cont.)	the nutrients that you will get from eating one serving of that food. The goal is to eat 100% of that nutrient daily, so that if a serving contains 55% of fat, then that food is providing you with 55% of your daily needs for fat based on 2,000 kcals/d. That means that you only need to eat 45% more of fats in other foods for the rest of the day to reach 100%, so you need to check food labels with lower DVs in fat calories for the rest of the day. The DVs can be used to make dietary trade-offs with other foods throughout the day. You don't have to give up a favorite food to eat a healthy diet, but instead can balance it with other foods that are low in fats. Generally, a food with 20% DV or more indicates that it is high in that nutrient while one with 5% DV or less is low. You want to limit foods such as fat, saturated fats, trans fatty acids, cholesterol and sodium, but want to consume foods with high DVs in fiber, calcium, vitamins and minerals. Always try to stay below 100% DV. If you want to find out what percent of DVs corresponds with a 1,300 mg of calcium given in a food, divide by 10, so it carries 130% DV calcium, a very high DV percentage. Conversely, a cup of milk contains 30% DV, the equivalent of 300 mg. Note that neither sugars nor proteins are given a DV value. This is because recommendations for these nutrients have not yet been established. The amount of sugars listed includes naturally occurring sugars found in fruit and milk as well as those added to food or drinks. Current scientific evidence indicates that high protein intake does not cause alarm for public health.

U.S. Food and Drug Administration, June 2000; updated July 2003.

based on whether you eat 2,000 or 2,500 kcal/d. This information is significantly important for public health and is required to be noted on food labels.

Nutrient	DRI for normal healthy adults.
Fats	No more than 30% of total daily caloric intake.
Saturated fats	No more than 10% of total daily caloric intake of fat.
Cholesterol	Less than 300 mg daily.
Sodium	Less than 2,400 mg daily.

This part gives the amount of recommended fat intake if eating a 2,000 kcal/d or a 2,500 kcal/d diet. For a 2,000 kcal/d diet, a female should eat less than 65 g of fat and for 2,500 kcal/d, a male should eat less than 80 g of fat in total for the day. By doing this, a person will be following healthy dietary advice by consuming no more than 30% of their daily calories from fat, keeping the total daily fat intake below 100% DV. The daily values of cholesterol—300 mg and sodium—2,400 mg, remains the same no matter how many kcals eaten, but the recommended levels of other nutrients do depend on the daily kcals consumed.

Comparison claims

The FDA defines 11 core items, terminology used most commonly in food labeling—free, low, lean, extra lean, high, good source, reduced, less, light, fewer and a few more. For example, a food may be described as a "good source of calcium" or an "excellent source of calcium" with each term having different meanings. The term "zero" cannot be used because it is impossible to measure below a certain amount. However, the regulation will allow a fat-free claim with less than 0.5 g of fat per serving, an amount that is physiologically insignificant even if several servings are eaten. "Free" also can be used in reference to saturated fats, cholesterol, sodium, sugars and calories. See **Definitions of Comparison Claims**, pages 207-208, for definitions about claims to a comparable or reference food considered the ideal measurements for that nutrient.

Food labels and health claims

Health claims in food labels cannot be made if the percentage of a nutrient is more than the DV, particularly in the case of foods such as fats, saturated fats, cholesterol and sodium that are positively linked to health problems. Any claims made such as "cholesterol-free" must be supported by scientific evidence and must be clear and honest. For example, a product must not claim to be low in cholesterol if it contains a high amount of fat; that is contradictory.

Definitions of Comparison Claims

Calories

Calorie free—No more than 5 kcals per serving.

Low calorie—40 kcals or less per serving.

Reduced or fewer kcals—At least 25% fewer kcals per serving than the reference food.

Light—1/3 fewer kcals than the reference food.

Fats

Fat-free—Less than 0.5 g of fat per serving.

Saturated fat-free—Less than 0.5 g per serving of both saturated fat and trans fatty acids per serving.

Low fat—3 g or less per serving.

Low saturated fat—1 g or less per serving.

Reduced or less saturated fats—25% less per serving than the reference food.

Cholesterol

Cholesterol-free—Less than 2 mg of cholesterol and 2 g or less of saturated fats per serving.

Low cholesterol—20 mg or less per serving and 2 g or less saturated fats per serving.

Reduced or less cholesterol—25% or less and 2 g or less saturated fats per serving than the reference food.

Sodium

Sodium-free—Less than 5 mg or 1 teaspoon per serving.

Low sodium—140 mg or less per serving.

Very low sodium—35 mg or less per serving.

Light in sodium—No more than 50% sodium than the reference food.

Sugar

Sugar-free—Less than 0.5 g per serving.

No added sugar—No sugars added during processing or packing.

Without added sugar—Processing does not increase the sugar content above its natural amount present.

Reduced sugar—25% less per serving than the reference food.

Fiber

High fiber—5 g or more per serving.

Good source of fiber—2.5 to 4.9 g per serving.

More or added fiber—2.5 g more per serving than the reference food.

Definitions of Comparison Claims *(cont.)*

Other terms

"Lean" or "extra lean"—Describes the fat content of meat, poultry and seafood. "Lean" means the food has less than 10 g fat, less than 4 g saturated fat and less than 96 mg of cholesterol per serving per 100 g. "Extra Lean" denotes less than 5 g of fat, less than 2 g of saturated fats and less than 95 mg of cholesterol per serving and per 100 g.

"High source of" or *"rich in"*—The food must contain 20% or more of the DVs for that nutrient in a serving.

"Good source"—A serving containing 10–19% of the DVs for that nutrient.

"Lite" or *"Light"*—Means it either contains 1/3 fewer kcals or 1/2 the fat of the reference food. If the food derives 50% or more of its kcals from fat, the reduction must be 50% of the fat. The sodium content of a low kcal, low fat food has been reduced by 50%. "Light" also can be used to describe the color or texture of food and not the kcal or fat content.

Labels in the past have been misleading—for example, the public misunderstood the meaning of "light" for kcals when it meant light in color and texture. The term "fresh" only can be used for raw foods while "freshly prepared" only can be made if the food has been made recently and has not been frozen or chemically preserved. Foods bearing health claims therefore must contain only 20% or less of the DVs of fat, saturated fat, cholesterol and sodium. As a result, whole milk that is high in calcium cannot bear a calcium-osteoporosis claim because its fat content exceeds the qualifying levels for a health claim; excess fats are high risk for heart disease. Therefore, one claim may disqualify the other. However, skim milk or lowfat milk can qualify for health claims.

A serving of a food with a "more," "fortified," "enriched" or "added" claim must have at least 10% more of the DVs for a particular nutrient than the food to which it is compared. The FDA recently issued a warning to some milk producers to remove the term "hormone-free" from milk products because the term was considered misleading to the public. Since all milk contains naturally occurring hormones, it cannot be processed in a manner that renders it free from hormones. See **Supported Health Claims**, page 209, for health claims that are supported by scientists and accepted by health authorities.

Supported Health Claims

The following health claims have been supported by scientists and accepted by health authorities. These claims state that there is a correlation between the two variables.

- High calcium is linked with low osteoporosis.
- High sodium is linked with hypertension.
- High lipids often are linked with cardiovascular diseases and certain cancers.
- High dietary fiber reduces cardiovascular diseases and certain cancers.
- High folate is linked to reduced neural tubular disorders.
- High antioxidants are linked to reduced cancer.
- High zinc is positively linked to immunity.
- High omega-3 fatty acids are linked to reduction in heart disease.

Exemptions

Many foods do not have information on them and may be exempt from food labeling. This includes food in restaurants, on airlines, in hospital cafeterias, food service vendors, food colors, bulk foods, additives and other foods that contain no significant amounts of nutrients.

Organic foods

The term "organic" refers to the how foods are grown and processed in a more natural way than conventional farming. Organic farming practices are designed to encourage soil and water conservation and reduce pollution. Following is a list of the different farming practices between conventional and organic farming.

Conventional farming

- Applies chemical fertilizers to promote growth.
- Uses insecticides to reduce pests and disease.
- Uses chemical herbicides to control weeds.

Food Safety Hints

1. Wash hands with soap before and after handling food.
2. Use brushes to clean fruits and vegetables instead of peeling them. Cruceriferous vegetables such as broccoli, cauliflower and brussel sprouts should be washed thoroughly and blanched with boiling water for a few minutes to kill the large amount of microorganisms lurking within them. Peel waxed fruits to remove traces of pesticides.
3. Trim all fat from meats and wash thoroughly. Minimal washing of red meats is recommended to avoid loss of nutrients.
4. Cook vegetables in as little amount of water as possible, or try steaming. Vegetables contain a great deal of water and do not require added water.
5. Use fresh foods as quickly as possible to avoid loss of vitamins.
6. Season with spices and herbs instead of high-fat sauces, butter or margarine.
7. Substitute high-fat sauces for blend-whipped low-fat cottage cheese or yogurt. This means that these foods can be placed in a blender and whipped on a high speed giving the texture of cream for sauces.
8. Keep raw meats and their juices away from other foods in the refrigerator.
9. Cooked meats should be eaten immediately because bacteria can multiply very quickly if left to cool at room temperature.
10. Slow cookers are not recommended for cooking large pieces of meat or frozen/stuffed products because the cooking temperatures may not be high enough.
11. Cooked foods such as meat casseroles or milk/milk products should not be left to thaw out for more than two hours to avoid salmonella poisoning.
12. Wash hands and cutting boards thoroughly before cutting up other meats and vegetables. A plastic board is better than a wooden one because bacteria tends to lurk in the grooves of the wood. If possible, place chopping boards in the dishwasher after use.
13. Wash and replace sponges and dishcloths regularly, and avoid hanging dishcloths near garbage containers.

- Gives animals antibiotics, growth hormones and medications to spur growth and prevent diseases.

Organic farming

- Uses natural fertilizers to feed soil and plants.
- Uses beneficial insects and birds, mating disruption and traps to reduce pests.
- Rotates crops, tills, hand-weeds and uses mulch to control weeds.
- Feeds animals with organic feed and implements measures to minimize disease such as rotational grazing, balanced diet and clean housing.

Should you buy organic?

Before choosing organic foods, consider these factors.

- Nutrition-wise, there is no conclusive evidence showing that organic food is more nutritious than conventionally grown food.
- The difference lies in how the food is produced, processed and handled. Due to non-usage of preservatives and waxes, organic foods spoil faster than conventionally grown foods. If there is a slow transfer of foods from the field to the marketplace, nutrient values may be reduced or lost.
- People with environmental concerns are more likely to buy organic foods because of their reduced exposure to pesticide residue, but large-scale

Text continues on page 215.

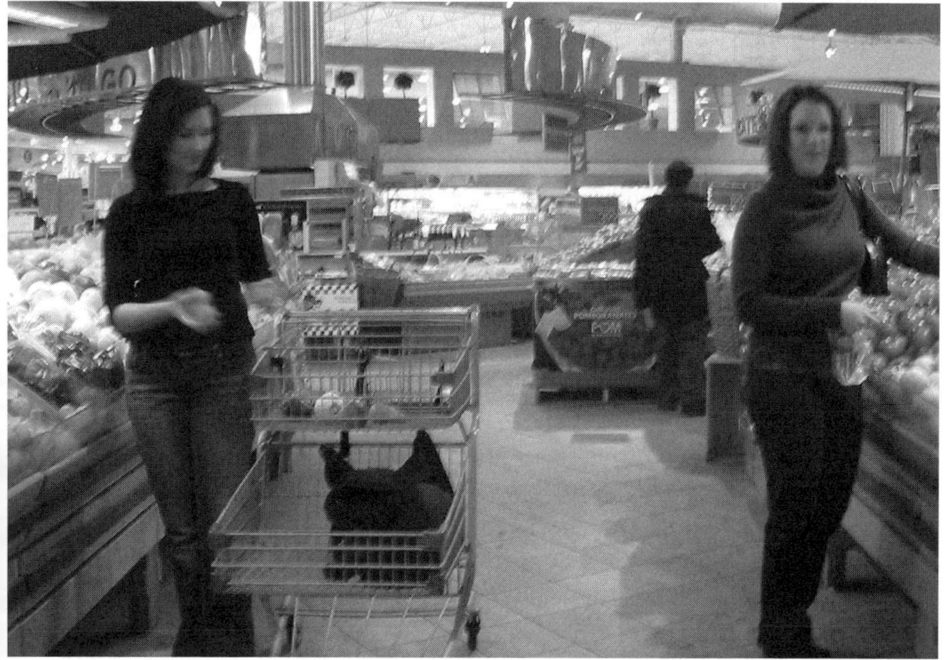

Food preparation and storage

One of the functions of the spa professional is to inform their clients how to prepare food safely. Food allergies and contamination are of particular importance today due to health epidemics such as SARS that have invaded the world. The correct choice, preparation and storage of food will provide a more nutritious product and also will give a positive psychological tone to an attractively prepared meal. Following are four guidelines to keep food safe.

Clean. Wash hands and surfaces often.
Separate. Don't cross-contaminate.
Cook. To proper temperature.
Refrigerate. As soon as possible.

Food selection. The key to healthy cooking begins with wise food selection and purchasing. A good strategy is to have a compiled grocery list. Avoid shopping when hungry because you are more likely to grab fattening foods that are attractively displayed or simply smell good. The freshness and overall quality of food depends in large part on the distribution and marketing systems.

Select foods in good condition—choose frozen foods that are solid. Seafood is one of the most difficult foods to keep fresh, and it harbors millions of bacteria. Inspect fish for color, resilience and sliminess, and also check the eyes for clarity and sheen. Most of all, smell it, if possible, for a final decision.

Avoid buying cans with dents, cracks or bulges because their contents may be affected. Avoid potatoes that have grown sprouts, turned green or are wilted. Freezing does not destroy the nutritional values of frozen or pre-cut vegetables, so pre-chopped garlic and dried onions are all good buys.

Check the expiration dates and choose low-fat versions of milk, yogurt, cheese and salad dressings. Stick to the leanest cuts of meats such as flank steaks, extra lean hamburger and skinless free-range poultry. Free-range refers to chickens that are free to run around the farm and were not brought up in a cooped cage. Therefore their thighs are more muscular and less fat than their breasts. On the contrary, duck breasts are more muscular than their thighs. Never choose meat or poultry in torn or leaking packaging, and check the expiration dates. To avoid contamination to other foods, place meats and poultry in plastic bags.

It is wise to purchase fruits and vegetables that are in season because they are fresher and more economical. Good additions are canned beans, peas and lentils because there is no preparation involved. Remember, the more variety of foods

Food preparation and storage *(cont.)*

eaten, the greater the chances of obtaining the needed nutrients. Do not be afraid to try new fruits and vegetables because they can open up exciting new tastes and even be a good topic of conversation. Purchase refrigerated or frozen foods last and plan to drive home directly. If the temperature outside is very high, do not leave groceries in a hot car for a long period.

Food storage. Meats should be refrigerated or frozen immediately upon arrival at home, perishable foods within two hours, and if the temperature is above 90 F, no less than one hour. Cook or freeze fresh poultry, fish and ground meats within two days and beef, veal, lamb or pork within 3–5 days. Perishables such as meat and poultry should be double-wrapped in plastic or foil to maintain quality and prevent contamination to other foods.

Eggs and milk have a shelf life of ten days and should not be used past their expiration dates. Fresh fruits and vegetables are good up to about one week. Frozen foods that are thawed and refrozen usually lose a certain amount of nutrients and cannot be held for long in the freezer. It is wise to separate the meats when they are unfrozen in required portions, and rewrap and freeze them. Better yet, ask your butcher to pack them in the required portions and if vacuum-packing is available, request this service because the meat remains fresher and lasts longer. In general, defrosted meats can be refrozen if ice crystals are present.

Thawing. Meats can be placed in the refrigerator for slow, safe thawing, but ensure that their juices do not drip onto other food. For faster thawing, they can be placed in a leak-proof plastic bag and submerged in cold tap water, but change the water often. Microwaving also is a quick and safe way to thaw foods. Cook immediately after thawing.

Cooking and serving. Meats should be cooked thoroughly and served hot or warm. If serving buffets, keep foot hot with chafing dishes, slow cookers or warm ovens. Cold food can be nestled in bowls of ice. Marinated meats should be placed in a covered dish in the refrigerator.

Preparing staple foods

Rice. Rice is a staple food for most populations, especially Asians. Brown or wild rice is better than white rice, but is more expensive. There are mixed grains available now even in bulk food stores, and this is reasonably priced for every day use. To maximize nutrient value, do not cook rice in an excessive amount of water and then

Food preparation and storage *(cont.)*

drain it because the nutrients will be lost. The rule of thumb is to use one cup of water to one cup of wet, washed rice. It is unnecessary to add salt when cooking rice.

Bread. Many healthier forms of bread now are found in most grocery stores and are enriched with thiamin, niacin, riboflavin and iron. When purchasing bread, choose whole grains over white bread, and check food labels for fiber and nutrient content. Try eating breads with good quality olive oils instead of using butter or margarine.

Potatoes. Potatoes are a staple food of Europeans. It is unnecessary to peel potatoes unless dirt is enmeshed into the skin. Instead, use a vegetable brush to clean and cook them in their skins to maximize the fiber and vitamin C content that is found just beneath the skin. Microwave cooking of baked potatoes is much faster than standard oven cooking. Baked potatoes contain about 25% more solids and contain higher levels of all nutrients than raw or boiled potatoes. If you boil the potatoes, the nutrients seep into the water instead reducing their taste and nutrient values. It is a good idea to keep the stock handy for making soups later. Instead of refrying, place frozen french fries in the oven without adding any fat. A healthier way of serving potatoes is to replace butter, cheese, mayonnaise or sour cream with olive oil, yogurt or cottage cheese. (See **Figure 14.2** below.)

Leftovers

Many people eat leftovers the next day, and this is fine if the food has not been left out at room temperature for more two hours or one hour if the temperature is over 90 F. Place leftovers in shallow containers and place in the refrigerator or freezer immediately.

Figure 14.2: *Nutrient content of different styles in preparing potatoes. Source: FDA, 1991.*

1 medium potato	Weight (g)	Kcal (mg)	Vitamin C (g)	Fiber (mg)	Calcium (mg)	Iron
Baked (with skin)	202	220	26	1.3	20	2.7
Boiled	36	115	14	2.0	9	0.4
French fries (10 strips, 2 x 3.5")	50	163	3	<1.0	6	0.8

studies suggest that pesticide residues are not necessarily an important risk factor for cancer. Most experts agree that the amount of pesticides in fruits and vegetables pose a very small risk. It is more important to eat fruits and vegetables regardless how they are grown to reduce health risks.

- Some people believe that organic foods taste better, but this is an individualized opinion. Freshness is probably a more important factor to consider than quality of taste.
- Organic foods cost much more than conventionally grown foods.

In the end, the major advantage of organic foods is less environmental pollution, but the real disadvantage is more expense for the consumer. If deciding to buy organic, look for the USDA organic seal because strict government standards are imposed to obtain organic certification.

CHAPTER 15

Physical Fitness

Fitness and nutrition are two components of wellness that people use to change their lifestyle and improve the quality of their longevity. Estheticians perform body treatments such as body massage, body wraps, and detoxifying and cellulite treatments with many spas advertising that a person can lose inches in one or more treatments. In order to get credible results in body treatments, estheticians need to acquire a sound knowledge of basic nutrition and exercise guidelines for acquiring a healthy body weight and improving body shape. A therapist does not need to be a nutritionist or fitness expert to know the basics of fitness and nutrition, but is expected at least to look the part by having clear, smooth skin and a trim, toned body. While pampering or stress-relieving treatments are psychologically effective in developing an improved frame of mind, proper advice on nutrition and simple exercises to correct postural faults will enhance results for body treatments and help fight the effects of aging.

Skin care and physical fitness

The first impression of the esthetician should be a positive one. Clients coming to a wellness spa expect the staff to have healthy looking skin and a trim, toned body with good posture. Proper posture exudes self-confidence motivating clients and others to admire and follow the therapist's advice. An attractive appearance lends credibility to a profession that is becoming more health-oriented. Having knowledge of physical fitness is important to recommend effective and corrective exercises that would complement body treatment programs.

Anti-aging therapy

Anti-aging health practitioners extol the virtues of physical exercise as one of the five pillars of anti-aging. Exercise is considered the fountain of youth, and the effects of aging are visible particularly in the musculo-skeletal system which includes the muscles, bones, joints, ligaments, tendons and cartilage. Early ancestors got their share of exercise by walking long distances and pulling carts and other heavy objects, but in today's modern society, advanced technologies have created such easy lifestyles with elevators, escalators and, of course, vehicles for easy commutes and transportation.

Many people do not even do the minimum of exercise on a daily basis lending to a sedentary society. To become active, people have to be pushed into joining gyms and fitness clubs. Many researchers believe that the current obesity epidemic found in Western societies has developed largely due to a sedentary lifestyle that also has spread to Europe and the Far East. This phenomenon has stimulated interest in several countries to return to developing programs of physical activity, starting in the early school years, to stem the epidemic.

Since nutrition has been discussed throughout this book, this chapter is focused on promoting a more active lifestyle.

Body alignment

As a body therapist, it is important to be able to detect proper alignment of the client in order to recommend exercises and to understand the contraindications to specific movements. Good posture results from a well-positioned, healthy skeletal system supported by a strong muscular system. There is a clear correlation between good posture and how a person views herself. For example, when depressed, people tend to slouch and drop their heads forward, giving the impression of a weak individual with low confidence. However, when pleased with life, people tend to hold their head and shoulders upright. Then, you are more likely to be viewed as a happy and confident individual and others listen when you speak. If a client can be made aware of proper body alignment, it paves the road to them feeling happier and more confident. Regular exercise activity, particularly isotonic exercises, also should be recommended.

Fitness terminology

Before learning about physical fitness, you should become more familiar with certain terminology used to describe movements of the body in exercise. **Movement** occurs when muscles contract. Muscles have two points of attachment—the **origin** is the fixed point where no movement occurs, and the **insertion** is where the muscle attaches to another muscle or bone causing movement at the joints. For example, in an abdominal curl, the origin is at the symphysis pubis, and the insertion is at the lower part of the ribs where the rectus abdominal muscles insert onto the ribs—that's where movement occurs. The **midline** is an imaginary line that passes through the middle of the body.

Proximal refers to nearest while **distal** means furthest to a point of reference.

Concentric refers to a movement that bends or flexes a limb at a joint and muscle fibers shorten and become thicker.

Eccentric refers to movements where the limbs are straightened or stretched and muscle fibers lengthen.

Isometric refers to the **tensing**, or toning of a muscle without any change in length and no movement occurs. No calories are burnt and isometric movements can be performed by anyone, even the disabled.

Isotonic refers to any free activity where muscles change in length and become shorter bringing about movement. Both concentric and eccentric movements are isotonic where movement occurs at the joint. Isotonic movements improve blood circulation, increase deep respiration, use energy and burn calories.

Abduct movement is drawn away from the midline.

Adduct movement is drawn toward the midline.

Rotation refers to turning on a long axis—the shoulder rolls at the shoulder joint.

Hyperextension refers to joint movement beyond the midline.

Inversion involves the limb turning inward toward the midline.

Eversion involves the limb turning outward away from the midline.

Range of Motion (ROM) refers to the flexibility or possible movement of muscles at a joint. For example, ball and socket joints such as hip and shoulder joints yield the greatest ROM of all body joints, while the wrist, a gliding joint, has the least ROM.

- **Full range** is the range where muscles work from full contraction to full stretch, causing movement at a joint. Full ROM gives the greatest power, flexibility and motion.
- **Inner range** is the range where muscles work from half-contraction to full-contraction and vice versa. Inner range is used to gain or maintain movement of a joint in the direction of the muscle pull.
- **Outer range** is the range where a muscle works from a half-contraction to full stretch and vice versa. Outer range is used to gain additional strength.
- **Middle range** is the contraction that occurs between inner and outer ranges and is the most commonly used range. This is also referred to as pulsing. Muscles are the most efficient in this range.

Planes of the body. In body alignment, this terminology sometimes is used for easy description of different sections of the body. A plane is an imaginary flat surface in relation to a reference point, such as the midline, and is used to divide the body into parts. (See **Figure 15.1**.)

Frontal, or **coronal** plane is a vertical plane that divides the body into **anterior** (front) and **posterior** (back) sections.

Saggital, or **lateral** plane is a vertical plane that divides the body into left and right sections.

The **transverse**, or **horizontal** plane, runs across the body parallel to the ground, dividing the body into **superior** (upper) and **inferior** (lower) portions.

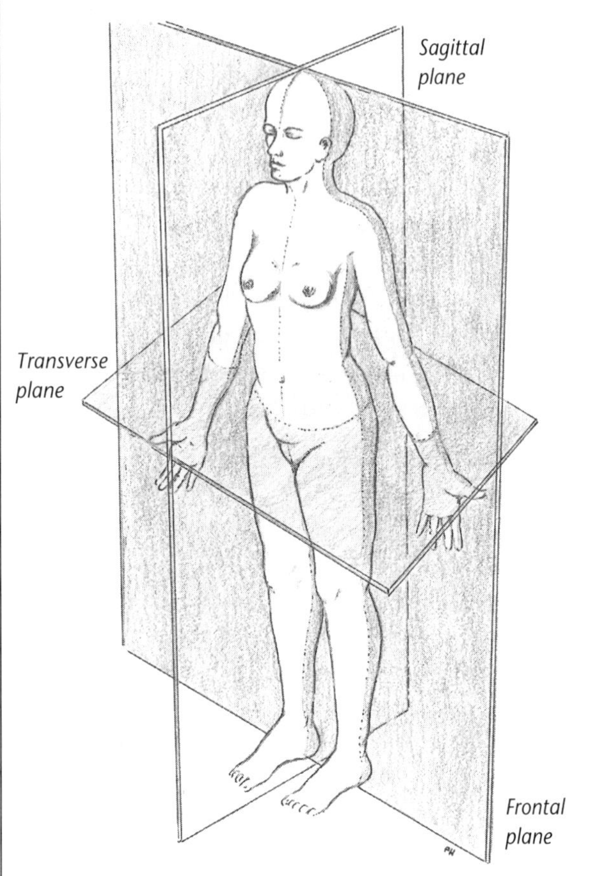

Figure 15.1: *The planes of the body.*
Source: Advanced Professional Skin Care, Peter Pugliese, MD.

Common postural faults. **Kyphosis** is an abnormally increased convex curve of the upper thoracic spine that can be seen when a body is viewed from the side. This condition often is associated with tight pectoral muscles. These individuals also exhibit forward head tilt, round shoulders and weak upper body. This postural fault is commonly found among the ectomorph, the thin, willowy body type which will be discussed further later in this chapter.

Lordosis is an exaggerated lumbar curve that may be associated with an anterior pelvic tilt and shortened hip flexors. Tall slender individuals, such as the ectomorph body type, usually suffer from lordosis. In these instances, the abdominal muscles are overstretched and the lower back muscles are tight resulting in lower back problems.

Kypholordosis is a combination of kyphosis and lordosis.

Scoliosis is a deviation of the spine resulting in uneven shoulder positions, scapular deviations, slight horizontal rotation of the pelvic girdle and uneven lengths of the legs.

Checking body alignment

Alignment is the proper positioning of body parts in relation to one another. Good posture is the result of a well-positioned, healthy skeletal structure held together by the muscular system. Muscular movement occurs as the result of neuro-muscular systems working together for proper coordination. Proper body alignment helps the therapist to recognize the overall balance of the body and observe deviations from the line of gravity such as an out of proportion figure and abnormalities of the spine or feet. Extreme deviations may imply more serious problems. An anterior pelvic tilt may indicate tight hip flexors, and round shoulders give clues to weak upper back muscles and tight pectorals. These observations can help the body therapist determine areas of weak muscles and program corrective exercises to improve body strength and body alignment. The use of a *"plumb's line"* or an imaginary line of gravity helps to assess various figure faults. It can be used from an anterior, posterior and side position to observe specific figure faults more clearly. Figure faults shown from these positions are indicated below.

Anterior or frontal view. For this view, use the saggital plane to divide the body into left and right parts.

- Overall shape of the body and how it moves in daily life—whether it is overweight or underweight.
- Proportion of figure—smaller upper body versus larger lower body, using the transverse plane to divide the body into upper and lower parts.
- One shoulder higher than the other.
- One breast higher than the other.
- Size of breasts—overly large, small, high positioned, inverted nipples.
- Sunken chest.
- Wide waist or thick trunk.
- Heavy thighs or thin legs.
- Cellulite deposits.
- Bowed legs or knock knees.
- Hammer toes, everted or inverted feet.

Posterior or ventral view. For this view, use the saggital plane to divide the body into left and right parts.

- Scoliosis or pelvic tilt.
- Cellulite or fatty deposits.

Side view. For this view, use the frontal plane to divide the body into anterior and posterior parts.

- Forward head tilt.
- Round shoulders, dowager's hump, scapular abduction.
- Back—flat, kyphosis, lordosis, scoliosis or kypholordosis.
- Breasts—sagging.
- Abdomen—protruding, loose, large or heavy.
- Buttocks—protruding, low slung, heavy and thick.
- Knees—hyper-extended.
- Feet—flat or highly arched.

Health benefits of exercise

Exercise should form an integral part of daily life, yet it appears to be so difficult for people to adopt. Research repeatedly has shown that those who exercise regularly live longer and healthier lives. The innumerable benefits of exercise include the following.

- Improves blood circulation and body metabolism leading to a stronger heart and reducing risk of cardiovascular disease.
- Controls body weight by reducing fat mass and increasing lean muscle mass.
- Improves muscular strength, body shape and posture.
- Increases energy levels.
- Reduces stress and promotes a sense of well-being.
- Improves sleep.
- Increases mobility, flexibility, balance and coordination.
- Increases growth hormone levels for an anti-aging effect.

When to avoid exercise

- Immediately after surgery.
- Injuries such as strains, sprains.
- Immediately after a meal, especially a heavy one, or on an empty stomach.
- Certain medical conditions are contraindicated for specific exercises such as high blood pressure, dizziness, migraines and weak lower back.

Physical activity and physical fitness

There is a difference between these two terms, and one of the functions of the health and beauty professional is to motivate the client to become physically active and fit.

Physical activity. This includes any exercises for either leisure or non-leisure activities and does not have be a structured or repetitive event, such as walking to the store instead of driving, taking the stairs instead of elevators or escalators, and having fun by playing any game that requires active body movements. The goal is to get the client to participate in any activity that will increase the BMR.

Physical fitness. This refers to body movements related to achieving health such as working out in the gym, or performance-related, such as improving sports skills.

Resting Heart Rate (RHR)

To improve physical fitness, it is important to understand the relationship between the heart and its heart rate. Your heart is a critical part of the cardiovascular system as it pumps blood to all parts of the body. A stronger heart reduces the risk of cardiovascular diseases. The resting heart rate (RHR) is the number of heartbeats recorded upon awakening and before you start moving. Record the number of heartbeats either on the pulse on your left hand or use the first two fingers of the right hand on the right side of the neck. Start the count at zero and count the number of pulses for 15 seconds. Multiply by four to get the average number of heartbeats per minute.

Normal RHRs vary from 50–100 beats per minute with women's RHR faster than men's. The heart rate is slowest during sleep, increasing slightly upon awakening and gradually increasing throughout the day. Smoking, drinking alcohol or caffeine, stress, excitement and high temperatures may increase the resting heart rate by as much as ten beats per minute. The maximum heart rate

(MHR) is the highest heart rate a person can attain. It decreases with age about one beat per minute per year after age 20.

When you first start your fitness program, record your baseline RHR. After you have been performing aerobic activity for about three months, take your RHR once again. If you have been working out at a moderate-to-hard intensity regularly, your RHR will be lower than your baseline RHR. This means that your heart is beating slower and has become stronger and does not have to work as hard as before to push the blood throughout the valves and arteries. This is important because a stronger heart reduces the risk of cardiovascular diseases, the leading cause of death today. This is a significant indicator for improving health in the obese, diabetic and those with a family history of cardiovascular disease. Those who are interested in participating in a fitness program should be aware of the various components of fitness—aerobic fitness, or cardiovascular endurance; muscular strength; and flexibility, balance and coordination.

Aerobic fitness, or cardiovascular endurance

This is the perhaps the most important component of physical fitness. Cardiovascular endurance refers to the ability of the heart, lungs and blood vessels to function at an optimal level at rest and during physical exercise. Aerobic fitness consists of continuous strenuous exercise movements to place stress on the circulation—heart and respiration—lungs for long periods of time. Stressing the cardiovascular system over time will lead to a stronger heart and a lowered RHR. Examples of aerobic exercise include brisk walking, jogging, skating, swimming and cycling. During aerobic training, the skeletal, or working muscles, work harder and require increased oxygen and greater supply of nutrients so deeper breathing is performed involuntarily to prevent buildup of lactic acid in the muscles that eventually leads to fatigue.

Target Heart Rate (THR). This refers to the maximum working heart rate aimed for at the peak of exercise activity, and usually depends on the level of physical condition of the individual. In aerobic fitness, the goal is to achieve a higher target heart rate (THR) or cardiovascular endurance. The intensity of training is measured by age and how hard you worked out at the highest intensity during physical activity. **THR Formula According to Age**, page 225, shows how you can work out the target heart rate with a formula according to age. The lower limit is 60%, and the higher limit is 85%.

Working Heart Rate (WHR). Learn how to listen to the body as the heart responds to physical activity. At the peak of aerobic activity, when your heart is

THR Formula According to Age

Heart rate formula = 220 – age x THR

For example, 220 – 40, or age = 180

To work out 85% maximum THR = 180 x 85 = 1,530

A-10 secs heart rate (a 10 second pulse reading taken at the highest point of exertion during aerobic exercise) = 1,530 divided by 6 = 25 (10 seconds is 1/6 of 1 minute)

To work out the 65% (lower limit) = 180 x 65 = 1,170

A-10 secs heart rate = 1,170/6 = 20

pounding the hardest, stop the activity for a few seconds, find your pulse quickly and take a ten-second count starting from zero. Keep your feet moving slower while taking your pulse, but don't stop completely. A lower limit of 65% would show that you did not work out with great effort while someone who worked out very hard would show the THR upper limit of 85%. Aim for the upper limit for the age group to achieve the highest level of cardiovascular endurance. Check to see if your pulse falls within the lower or higher limit of the target zone according to your age group.

When first starting aerobic activity, stay within the lower limit. As you progress, your heart muscles become conditioned and gradually your THR will approach the upper limit. Remember, MHR decreases with age so don't beat your body up by trying to get to the THR of a younger individual. Proper and safe training requires a warm-up period—longer for sedentary people to prepare for the more intense aerobic workout. A cool down at the end should include stretches for the main muscle groups worked on such as quadriceps, hamstrings, gastrocnemius and particularly the Achilles tendon and shoulder girdle stretches.

Strength training, or resistance training

Weight training increases muscular strength and converts fat mass to lean body mass. *Muscular strength* refers to the maximum tension that a muscle can exert in a single contraction against a resistant object, such as free weights, weight machines, water or even the body, as in push ups. Weight training uses resistance for the targeted muscle to contract and bulk up. It is a form of anaerobic training where, during the concentric movement, the muscles shorten and become thicker and the breath is held for brief movements against the resistance (concentric movement), then lowered to relax and stretch the muscle (eccentric movement). Remember that when weight training is performed on one major muscle group, the antagonist muscle also must be worked on in order to stabilize the muscles worked. For example, if you performed bicep curls, the triceps also must be exercised, and to maintain core strength, when abdomen curls are performed, the opposing muscle group, erector spinae, also must be exercised.

Before beginning strength training, it is important to warm up the body, in particular, the large muscle groups, for 5–10 minutes using any type of light cardiovascular activity such walking, twisting, dancing or stretching movements.

It is equally important to stretch each muscle group after strength training because the muscles will remain tight and contracted leading to discomfort and fatigue later. Hold each stretch for 10–20 seconds. When using heavier weights, hold the stretch longer to allow the muscle fibers to return to their former length.

Each person uses different muscle groups more than others according to daily lifestyle. For example, some individuals use their thighs in biking to work daily, while others such as a gardener or mechanic use their arms more than their legs. Of course, there also are those who just camp out in front of the television and don't use any muscular effort. Men possess larger muscle mass and high testosterone levels to build muscle strength more easily than women who possess more body fat and less muscle mass. Therefore, it is more difficult for women to lose fat and gain muscle bulk.

Increasing muscular strength. To build muscle strength, increase volume of weights, reduce the number of repetitions and take more rests between sets. When first beginning to weight train, perform more repetitions with less volume of weights. For example, perform one set of 15–20 reps using light weights (1 set/15 reps/1–3 kg) and take a minute between each set to stretch those muscles before proceeding to the next set. If someone now is starting to weight train, they should focus on technique—not how much weight they are lifting. If weight training regularly, you will notice that approximately one month after beginning, the muscles you are working have become stronger, and the workout can increase to 2 sets/10 reps/4 kg with approximately one to three minutes between sets, and in another month, possibly 3 sets/10 reps/5 kg. As the weights begin to feel lighter for you, increase the volume to 3 sets/8 reps/6 kg, then 3 sets/8 reps/8 kg and so on, but take more rest time between sets because the muscle will fatigue under the pressure of the weights. In other words, perform fewer reps when the weights are increased, but increase rest between sets to give the muscle groups time to relax and recover. At this phase, you will feel stronger, more powerful and experience exhilarating feelings. You will feel lighter and bouncier on your feet, move effortlessly, not tire easily and always feel full of youthful energy. You will be in peak form, feel self-confident, have higher self-esteem and feel so much healthier.

Improving muscular tone. Muscular tone refers to the ability to perform repeated contractions, or reps. To improve muscle tone, reduce the volume of weights, increase the reps and the number of sets. Take less rest time between sets such as 3 sets/15 reps/2 kg with approximately 30 seconds of resting time between sets. With good muscular tone, the muscles do not become bulky but acquire better shape. Good posture is achieved and less fatigue will be experienced. Muscular tone maintains muscle strength, and improves body shape and good posture.

There are many ways of organizing your workout to optimize physical fitness. A good training program consists of workouts on alternate days for various muscle groups. For example:

Monday—upper body
Tuesday—lower body
Wednesday—upper body
Thursday—lower body
Friday—circuit workout

Flexibility, balance and coordination

Balance refers to maintaining equilibrium while **coordination** is the ability to integrate body movements involving several muscle groups at the same time, such as grapevine movements where both arms and feet move simultaneously. **Flexibility** is the ROM at joints—the greater the ROM, the better the flexibility. Examples of movements to increase flexibility include backward-forward, circular or rotational movements.

Although sedentary individuals and the elderly suffer from poor flexibility and balance, this can be improved at any age. Stretching before and after exercise particularly is important for those individuals with tight muscle groups in the gastrocnemius, hamstrings, hip flexors and arms to elongate them since they were tightened and shortened during exercise. Yoga and Pilates are excellent forms of exercise that improve both flexibility and balance.

In designing a fitness program, the FITT principle—Frequency, Intensity, Time and Type—is used by fitness professionals.

Frequency. Most fitness professionals recommend that it is best that everyone exercise daily, but a minimum of least 3–5 times a week is essential for maximizing fitness potential. So many people do not make it a priority and make frail excuses not to exercise, but this regular activity should be viewed as a set appointment for the body that has to be met without any excuses.

Intensity. Try to reach a THR between 70–85% every time you work out. Low intensity exercises such as brisk walking for a longer period of time are excellent for improving cardiovascular training and can be carried out for a much longer duration than high intensity exercises. As discussed earlier, heavier volume of weights is high intensity exercise and would require more rest between sets. It is important to remember that the higher the intensity of your workout, the more stretching should be done after each set of exercises.

Time. A minimum of 20 minutes of continuous aerobic exercise is needed to reach your maximum THR. Some fitness experts even suggest it is better to try ten minutes, three times a day throughout the day, if it all cannot be done at one time. This is better than not to exercise at all. For preventive care, the longer the duration of the exercise, the better the protective benefits.

Type. What type of exercise is being performed? Is it aerobic, anaerobic, yoga, Pilates? The longer the exercise is being performed, the higher the endurance developed; the greater the volume of weights used, the more the muscle hypertrophy. Some fitness professionals suggest that certain body types should concentrate on particular exercises more than others. For example, the endomorph needs to perform aerobic exercise for at least 30 minutes at one session to burn fats, while the ectomorph needs to concentrate on weight training and do less aerobic activity. Yoga and Pilates are best for muscle toning and flexibility, and are particularly good for the mesomorph, who already is quite muscular, but lacks flexibility.

Use it or lose it!

This old adage appears to be true. In aging, the body is susceptible to cardiovascular diseases and the neuromuscular systems degenerates making it more difficult to maintain proper balance, coordination and flexibility. It is common to see the elderly shuffling their feet as they walk because they are less oriented, and their bones and muscles have become weakened as they become more vulnerable to osteoporosis. This may result in breaking the hip bones eventually leading to disability.

Anti-aging or preventive exercises concentrate on three main components: cardiovascular, strength and flexibility training. Many baby boomers have become very aware that physical exercise can prevent these aging effects and have become very active in the gyms. Therefore, it is not uncommon to find more than 50% of gym memberships consisting of men and women over 50 working out on treadmills, elliptical machines, stationary bikes and weight machines. Mind and body exercises such as yoga, Pilates and meditation also have become popular with this generation who do not have the same strength and energy as they did in earlier years to continue performing high impact exercises. The message is clear. By beginning an exercise program early in life, people can take control of their bodies and preserve what they had in earlier years.

The exercises in **Exercises for Main Muscle Groups**, pages 238 - 243 can be performed standing, using free weights or a body bar. The muscle groups that are being worked are listed, and each exercise is described and demonstrated. However, it should be noted that these exercises are more effective when resistance, such as weights or gravity, is used. It also is important to know when to breathe in and out during the exercise. For instance, breathe out when the muscle is exerted, and breathe in as the muscle relaxes. Note that the exercises described below should be repeated on both sides of the body.

Anti-aging exercises

Anti-aging health practitioners strongly recommend the following exercises for strengthening the upper back, hip and knee joints, and core muscles—abdomen and lower back, all of which improve flexibility and posture.

1. Squats, or alternative lunges—strengthen joints at shoulders, abdomen, knees and lower back.
2. Lats pull-downs—strengthen upper back. Lats is the latissimus dorsi muscles at the mid-back.
3. Abdominal curls—strengthen core muscles.
4. Hip extensions—strengthen hip joints.
5. Knee extensions—strengthen knee joints

Monitoring for self-improvement. To find out if any progress has been made in the fitness program, monitor yourself or your client by taking the following measurements at consecutive periods during the training program.

First, a fitness appraisal should be conducted before you begin a fitness program. Baseline measurements should be taken for the various components of physical fitness—aerobic fitness, muscular strength, endurance, energy levels, flexibility and posture. Girth measurements of the waist, hips, bust and thighs also must be recorded. A fitness assessment to monitor progress usually is taken after one, two, three and six months. This monitoring keeps the client motivated, and they will find it encouraging as they see some visible results. The following are areas where improvement is usually seen.

Cardio assessment. If you have a lower RHR than the baseline RHR, it is indicative of a stronger heart. Check if your WHR has increased—closer to 80-85% of THR. Also measure the distance you usually walk, whether on a treadmill or outside, to see if your speed has improved. Alternatively, has your endurance improved? Can you walk a longer distance in the same time frame?

Results. The heart beats slower but stronger with increased oxygen for the heart. The RHR is lower, improving cardiovascular health.

Muscular strength. You can measure if strength has improved by the volume of weights you now can lift. For example, after one month, you probably can lift an 8-lb weight instead of 5 lbs, without fatigue.

Results. Muscles have bulked, giving more shape to body, and lifting heavy items is effortless.

Endurance. You now can exercise for longer periods before getting fatigued, whether it is aerobic or anaerobic exercise. For muscular endurance, check the number of repetitions you now can perform.

Results. You can walk or run for longer periods before getting tired and can perform 2 sets/10 reps, up from 2 sets/8 reps. After three months, you should be able to perform 3 sets/12 reps without fatigue.

Flexibility. You can bend in different positions and stretch deeper, a feat that was not possible before the program began.

Results. Using a measuring device, you can reach out to 10 instead of 8 inches. Now you even can touch your toes.

Posture. Check line of gravity to see if body alignment has improved.

Results. Posture will be straighter and more upright. You appear taller and leaner, and any conditions dealing with forward head tilt, abdominal protrusion, shoulders, lower back and locked knees will be improved, giving a more confident appearance.

Girth measurements. Inches are lost or gained. This is where everyone feels happiest!

Results. Use tape measurements for the bust, waist, hips and thighs to see if they are slimmer. Your clothes should fit looser as well. Sometimes there is no weight loss, but the girth measurements show improvement. The body is more toned and firmer, resulting in a better body shape. The weight loss does not have to occur to show improvement in health status. More importantly, there is less fat and more muscle, which weighs more. Remember that the more muscle cells you have, the more energy is burned or expended even at rest. That is why men who have more muscle mass can lose their abdominal fat faster than women. Nutritional factors also need to be considered for weight loss to occur.

Results of fitness program. Overall, at the end of the fitness program, you will feel younger, lighter and walk quicker with a bouncier step. Improved posture allows you to breathe better and infers confidence as you walk with more powerful steps. Best of all, you always will feel energetic and won't feel tired even after a long day. Studies have shown that people who exercise regularly are more health conscious and more careful of what they eat. Good results usually lead to buying a new wardrobe to show off your new figure, and this instills even more confidence in your work and social life.

Mind and body fitness

Despite sociologists' prediction of an earlier retirement of leisure, today's world is a more stressful one. Never has there been so much documented research on sedentary lifestyles, stress and their relationship to diseases. A resurgence of mental fitness in spas and fitness clubs is indicated with the emergence of the baby boomers participating in yoga, meditation and Pilates. They are finding that their energy levels are not as high as they used to be to keep up with the heavy aerobic classes such as jogging and stepping. Yoga and Pilates have been found to be quite effective in helping people achieve their body form without stressing their joints. In addition, they enhance body posture, strength, flexibility, coordination and balance, and simultaneously create more awareness of the various muscle groups and how to control them voluntarily leading to reduced stress and relaxation. The deep breathing involved in these exercises helps to control the heartbeat reducing hypertension. Both yoga and Pilates have been found to be very effective in increasing muscle tone, improving flexibility, and improving mental and physical health.

Yoga—"to unite." Although yoga has been practiced for hundreds of years in Asia, today it has become one of the hottest trends in fitness. This Eastern philosophy originating in India is viewed as a religion in the Far East, but actually is a system of living designed to promote health, peace of mind and deeper awareness of the body. Yoga teaches that the body can heal by releasing **prana**, the body's vital energy. When prana is blocked, illness can set in. The practice of yoga allows the body's natural healing ability to take over.

There are several branches of yoga, each with different philosophies toward self-improvement. **Hatha yoga**, the most popular form of yoga in North America, concentrates on physical health and mental well-being. It focuses on poses, or **asanas** that involve deep breathing, stretching and meditation. Yoga is good particularly for those body types that tend to have tight muscles such as the mesomorph and, of course, is excellent for stress reduction. Most spas, particularly destination spas, have incorporated yoga as an integral part of their spa menu. There are hundreds of yoga poses, the most common asana being the **sun salutation** since it stretches numerous muscles.

Pilates. This incredible form of exercise has been used in medicine, top-level sports and performing arts since 1920. Developed by Joseph Pilates, it is a form of fitness used to develop deep core muscular strength, balance, flexibility, endurance and coordination of body movements. It is a unique regimen of body conditioning that can change both your appearance and the way you move.

Working on the deep postural muscles of the body, Pilates helps to rebalance muscle groups, improve body alignment and restore natural movements. Emphasis is placed on building **core strength**, considered the body's powerhouse. The aim is to stabilize the torso by stimulating a contraction between the abdominal and back muscles. Arm crosses, arm sweeps, shoulder circles, rollups, pushups and swimming types of movements also are used to develop the whole ROM.

Stretches are a vital part of Pilates, especially spine stretches and twists. They all involve deep breathing and postural balance simultaneously. The exercises can be performed on a mat or with special equipment wearing comfortable cotton clothes that contour to the body. Baggy clothing and tight elastic bands should be avoided. Pilates is performed barefoot to avoid slippage on mats. Practicing Pilates regularly will lead to suppleness and a natural grace that is evident even in the way a person walks. People will develop strong muscular strength, and aerobic endurance to walk, run or travel for long distances without undue body fatigue or mental strain. With postural improvement, the spine is lengthened to its maximum potential, making the body appear longer and slimmer.

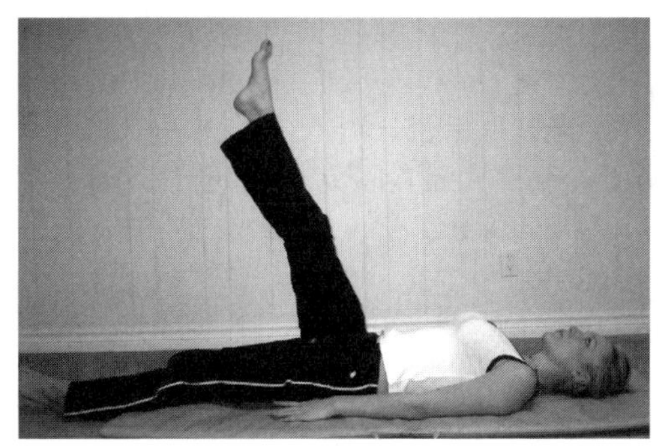
Figure 15-2: Leg circles.

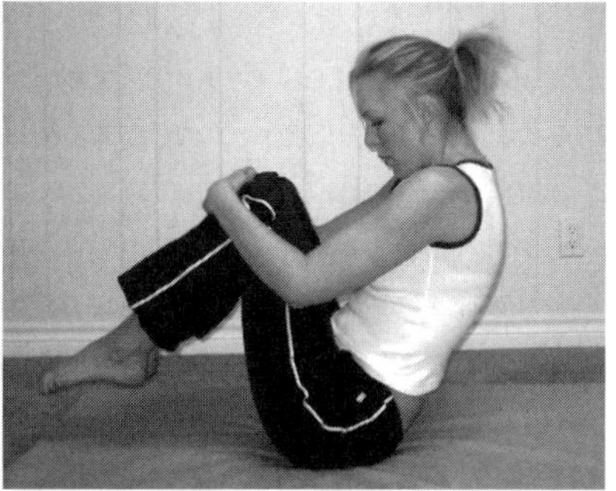
Figure 15-3: Rolling.

Today there are numerous Pilates studios found in major cities throughout North America, and Pilates classes are in high demand by health and fitness clubs. Each Pilates movement is designed to strengthen and stretch complementary muscle groups simultaneously in order to enhance articulation and muscular support of the spine; increase ROM movement; and optimize the relationship between mobility and stability in all movements.

These three Pilates mat exercises strengthen core muscles. Each exercise works on primary and secondary muscles.

Leg circles. Primary muscles worked on include hip flexors, hamstrings, adductors, abductors and hip rotators. Secondary muscles include arm extensors and the trunk muscles are the stabilizing force. (See **Figure 15-2**.)

Rolling. Primary muscles worked on include iliopsoas, rectus abdominus and obliques. Secondary muscles include hip and arm flexors; the trunk muscles are the stabilizers. (See **Figure 15-3**.)

Single leg stretch. Primary muscles worked on include iliopsoas, rectus abdominus, obliques, hip flexors and extensors. Secondary muscles include arm flexors; the trunk muscles are the stabilizers.

Body types

As illustrated and described in **Chapter 12**, most people can be placed in three basic body categories according to their human physique. These categories correlate with certain physical and physiological characteristics. However, some individuals may be a combination of more than one body type. The three basic body types are endomorph, such as Marilyn Monroe and Oprah, mesomorph such as Arnold Schwarzeneger, Demi Moore and Jennifer Aniston, and ectomorph, such as Twiggy, Calista Flockhart and Tom Hanks. Knowing your body type can help design nutritional and exercise strategies to achieve a healthier BMI for weight control and optimizing health. The following chart lists common physical characteristics and dietary strategies for these body types.

Body Type: Endomorph

Theory. Body type formed from endoderm layer in embryo giving rise to overdevelopment of internal organs including the digestive organs and subcutaneous tissues. Endormorphs have thicker adipose tissue and overdeveloped digestive systems leading to overeating.

Physical Characteristics

- Tendency to be short in stature with a full, round, voluptuous body.
- Short limbs and neck with fatty deposits.
- Forward head tilt, round shoulders and abdominal protrusions.
- Gains weight easily.
- High BMI, low BMR.
- Poor posture with a tendency to stand with locked knees resulting in hyper-extended knees.

Common Goals

- Increase lean body mass.
- Reduce body fat.
- Improve posture.
- Increase physical activity.
- Increase mobility.
- Decrease BMI, increase BMR.

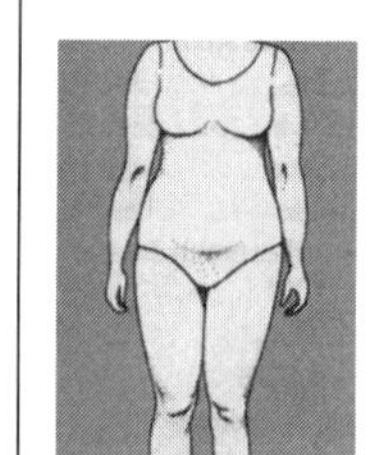

Endomorph.

Dietary Recommendations

- Reduce approximately 500 kcal/d to lose 1 lb/wk.
- Low fat, unsaturated fat diet.
- Avoid or reduce fried foods and eat more grilled or steamed foods.
- High fiber diet.
- Avoid salt.

- Drink one 8-oz. glass of water before and after each meal for improved digestion, absorption and elimination.
- Smaller, more frequent meals throughout day instead of three main meals.
- More fresh, wholesome foods.
- Minimize starchy and sugary foods.
- Eat less meat, eat more fish and soy foods.
- If eating meat, choose smaller amounts of lean meat.
- Choose organic, skinless poultry, especially dark meat over white meat.
- More low glycemic index foods to maintain satiety and avoid overeating.
- Increase antioxidant foods.
- Increase phytochemical foods.
- Supplements. Antioxidant supplements such as vitamins A, C and E.
- Omega-3 to combat free radicals formed from adipose cells.
- Vitamin B to release energy and reduce stress.

Body Type: Mesomorph

Theory. This body type rises from mesoderm layer in embryo, giving rise to increased muscle development.

Physical Characteristics

- Usually medium height.
- Strong, muscular, toned athletic-type of body.
- Wide well-developed shoulders with slim, boyish hips.
- Medium to high BMI.
- Moderate to high BMR.
- Good upright posture.

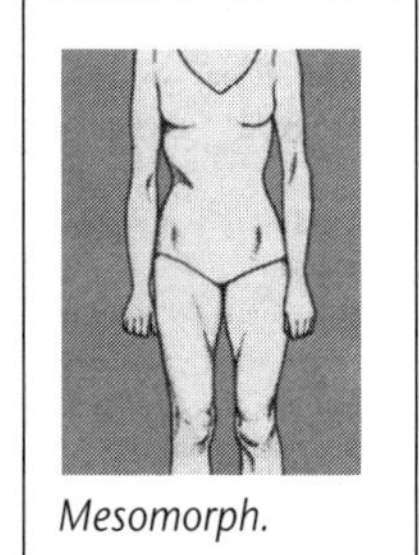

Mesomorph.

Common Goals

- Increase or maintain lean body mass.
- Increase flexibility.

Dietary Recommendations

- Consume 1 to 1.5 g protein per kg/body weight.
- Fats: <30% of total daily kcals.
- Eat approximately 60% complex carbohydrates.
- Consume low to moderate glycemic index foods for sustained endurance for longer workout.
- Eat omega-3 foods after heavy exercise to combat free radicals.
- Take antioxidants and supplements.
- Whey protein and creatine for building lean muscle mass and extra energy.

- Flavonoids.
- Flaxseed oil.

Body Type: Ectomorph

Theory. Body type arises from ectoderm layer which develops the skin and nervous system resulting in high nervous disposition and thinner skin.

Physical Characteristics

- Long, slender, fragile-looking body.
- Small bones, lacks muscle bulk, winged scapula.
- Likely underweight.
- Bent-over posture infers lacking energy.
- Likely suffers from lordosis.
- May have hyper-extended knees.
- Low BMI, high BMR.

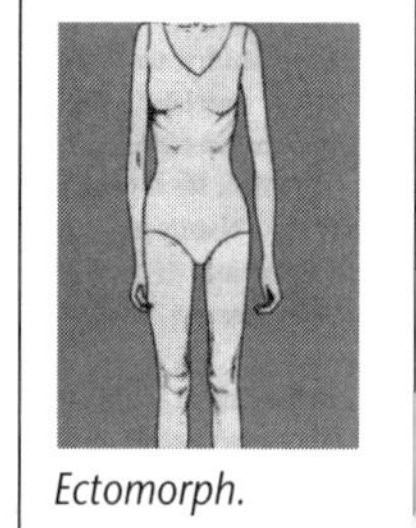

Ectomorph.

Common Goals

- Increase lean body mass.
- Increase body weight.
- Improve posture.
- Build up pectoralis muscles.
- Strengthen and stretch lower back muscles.
- Strengthen arm muscles and soften knees.

Dietary Recommendations

- Increase daily kcals by approximately 500 kcal/d.
- Increase meal portions.
- Consumer frequent healthy snacks 5–7 times day such as protein shakes.
- Increase protein to 1.5–2 g per kg of body weight.
- Supplements.
- Omega-3.
- Flavonoids.
- Flaxseed.
- Glucosamine sulfate.

Workouts for different body types

Several health and fitness experts believe that certain general exercise routines work best for these body types. However, it must be pointed out that this may not apply to everyone—each person should be assessed individually.

Recommended exercise routines for the endomorph.

- Since there is a predisposition to weight gain, focus on enhancing BMR to burn energy.
- Perform more than 30 minutes, and no less than 20 minutes, of aerobic exercise daily. Aim at THR of 75–80% of MHR.
- Follow with resistance training with emphasis on muscular endurance with a goal of more repetitions with shorter rest periods between sets. Increase volume of weights slowly as you get stronger.
- Train everyday or at least 5–6 times a week, but avoid training too heavily and too often.
- Exercises to improve posture include squats, upright rows, abdominal crunches, back extensions, knee extensions, hamstring curls, lateral pull downs, pectoral flies, biceps curls and triceps extensions.
- Pilates and yoga are very beneficial for the endomorph to rebuild muscle groups, improve posture and reduce stress.

Contraindications.

- If suffering from hypertension, avoid exercises over the head such as chest press.

Recommended exercise routines for the mesomorph.

- Genetically predisposed to gaining muscle bulk and losing fat easily, particularly men who continue athletic activities and cardiovascular exercises at least 2–3 times/week for 20–30 minutes, not only performing strength training.
- Overweight mesomorphs, usually middle-aged men, tend to accumulate excess fat in the abdomen and will need to perform cardiovascular exercises 4–5 times/week.
- In weight training, allow more recovery time between heavy sets and use a variety of exercises on different muscle groups.
- Try circuit training—five minutes aerobic, followed by weight training, back to aerobics and repeat weights finishing with five minutes of aerobics to remove buildup of lactic acid in muscles.
- It is very important to stretch muscle groups after each set because the mesomorph usually suffers from tight muscles and lacks flexibility. Yoga and Pilates are very beneficial to the mesomorph.

Recommended exercise routines for the ectomorph.

- Generally underweight and has difficulty gaining weight.
- High metabolic rate burns energy quickly—can eat anything and not gain weight.

- Should limit high-intensity cardio, only 20 minutes 3 times/week instead of daily.
- Concentrate on weight training to increase muscle mass. Use free weights to bulk major muscle groups for improving strength and posture. Start slowly with less weights and more sets then increase slowly to heavier volume and fewer sets to build bulk and improve body shape. Rest and stretch more between sets.
- With resistance training, use full ROM.
- Exercises should strengthen upper body such as lateral pull downs, push ups, pectoral flies, upright rows, incline chest presses and lateral raises. Strengthen the lower body with squats, back extensions and abdominal crunches; build muscle bulk on thighs with alternate leg lunges, knee extensions and hamstring curls. The ectomorph will benefit greatly from Pilates and yoga to correct postural alignment.

Why not?

Nutrition and fitness go hand-in-hand and adopting a lifestyle that integrates both will make you feel more energetic, healthier and keep you in a good mood. Best of all, your body's shape will improve significantly, you will feel more energetic, look and feel younger, and best of all, develop overall self-confidence and self-esteem.

Myths and Misconceptions about Fitness

1. *You have to look good first before joining a gym.*
   You join a gym in order to improve your fitness, body shape and body weight.
2. *I want to look good but am afraid to get big muscles.*
   Women will not get big muscles because they have less testosterone hormones that develop big muscles.
3. *I want to have a body like someone else's.*
   Everyone's body is different, but your body's appearance will improve with regular exercise, and you will feel better about yourself.
4. *Strength training is only for men.*
   Muscular strength and endurance is for everyone who wants to become stronger and more independent, so women do not always have to rely on men to help them. Let us do away with the term the weaker sex.

Exercises for Main Muscle Groups

THIGHS

Quadriceps.

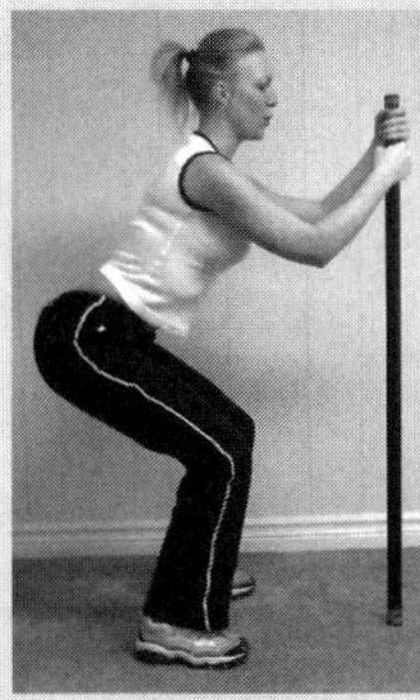

Figure 15-4A: Squats for the thighs.

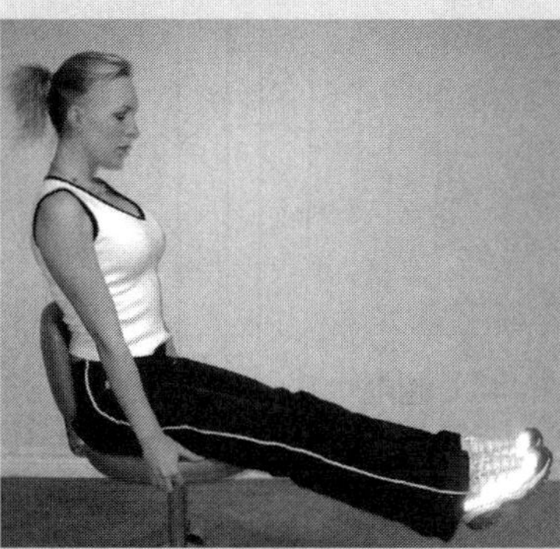

Figure 15-4B: Knee extension for thighs.

1. *Squats.* Pressing feet firmly into floor, hold body bar, tighten abdominals, keep chest up and bend knees slowly, ensuring that knees go past the toes, breathing out. Breathe in as you come up. (See **Figure 15-4A.**)
2. *Knee extension.* Sitting with back pressed against back of chair, press sitting bones, or pelvic bones, into the chair. Grasp sides of chair with arms and tighten abdominals, breathe out, and lift feet slowly off floor to extend knees. Keep knees soft and, breathing in, lower feet slowly to floor. (See **Figure 15-4B.**)

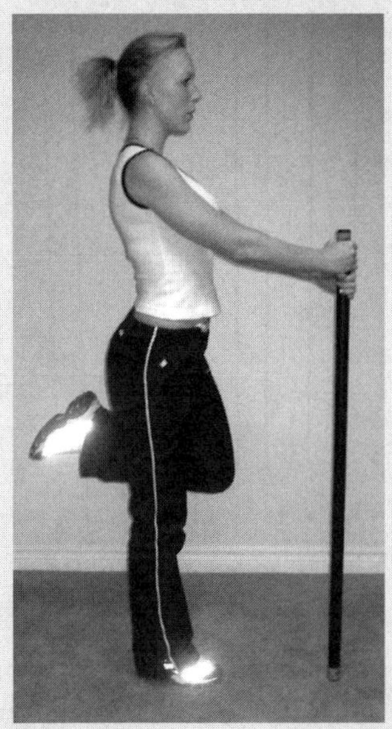

Figure 15-5: Hamstring curl.

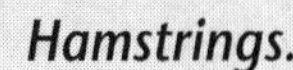

Hamstrings.

1. Holding the wall or body bar with both hands, press one leg firmly into the ground and lift other leg toward the buttocks, emphasizing the hamstring contraction. Lower the leg slowly and repeat on other side. (See **Figure 15-5.**)
2. Lying on your back with your knees bent, place feet firmly on ground at hips width apart, tighten abdomen, breathe out slowly as the lower back is lifted slowly, vertebrae by vertebrae, lifting thighs to knee level. Breathe in and slowly lower the back, vertebrae by vertebrae, to floor.

Exercises for Main Muscle Groups *(cont.)*

Abductors.

1. Holding onto body bar or chair with one hand, lift right leg with toes pointed straight, away from midline, the imaginary line that runs through the body dividing it into two equal parts. Repeat on other side. (See **Figure 15-6.**)
2. Lying on the side, lift upper leg outward away from midline. You also can use body bar as a resistance. Repeat on other side.

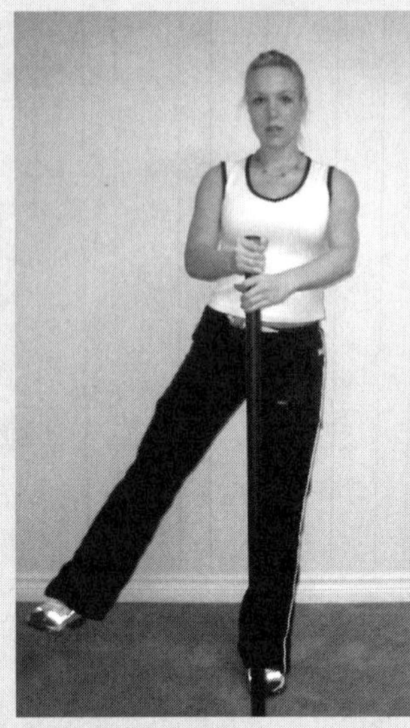

Figure 15-6: *Abductors.*

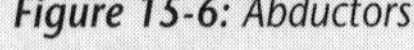

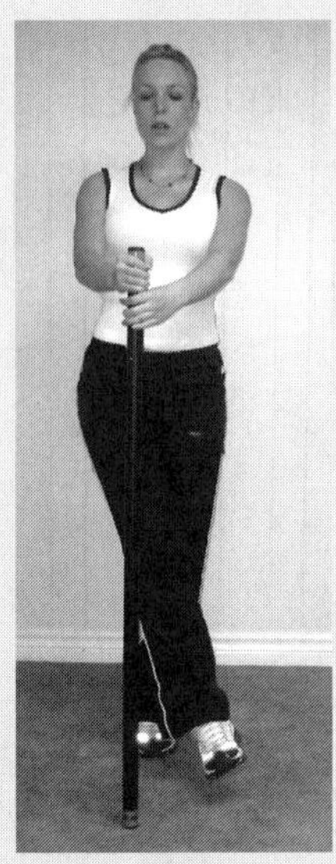

Figure 15-7: *Adductors.*

Adductors.

1. Holding onto body bar or chair with one arm, breathe out and move opposite leg toward the midline. Repeat on other side. (See **Figure 15-7**.)
2. Lying on right side, bend left leg and place foot firmly on floor, lift right leg upward, keeping foot parallel to floor. Body bar also can be used for added resistance.

HIPS

Gluteus Medius.

1. Stand in boxing position with arms bent at elbows, press both feet into ground, tighten abdominal muscles, take a deep breath and turn body slightly inward toward the midlines so it is turned somewhat sideways. Breathing out, bend knees and lift the leg that is turned inward to kick outward. (See **Figure 15-8.**)

Figure 15-8: *Working the gluteus medius.*

BUTTOCKS

Gluteus Maximus.

1. *Step-Up:* Step onto a step with the left leg. Using a straight back, tighten abdominals to stabilize the left knee, then shift body weight on to left leg. With a soft left knee, lift the right foot to push off onto the steps, but do not place it directly on the step. Rather, hold for a few seconds and return the right foot to the floor slowly and under control. Repeat on the other side.

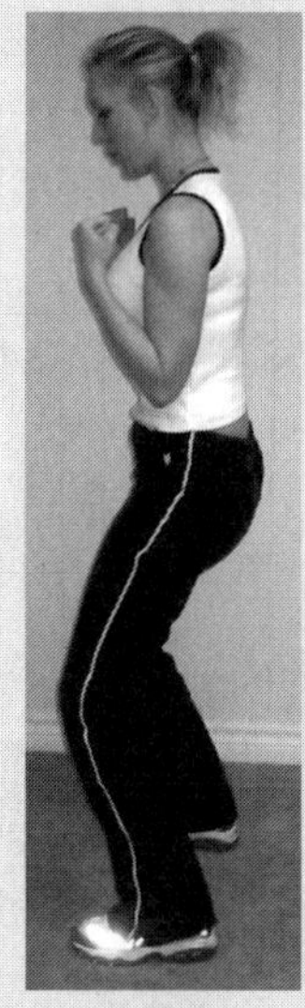

Figure 15-9: *Abdominal crunch.*

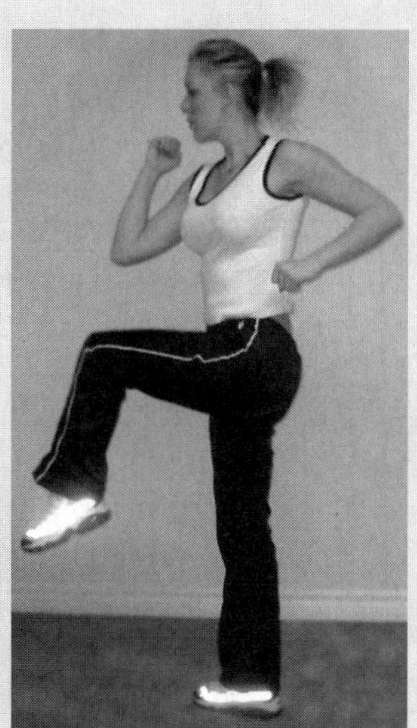

Figure 15-10: *Obliques.*

2. *Squats.* Holding onto body bar or chair, lower body in a squatting position, ensuring that the knees do not go over the feet. The most effective squats are when the body can be lowered to a position with thighs parallel to the floor. Keep shoulders and chest lifted and abdomen tight For those who have difficulty performing squats, try lunges instead.

ABDOMINALS

Rectus Abdominus.

1. Standing, perform abdominal crunch: breathe in, tighten abdominal muscles. Hold and breathe out as you release. (See **Figure 15-9**.)
2. Lying on back, press lower back and feet into floor. Tighten abdominals, and lift head and shoulders simultaneously. Keep head tucked in slightly to prevent neck from becoming tired, and breathe out as you come up. Breathe in as the body is lowered to the floor. To contract lower and upper abdominals, lift both legs simultaneously off floor at a 90 degree angle, and perform same movement.

Exercises for Main Muscle Groups *(cont.)*

Obliques.

1. Standing or lying, tighten abdomen. With palms placed at ears, meet elbows to opposite knee. (See **Figure 15-10**, page 232.)

Transverse Abdominus.

1. Standing with knees slightly bent, tighten abdominals, flex elbows and perform trunk twist. (See **Figure 15-11.**)

LOWER BACK

Erector Spinae.

1. Standing, feet together and holding onto body bar or chair, bend slightly forward and breathe out, lifting one arm straight upward and opposite foot backward simultaneously in a hyper-extended motion.

Dead lift.

1. With feet planted firmly into ground at hips distance apart, bend with flat back to pick up free weights or body bar. Maintain flat back, soft knees, keep arms close to body and slowly lift weights to standing position. Lower weights slowly to floor with soft knees and repeat.

Upper back

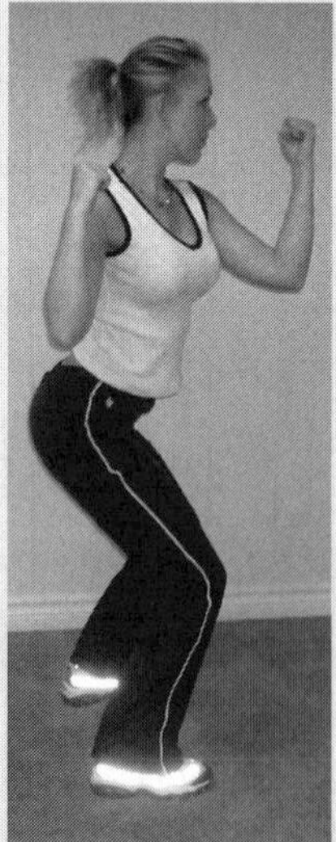

Figure 15-11: *Trunk twist.*

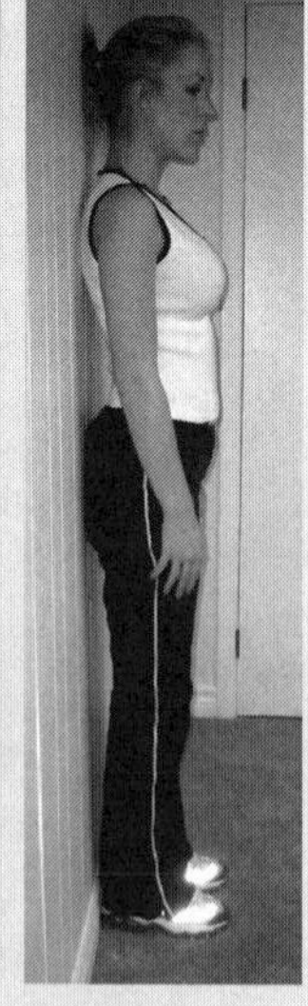

Figure 15-12: *Shoulder roll against the wall.*

1. Standing against a wall, place head, shoulders, lower back and back of heels against wall. With shoulders pushed against wall, breathe out. Relax shoulders and breathe in. (See **Figure 15-12.**)
2. *Yoga stance.* Standing, feet pressed into floor, abdomen tight, open up chest and turn shoulders outward, place palms of hands on the back of the upper hips and slowly slide to lower hips. This movement will push head and shoulders backward. Hold, breathe out and breathe in to come out of the movement in an upright position.

3. *Shoulder shrugs.* Standing erect, arms at sides, lift both shoulders up and then lower them.

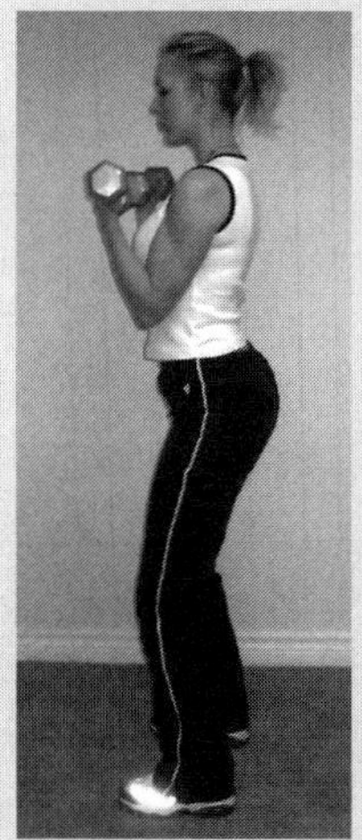

Figure 15-13: Bicep curls.

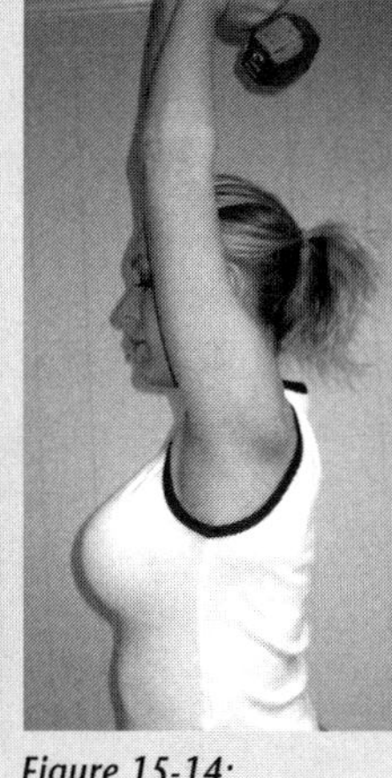

Figure 15-14: Triceps.

ARMS

Biceps.

1. *Biceps curl with free weights.* Can use full range, midrange or outer range to perform movement. (See **Figure 15-13**.)
2. *Hammer curl.* Lift weights using hammer-like movement.

Triceps.

1. Standing feet apart and firmly planted on floor, use both hands to hold free weights close to and above the head, bend elbows and lower weights to upper back between both scapulas, breathing out. Lift upward above head keeping arms close to head and breathe in. (See **Figure 15-14**.)
2. *Triceps kickbacks.* Stand at staggered position with left knee bent. Using left elbow pressed to left knee, lean forward, and bring right elbow up to shoulder level. Breathing out, extend the arm backward but keep it close to the sides of the body. Repeat on other side.

Deltoids

1. Standing, feet at hips width, tighten abdomen, soft knees, extend arms to lift light weights forward and upward to chest level breathing out. Breathe in as arms are lowered. (See **Figure 15-15**.)
2. Standing with feet closer together, soft knees, lift arms outward away from the midline.

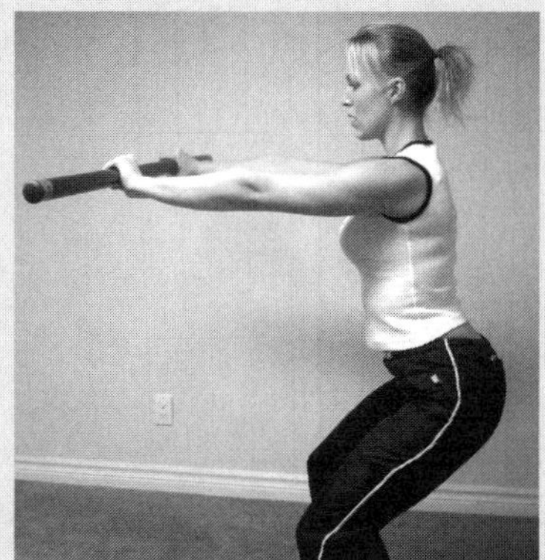

Figure 15-15: Deltoids.

CHAPTER 16

Cultural Foods

You always have been told not to talk politics and religion to clients because they are very controversial topics that may stimulate strong psychological reactions. On the other hand, food is a neutral and interesting subject that can bring people together, and the cultural perspective of various ethnic foods will not only greatly benefit the therapist, but also open up a wealth of information about food and culture. This chapter deals with information on the cuisine of some of the most common ethnic groups found in westernized societies. Within this chapter, you will learn about cultural tips, traditional values that have an impact on ethnic cuisine, some of the popular foods associated with these groups, key ingredients and traditional spices. At the conclusion of each ethnic food, general comments on the food's nutritional status are given.

Social and cultural aspects of food

Culture refers to beliefs, attitudes, values, customs, rituals and habits accepted and practiced by a community. Every country or region of a country has its own traditional or cultural ethnic diet. Social and political forces during the past decades have increased mass migrant flow throughout the world. Refugees from war-torn countries such as South Asia, certain European countries, Russia and certain South American countries have flooded developed nations such as the United States, Canada and Europe, changing the face of society forever.

The use of common foods among ethnic groups infers a sense of belonging, and they may represent comfort and happiness during stress or illness. **Assimilation** occurs when individuals from a culture shed their ethnic identity and fully merges with the mainstream culture, adopting most beliefs and behavioral patterns. As the new immigrant becomes acclimated into a new society, health perspectives and food habits may change as she becomes affected by new social and economic influences.

The first generation tries to maintain cultural heritage and eating patterns within the family, but as the second and third generations become acclimated, they adapt to their new environment, adopting the lifestyles of their peers and friends. Over many decades, the ethnic composition of cities has changed as did the clientele of the health and beauty profession.

In order to help treat people from other cultures or religions, therapists should learn more about their traditions and respect or honor their eating behaviors. Food is an excellent neutral topic that tends to create a close rapport between the client and the therapist. You need to know more about the composition of their traditional foods and how they are prepared. What are some of their traditional values and how do they affect health and eating behavior? Does their diet contain a high amount of fat or fiber? Do they eat meat or are they restricted from certain types of food? What are the typical seasonings used in the cooking their foods? Knowledge in these areas can help the skin care therapist advise their ethnic client more effectively without causing any unnecessary embarrassment.

Melting pot or multiculturalism

The proliferation of ethnic restaurants in cities such as New York, San Francisco, Toronto, Vancouver, London, Amsterdam, Capetown and Johannesburg, reflect the multicultural diversity of modern society. In the United States, the term **melting pot** is used to infer that numerous cultural groups have "melted" into the mainstream group—the American culture practiced by everyone. Also in the United States, as well as Canada, the term **multicultural** is forged to suggest that each ethnic group can exist peacefully alongside one another and carry on their individual cultural norms without restrictions.

For example, a survey in Toronto indicated more than 80 ethnic groups lived in the city and surrounding areas. The cultural mosaic is reflected in the large number of ethnic enclaves that have evolved from the large ethnic communities such as Chinatown, Little Italy, Greektown, Little Korea, Japantown and huge German populations that dominate some cities.

Cuisines that were confined to large cities are working their way into smaller ones, acquiring new prominence as second and third generations of immigrants who are firmly entrenched in their adopted country begin to take time to rediscover their cultural roots. These new generations also are developing exciting tastes in foods and making new social friends in the undertaking. Cookbooks about ethnic cuisine are plentiful in bookstores and cooking classes while multicultural food festivals are quite popular in the summer when people of all nations come out to investigate and try new foods and flavors. Many shelves in supermarkets are devoted to ethnic food products, and a wider selection of herbs and spices now are more available than ever before.

New world cuisine

The impact of cultural, social and economic factors on traditional foods therefore is dependent on complex and dynamic factors. Subcultural diets of "American-style" foods such as egg rolls, spaghetti, tortillas and pita breads have evolved over time. This phenomenon is the result of influence of environment and the availability or lack of certain ingredients necessary for making the traditional food.

In recent years, several cultural foods that had been modified to local tastes are now re-emerging in far more authentic and satisfying forms as the imports of these foods became more available. Food also can be used to express social status. For example, champagne and caviar imply wealth, and sushi is the new trend among the middle to upper class.

The explosion of Pacific Rim trade and the emergence of a black entrepreneurial class in North America, the Caribbean and West Africa also have inspired new tastes in restaurant foods. Because of closer social interaction in a new environment, traditional diets of various cultural groups begin to blend, resulting in several different cuisines over time, referred to **fusion foods**.

Dominant ethnic foods

The three main factors that differentiate cuisines of the world are spices, cooking methods and, to a lesser degree, specific local food components. Although many European countries form the base of the American cuisine, at the current time, the most popular ethnic cuisines in Western societies include Asian, particularly Chinese and Japanese, in addition to Italian and Mexican foods. The following information may lead to a better understanding of various ethnic foods and their traditions.

Asian—Chinese. Asians are the fastest growing ethnic group in America. Asian foods include those of the Far East, such as Chinese, Thai, Japanese, Korean, Vietnamese and Filipino. Almost everyone loves Chinese food, and it is the most common and popular Asian food. Chinese restaurants are found in almost in every town or city in the world.

Chinese cuisine varies depending on which part of China it originated. For example, noodles, buns and pancakes made from wheat and grains are popular for those who come from Northern China, rice and lightly seasoned Cantonese food come from southern China, and hot spicy Szechwan and Hunan dishes come from inland China.

In North America, Chinese-American foods dominate in most communities because they are comparatively inexpensive and quick to prepare making them very popular even among other ethnic groups. The Chinese diet is perhaps the most balanced of all ethnic foods since it incorporates a wide variety of fresh vegetables and small portions of meat in bite-sized forms. Rice is the main staple that originated in China and is washed and steamed with no salt. Although the Chinese eat fruits, they do not use a large variety.

Traditional health beliefs and practices. The Chinese maintain health through a properly balanced diet, adequate sleep and moderate activity. Chinese medicine includes a complex system of using the services of both physicians as well as folk remedies used at home. Health beliefs and practices developed over generations incorporate the teachings of Confucian, Taoist and Buddhism.

The concept of harmony involves the balance of **yin**, or cold, and **yang**, or hot. The Chinese believe that symptoms of diseases usually reflect an imbalance between yin and yang. This includes acne, rashes, hemorrhoids, constipation, weight loss and various infections.

The vital energy force is **chi** which flows along meridian lines in the body—some conditions are believed to be related to the disruption of this force. The Chinese believe that chi must flow freely and blood must be strengthened through nourishment. The theory holds that foods should be chosen to help balance the body in the cosmic scheme—hot foods should be consumed in the winter, and cold foods in the summer. Hot to warm-humored foods such as lamb, beef, shrimp, peppers and garlic increase circulation and energy, while cool to cold-humored foods such as bean curd, green vegetables and crab, relax and detoxify the body.

In addition to yin and yang, they believe that some foods affect the blood and promote wound healing. For example, yin is a negative force associated with "weak blood" that occurs during pregnancy, postpartum and post-surgical procedures, and is treated with yang, associated with hot, protein-rich foods made of whole chickens, port liver, eggs and wine. They also use large amounts of medicinal herbs such as ginseng, royal jelly and garlic to restore harmony.

Cultural foods. A variety of animal protein foods are consumed, but only small amounts in one meal, as compared to Westerners. In fact, 8-oz. of meat will be chopped up into numerous small pieces and stir fried with large amounts of vegetables or noodles for a family. Pork is the favorite meat, and most foods either are stir fried, steamed or boiled.

Chinese cuisine thrives on the freshest ingredients, and a huge variety of fresh vegetables are used so that the Chinese diet is high in vitamins, minerals and fiber. Many Chinese are lactose intolerant and do not consume many dairy products. However, Chinese-Americans have adapted and are consuming dairy products. Calcium is obtained from the daily consumption of soybean curd, small boned fish and poultry. In addition, calcium in various forms such as plain boiled beans, dried beans, bean sprouts, fermented bean paste and oy milk are popular.

Chinese foods in America tend to be overly greasy and not as healthy because they incorporate the usage of cornstarch, sugar, salt and monosodium glutamate (MSG) in the less expensive restaurants. However, the opening up of trade with China to the world has enabled traditional Chinese foods and spices to be brought into America so that authentic Chinese foods are returning to healthier states.

In comparison to other ethnic groups, the Chinese use an extensive assortment of vegetables including bamboo shoots, water chestnuts and a large variety of greens such as spinach, mustard and bok choy.

Tea time for the Chinese is very popular for lunch on the weekends when entire families meet at restaurants for the traditional lunch get-together called dim sum. Hundreds of different dumplings stuffed with meats or vegetables are either steamed or deep fried, placed in small bowls and rolled around on trolleys, and the number of bowls taken from the trolleys is charged to the table. Even non-Chinese diners enjoy dim sum, and it has become so popular that it is now offered every day instead of only on weekends.

The Chinese do not normally eat a lot of pastries, but instead prefer fresh fruit such as sliced oranges for dessert after dinner. However, in the past decade, many pastry shops have emerged to appease the American taste for sweetness even in Hong Kong. Hot soup or tea usually accompanies meals. Tea, particularly jasmine, black and green tea, is taken with all meals.

Nutritional status. The traditional Chinese diet is low in fat, cholesterol and dairy products, and high in complex carbohydrates. Due to the high consumption of soy, sodium also is high. However, over past decades, the Chinese-American diet has changed considerably with an increasing amount of fats, protein, sugar, cholesterol, salt and less complex carbohydrates.

A study by Scultz et al in 1994 found that American Chinese possessed higher levels of knowledge about nutrients, and their diet contained more nutrients than their foreign-born counterparts or white Americans. They also onsumed milk and milk products. Cardiovascular disease is low among the Chinese in China, but the risk of cancer has been found to increase among cculturated Chinese. Living a long and healthy life is a priority for the Chinese.

Asian—Japanese. A 1990 Census indicated that more than 866,000 Japanese-Americans live in the United States, of which approximately 70% live in California and Hawaii. A large Japanese population also lives in Brazil. In the past decade, an influx of Japanese restaurants has developed in almost every large modern city in the Western world. It is trendy to eat sushi, and people appear to love Japanese food. In Vancouver and San Francisco, Japanese fast food restaurants have appeared everywhere, many of them being run by non-Japanese chefs who see tremendous potential in serving Japanese food. Many of Japan's staples include tea, soy products, noodles and chopsticks, all proof of its deep cultural roots to China.

Traditional values. The Japanese come from a very high context culture and place high priority on preserving harmony with society. Formality and politeness are important in effective communication. They do not use prolonged eye contact and avoid physical contact with other people, therefore, it is very important to use appropriate communication when dealing with them. They do not believe in showing any display of emotions, especially anger, and older Japanese-Americans should not be addressed by their first names. The Japanese do not like to be criticized in their health habits because any loss of accomplishment is a form of "losing face." Using an unhurried, in-depth interview to determine the amount of acclimation will help to determine the best form of communication with them.

Cultural foods. Japanese cooking is noted for its simplicity of flavors and minimal use of sauces. It consists of a variety of nutrient-rich seaweed, fresh and dried fish, a wide use of soy-based foods and little oils attract health conscious diners. Fresh fish include salmon, mackerel, eel, clams, crab—real or imitation, yellowtail, octopus, shrimp and oysters. Fish eggs are a very popular sushi ingredient. Rice, miso soup, **sashimi**—plain raw seafood and seaweed, all are Japanese staples and commonly served with **sake**, or Japanese wine. Although **sukiyaki**, or thinly-sliced meat stew, and **tempura**—fried foods, have been around North America for more than 50 years, it was **sushi** that made a breakthrough for most Americans as the most popular ethnic lunch since pizza.

The difference between sashimi and sushi is that sashimi is served by itself, whereas sushi is draped over a bite-sized roll of seasoned rice called **nigiri** and then rolled with **nori** sheets—dark green paper made from algae rolled into logs then sliced. This is then called **maki**, or rolled sushi, and also can be served as a hand roll. Not all sushi is raw, and some of the seafood is precooked. (See **Figure 16-1**, on page 251.)

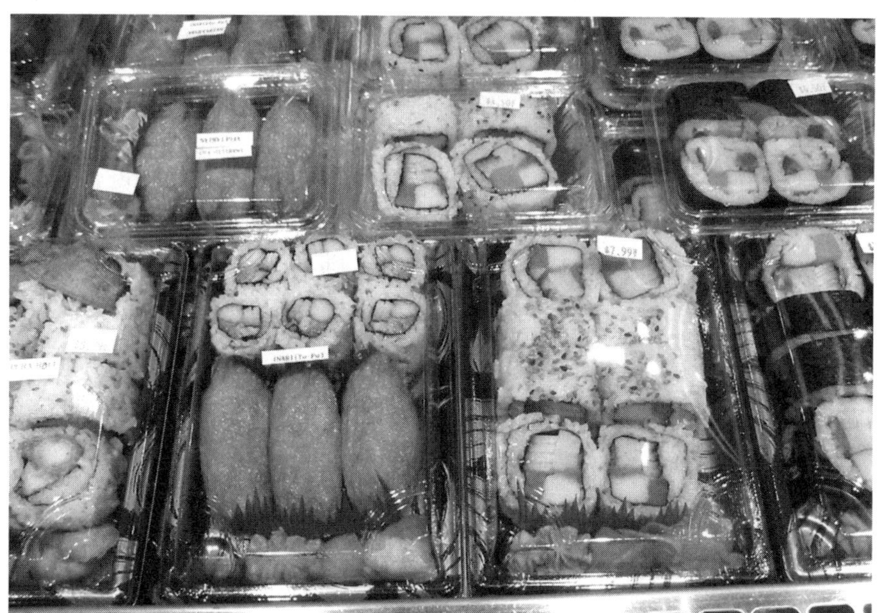

Figure 16-1: Popular sushi dishes.

Condiments served with Japanese food include soy sauce, pickled ginger and **wasabi**—a hot green paste that tastes like horseradish. Recent trends in Japanese restaurants appear to be using American ingredients such as mayonnaise, chili sauce and other sauces for a larger effect. Here again is the never-ending American effect on a healthy diet!

The Japanese utilize soybeans and its by-products in various forms of tofu, such as bean curd cakes, **miso**, or fermented soybean paste, and a liberal use of soy sauce. Soybeans, served fresh in their pods, called **edamame**, usually are lightly salted as appetizers or snacks. Pickled vegetables such as cucumbers, eggplant, cabbage and radishes are essential in the Japanese diet, but fresh vegetables are limited and served grilled and fried.

Noodles are very popular with the Japanese and are offered as **soba**, or buckwheat, or **udon**, soft, fat and plain. The Japanese do not eat a large variety of fruits, except for persimmons, grapes, melons and pineapples. Healthy green tea is served with most meals. Desserts are limited in the Japanese diet except for ice cream and sliced fruits.

Nutritional status. Japanese cooking does not use many dairy products, and many Japanese are lactose intolerant. They obtain their calcium from high consumption of soy foods, small bony fish and seaweed. However, traditional diets are high in sodium consumed from soy sauces and pickled vegetables. Like the Chinese, their diet is low in fat and cholesterol. However, in recent years, second generation Japanese have now adapted to the American diet of eating more rice, fat and dairy products, and this change may contribute to increased incidence of several diseases such as colon cancer, type II diabetes and heart diseases. It would be beneficial if they used semi-sweet dipping sauces instead of soy sauce to reduce their high sodium consumption, and eat a wider variety of fruits and vegetables to increase vitamin and mineral intake.

A comparison of Asian alcohol drinking habits showed that Japanese-American men and women drank quite heavily.

Hispanic. The terms *Hispanic* and *Latino* refer to the Spanish language of the conquistadors that underlies the language of Mexico and Central America. However, the cuisine of this region still is dependent on the Indians who dominated the population at that time. As a result, the staples of chilies, tomatoes, beans, avocados, nuts, sweet potatoes and corn form the basis of the Hispanic diet. The vast migration of Mexicans into United States over past decades have demographers predicting that the Hispanic population will dominate America during this millennium, even surpassing African-Americans as the largest United States minority. As a result, many demographers have begun to study the economical and social impact of this ethnic group in the United States.

Understanding the beliefs and values of this population would help the health and beauty professional to communicate more effectively with them. Hispanics constitute a large segment of the population in the United States, particularly in California and Texas, while Cubans dominate the state of Florida. Hispanics are moving up in society, and there are many signs that their socioeconomic status has improved significantly.

Traditional health beliefs and practices. The well-being of the family is placed before the needs of the individual in Hispanic culture, and the father is the head of the household. Hispanic families are large and children are cherished. Mexicans are traditionally superstitious people and often use home remedies for treating illness before a healer is sought for further help.

Cultural foods—Mexico. The majority of Mexicans come from lower socioeconomic class and mostly eat vegetable protein, although some eat pork, goat and common meats. The main staple of Mexican food is tortillas or flatbread with corn and rice products used throughout Mexico. True Mexican food is either grilled, stewed or braised in clay pots with rice, beans or meat stews. Although

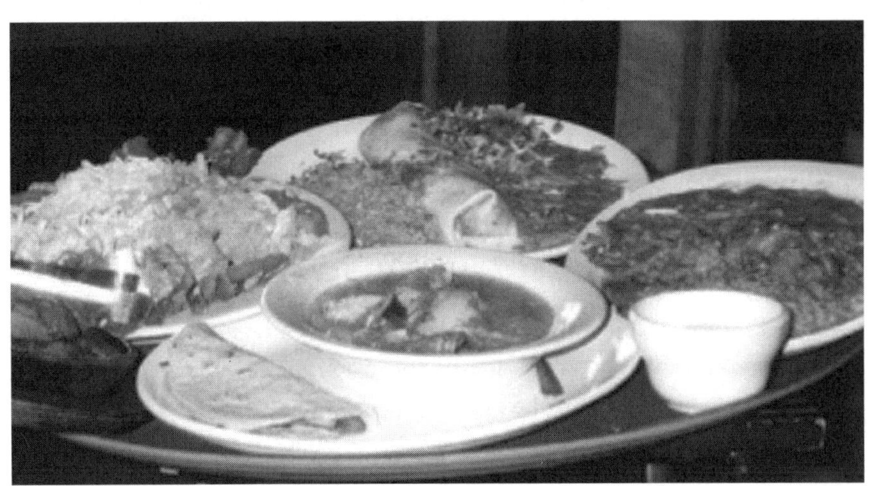

Figure 16-2: *Mexican food.*

more than 92 varieties of chilies are used in Mexican cooking, not all Mexican foods are hot and spicy. Mexicans, many of whom are lactose intolerant, do not consume many dairy products. Pork is the main meat, and organ meats are extremely popular. Cheese is used liberally in most dishes and **chorizo**, a spicy, unsmoked pork sausage, is a common item found at the street vendor. Fruits and vegetables are served as part of a dish, the most popular ones being avocado in the form of **guacamole** where it is mashed and seasoned, bananas, guava, papaya and mangoes.

Legumes constitute many Mexican specialties and include black, garbanzo, pinto and kidney beans, and are stuffed in pancake-like flatbreads such as tacos, enchiladas, tamales, quesadillas and burritos.

Eggs commonly are used in tortillas that are popular not only among Mexican-Americans, but other ethnic groups as well. The most common beverages are coffee and soft drinks. Popular desserts such as **flan** and **huevos reales** contain eggs with sugar, as well as fresh fruit blended with sugar and water. Alcohol is consumed at all occasions. (See **Figure 16-2.**)

Cultural foods—Puerto Rico and Cuba. Puerto Rican cuisine adopted more of the Spanish heritage. It contains more meat than other Caribbean countries because of it being influenced by Europeans who were their trading partners early in the 19th century. Paella, a rice casserole studded with shellfish and ham, is a very popular dish in Puerto Rico. On the other hand, Cuban food is not as highly spiced as that of Puerto Rico, and their national dish is black beans. Cubans rarely use fresh fruit or fruit salsas in their meals, but tend to drink juices or eat fresh fruit separately.

Nutritional status. Many Mexican-Americans eat a diet high in protein that is similar to that of their homeland, but acclimated Mexicans often adopt an American-like diet. A study by Bartholomew et al in 1990 found that in general, Mexican-Americans eat fewer beans and prefer sweetened fruit drinks to blended fruit drinks. They consume more fat, especially fried foods, and fewer fruits and vegetables than other Anglos of similar backgrounds. The obesity rates among people of Mexican descent have risen significantly, and they are two to four times more likely to be overweight than Caucasians. In addition, their consumption of alcohol generally also is high and may lead to liver problems. However, many Latino women believe that extra weight is a sign of health and well-being, especially after marriage, and obesity often is perceived as a status symbol. Researchers also have noted that deficiencies of calcium and riboflavin exist among many second generation Mexican-Americans.

Caribbean. These 1,000 islands of the Caribbean stretching from Florida to Venezuela are a tropical paradise attracting vacationers from all countries, particularly North America and Europe. Caribbean cuisine has been influenced by people who settled there from Africa, Britain, France, India, Portugal and Spain. Although each island has its own particular traditional food, the foods from the various islands can be classified as Caribbean cuisine. People from the Caribbean, especially Jamaica and Trinidad, have settled in different parts of North America and formed several small enclaves in larger cities where they have access to traditional spices and foods. Most Caribbean people are lactose intolerant.

Cultural foods. The daily fare in the Caribbean is three meals a day, where both lunch and dinner are heavy, usually consisting of meat, rice and peas. Caribbean fare consists of assorted meats, often stewed together with legumes and special spices. The most dominant Caribbean food is Jamaican which uses many spices including jerk that is rubbed on beef, goat, poultry and fish, which then is grilled or stewed. **Ackee**, a signature dish of Jamaicans, is a peapod containing yellow flesh that looks like scrambled eggs when cooked, but has a lemony flavor. Food is well seasoned with onions, peppers, garlic and all spices, and therefore usually is spicy. There is a tendency to use coconut oil that is high in saturated fats in cooking, posing a high risk for coronary disease.

Goat, pork, mutton and oxtail are popular and usually curried. Savory patties are very popular as snacks. The population uses a lot of salted meats, particularly salted codfish, in cooking. The Caribbean diet is very starchy, the main staples being corn, bread, fruit, cassava, rice, sweet potatoes and yams, with pumpkin as the most common squash. Plantains, a vegetable from the banana family, as well as green bananas are either fried or boiled and served with rice. Soups are very hearty and filling such as **calalloo**, or **pepperpot**, a vegetable and Creole soup containing salted meats and a wide variety of different vegetables. The Caribbean's diet is colorful and varied—often based on home grown organic fruits and vegetables. The emphasis is on heavy starches so that leafy vegetables and fresh fruits are limited fare. Milk is not used much in the Caribbean islands except for cow's milk, but Caribbean people living in North America now have adapted to drinking more milk. Rum is cheap and popular in the islands. Some of the most popular desserts are various puddings, mixed fruit salads, coconut custard and ginger cakes.

Nutritional status. The overall daily intake of high saturated fats, high sodium and heavy, starchy foods have resulted in high rates of obesity among the Caribbean people. Many of them suffer from high rates of coronary diseases, including high blood pressure, high cholesterol levels and type II diabetes.

Inadequate intake of leafy vegetables and fruits result in deficiencies of vitamins A, C and water-soluble fiber. Calcium deficiency results from low intake of milk and milk products. It would be healthier if sodium was reduced in food preparation, the use of coconut oil was eliminated and less meat, particularly salted meat, was consumed. A variety of green, leafy vegetables and fresh fruit should be added in their daily diet to reduce important vitamin deficiencies.

Indian. Asian-Indians are one of the fastest growing immigrant groups in the North America, coming from numerous states and regions of India. This ethnic group recognizes the importance of higher education in their advancement in the new society, and they sacrifice a great deal to send their children to universities. As a result, many of them have improved their financial and social status in their new homeland.

The cold weather in the United States, Canada and Europe play havoc with their skin and bodies, and, consequently, many of them seek treatments and products to improve their complexion by visiting skin care centers. The skin care therapist can make this ethnic group feel welcome by using food as a neutral topic to create a bond with them.

Traditional values. If you are dealing with Indian culture, it is necessary to have some knowledge about the influence of religion on dietary patterns. In addition, the caste system that placed Brahmins—physicians and professionals—at the top of the hierarchy and the Untouchables at the lowest level that existed for centuries, presently is outlawed, but still affects many individuals. The great majority of Indians are Hindus, followed by Muslims. One of every nine Asian-Indian is Muslim and the influence of Islam is seen, particularly in Northern India. Buddhism is a religion that is followed by less than 1% of Indians.

The husband is the head of the household, and the wife does not work, but is expected to perform all household duties as well take care of the children. When Indian families migrate to North America, conflicts may occur when the wife goes out to work and enjoys more freedom. In several cases, when the wife wants to have beauty treatments, the husband is willing to take her to the health and beauty center and wait for her. It is interesting to note that in many instances, the wife saves a portion of her household money to buy beauty products, sometimes without her husband's knowledge.

Hindus celebrate many festivals. The most important etiquette in India is that food is eaten with the hands, so cleanliness is important when handling food. Indians never offer food from their plates to another person, and rarely save leftovers in order to maintain sanitation. These practices are important symbols of the Indian relationship with food.

Cultural foods. About 30% of Asian-Indians are strict vegetarian, but others vary depending on the religious sect, caste group or the part of the country from which the individual hails. Ayurvedic medicine has emphasized the role of diet in health maintenance and, like all Asians, Indians also believe in the hot and cold classification system used for foods and their effects on the body.

For example, a balance of hot and cold foods is necessary for good health. Asian-Indians believe that a person should eat in a quiet atmosphere, sip warm water throughout and sit for a short while after dining. The different religious groups in India follow different dietary practices, but all of an Indian flavor. Cattle are the main economic power in India, since most people make their living from farming. Indians have a reverence for all life, and the cow is viewed as a sacred symbol.

Indians from the northern and southern parts of the country have different dietary patterns. The main Indian staple is rice, particularly the aromatic one called *basmati.* In general, those that come from the north of India eat more meat, drier dishes and breads, more wheat and use seasonings with Persian flavorings such as nuts, sweets, rosewater and saffron. Indians from the south consume more vegetables, wetter stews and rice, lentils and rice for dough and use seasonings such as ginger, garlic, chilies, cardamom, cinnamon, cloves and coconut milk. *Marsalas* are mixtures of spices and herbs that can be either fresh or dried. In other words, the food is spicier in the south than north. Pork is considered "unclean," and Muslims avoid pork and pork products, but are not vegetarians. (See **Figure 16-3.**)

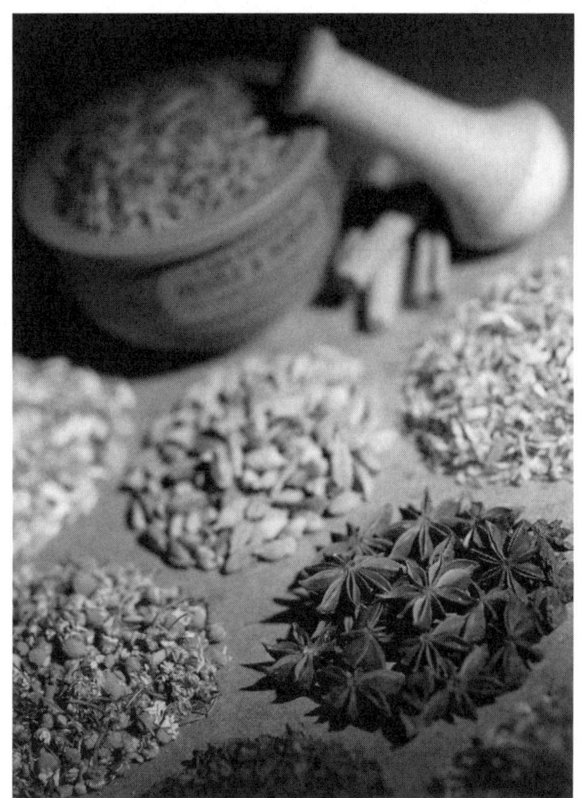

Figure 16-3: *Indian spices used for healthy cooking.*

Hindus and Buddhists do not eat any beef or pork. Beef is limited, but lamb, goat and chicken are the most popular meats, particularly in the north. Northern Indians drink tea, while coffee mainly is consumed in the south. Various cooking oils give flavors to Indian food. Small portions of meat are used, and many dishes are steamed, roasted, grilled or baked. Grains and legumes, especially lentils and beans, are used and little dairy is used except for low fat yogurt.

The most common breads are the flat, pita-like **chapatti** and **naan**, a flaky leavened bread from white or whole wheat flour that looks like a popover. Meat is placed in the rotis, rolled, and then eaten with the hands.

The most important dairy products are ghee, cheese and yogurt. **Ghee** is clarified butter that is boiled, the surface fat skimmed off then filtered, resulting in a finer, smoother form of butter. However, it has become too expensive, and other vegetable oils now are being used. Cheese or yogurt usually is mixed in curries; yogurt being used as an alternative to coconut milk or cream.

Dal refers to the different kinds of lentils that are usually pureed or stewed, sometimes with potatoes and peas that are very popular in Indian cuisine. **Samosas** are deep fried turnovers filled with spicy lamb, potatoes or vegetables.

Tandoori cooking is using a special clay oven heated with charcoal to cook meat or bread. Common vegetables such as okra, broad beans or spinach are pureed, stewed or fried with spices such as onions, tumeric, salt, mustard, cumin seeds and coriander.

Fruit is plentiful, especially mangoes, papayas and coconut, one of the building blocks of Indian cuisine. The most common relish is **chutney**, similar to salsa, and is a combination of fruit and vegetables mixed with spices eaten with main dishes.

Indians do not eat many sweets except on special occasions. Desserts include various puddings and sweetbreads, and beer is the most common beverage due to the spiciness of the curries.

The majority of Indian restaurants in the United States are described as either northern or southern style cooking. Indian-Americans accept American foods when eating out, but prefer Asian-Indian foods at home. However, young Asian-Indian-Americans, especially students, eventually become vulnerable to the fast food lifestyle of America and eventually suffer the same health problems, such as coronary disease and type II diabetes.

Nutritional status. Indian cuisine is quite healthy with little meat, a high proportion of grains and legumes, and little alcohol consumption. The diet mainly is vegetarian based, with low intake of dairy products. However, the diet is low in quality protein, and Indians will find difficulty in building larger muscle mass and strength in weight training. Perhaps that is why most Indians are of small stature—mainly ectomorphic body type. The high amount of vegetables and legumes, although mostly pureed, contain high fiber and most vitamins and minerals.

With their low consumption of meat, B-12 will be a nutritional consideration for many Indians since this vitamin only is found in meat products. Without this vitamin, homocysteine levels may be high, leading to higher risk of cardiovascular disease. Iron deficiency also may be expected due to the low levels of red meat consumed. Several studies have indicated that rates of heart disease and diabetes are higher among Asian-Indian immigrants than among Caucasians, regardless of religious background or vegetarian diet. This finding is hypothesized to hereditary differences in lipid metabolism, according to Thomas et all, 1986.

Europeans—Greeks. Current demographics indicate that the largest Greek concentrations are located in the urban areas of New York City, California and Florida in the United States, as well as Montreal and Toronto in Canada. Greek food has become very popular in western societies because it is considered one of the healthier diets of the Mediterranean cuisine. It is covered in this chapter because many North Americans partake in Greek cuisine regularly and, in some cities, Greek cultural festivals draw thousands of people to visit, eat their foods and enjoy their culture.

Traditional values. The traditional Greek family believes in a solid patriarchal base with strong family ties to extended families. Greeks predominantly are Eastern Orthodox in their religious beliefs, and traditional Greeks use home care remedies such as herbal teas when they are ill.

Food plays an important role in celebrating special occasion such as weddings or religious events, and there are numerous feasts and fasting days throughout the year. The most important festival is Easter where families get together to celebrate with red dyed Easter eggs and lots of food. Greek Americans also celebrate Greek Independence Day with folk dancing, songs and traditional dress. At celebrations such as weddings, it is traditional for men to perform special dancing such as saltatio during which you may hear the cheer "opa" when platters are thrown and broken.

Historically, Greek women have always been extremely interested in beauty because of *Aphrodite*, the Goddess of Love and Beauty, and they constantly are seeking opportunities to enhance their appearance.

Cultural foods. Many ingredients essential to Greek cuisine include grape leaves, goat cheese and olive oil. The olive tree is a key element in cooking and extra virgin oil is a staple, even in chain supermarkets. There is a high incidence of lactose intolerance among Greeks. Although fresh milk is used in puddings, it is not widely consumed in Greece. Most dairy products are derived from fermented milk such as yogurt, and cheese usually is made from goat, sheep or camel milk. **Feta cheese**, a sharp, salty, semi-soft cheese commonly is used in salads.

All meats including beef, baby goat, lamb and pork are eaten, but the most popular meat is lamb. It usually is marinated, grilled or roasted as **kebabs** on a spit called souvlas from which the name **souvlaki** developed, a common feature seen in Greek restaurants and shops.

Greeks are well known for the liberal use of fresh herbs and spices such as garlic, parsley, mint, bay, rosemary and oregano. Lemon often is used for flavoring, as well. Garlic is associated with antibiotic properties to boost the body's immunity. However, some individuals must be aware that the liberal use of this herb permeates the skin emitting a powerful odor that may be distasteful to people around them.

Bread and grains are eaten at most meals, particularly **pita** bread, a thin, round, Arabic bread with a hollow center which has become very popular in North American cities. Legumes form a regular part of Greek cooking and **hummus**, cooked, pureed chickpeas, popularly is used as a dip or appetizer. Although many vegetables are eaten, eggplant is the most popular. **Moussaka** is a cultural casserole made from eggplant or potatoes.

The most famous dessert is **baklava**, a phyllo pastry drenched in sugar, syrup and nuts and served on all occasions. Coffee and tea often are flavored with cardamom, mint and heavy sweeteners.

Nutritional status. Greek food generally is inexpensive, and many large cities have developed a Greektown where their cultural foods and customs are practiced and maintained. The traditional Greek diet is considered healthy because a lot of fish and more monounsaturated fats such as olive oil, are consumed. Greek salads with feta cheese and vegetables followed by a variety of fruits, especially watermelon and grapes, are very high in vitamins A and C, and fiber.

In general, Greeks consume a greater amount of food than Americans, but do not seem to gain weight because their meal portions are small. However, Greek cuisine in America may have changed with the second generation adopting the American lifestyle of high sugar, high fat foods. Olive oil still is entrenched in their cooking, and they still eat salads and fresh fruits with their meals. However, beef and pork are eaten more often, and the consumption of legumes has decreased.

Greek-Americans drink more milk and ice cream is very popular. Studies have indicated that because Greek-Americans respect authoritative figures, they are more receptive to verbal rather than written communication, and if they do not understand the question, they may provide answers just to please the therapist. They value privacy and are hesitant to disclose personal history until a trusting relationship has been established. Knowledge of their traditional values and cultural foods can help to establish that trust, and they can become very good clients for the health and beauty profession.

Europeans—Italians.

Traditional values. Historically, Italians are of strong Roman Catholic faith.

Italian food has been referred to as "Mama's cooking" and typically is depicted by an image of an Italian "mama" spoiling her son by always dishing out a feast for him. Italian cuisine actually is multicultural, and Italian restaurants proliferate throughout many cities around the world. In North America, Italian cuisine often is thought of as olive oils, salads and crusty breads.

Cultural foods. In Italy, cuisine varies from the north to the south. In northern Italy, more dairy products are used while in the south, little meat and more beans and vegetables such as artichokes, eggplant, bell peppers and tomatoes are consumed.

For example, in the north, pasta for which the Italians are famous is made with eggs in the shape of flat ribbons, filled with cheese or meat, such as *ravioli*, and served with cream sauce, while in the south, pasta is not made from eggs, but is tubular shaped and topped with tomato sauce. Pastas are named for their shapes. For example, spiral pastas are called **fusilli** and **rotelle**, tubular noodles can be smooth but angle-shaped such as **penne**, or grooved, **rigatoni**. Stuffed pastas, such as dumplings, can be little rings, such as **tortellini**, while **manicotti** is a square with a filling. When it is rectangular and stuffed with chicken, it assumes a new name—**cannelloni**.

Typical seasonings include fresh garlic, parsley and basil. Southern Italian food is therefore low fat until sauces containing high fat and high sodium cheeses such as parmesan are added. Italians are famous for the production of cheese that may be made from the milk of the cow, goat, sheep or buffalo. Italians produce both hard cheeses such as **parmesan** and **romano**, and soft cheeses such as **mozzarella**, **ricotta** and **fontina**.

The controversy about who first invented pizza never goes away, but many people believe that it started with the Greeks, who passed it on to the Italians. Italians make bread from a huge array of flours, such as hard wheat, semolina, soy, barley, bran and cornmeal, also used to make pizza. They do not use butter, but instead dip their breads into a small bowl of extra virgin oil that sometimes is mixed with a little balsamic vinegar. This is a healthy way of reducing the consumption of butter or trans fatty acids.

The crusts of traditional pizza are thin, but in **focaccia**, the crust is thicker. **Gnocchi** are dumplings made from semolina wheat, and **pesto** is a paste made from cheese, among other things. **Gorgonzola** is a fine blue cheese, and ricotta is a mild, slightly grainy, but very soft cheese made from reboiling cow's milk. **Antipastas** are appetizers which can be cold or warm such as **bruschetta**, toasted bread crusts liberally rubbed with olive oil, garlic and sometimes tomatoes. **Prosciutto** is raw, salted, air-cured ham that is a popular antipasta served hot or cold at social events such as weddings.

This Mediterranean diet favors fish, roast veal and chicken, with **cacciatore**, chicken stewed in wine with onions and tomatoes, a favorite on Italian menus. **Risotto**, a creamy rice dish cooked in butter and chicken stock, is the most popular way of serving rice. **Anchovies** are commonly served with meats, while balsamic vinegar and green olives are used as condiments.

The mixed greens with a touch of bitterness include **radicchio**, **escarole**, **arugula** and **romaine**, and they often are served with fresh mozzarella cheese and extra virgin olive oil. Cruciferous vegetables such as broccoli, cauliflower, brussel sprouts, artichokes and wild mushrooms are served very simply with no sauces. The inclusion of fresh fruits and wines, particularly red wine, with meals makes this Mediterranean diet a very healthy and popular one. Desserts often consists of fruits and cheese, and like most Europeans, Italians love their strong espresso coffee made from very finely ground beans that have been pressed and forced with steaming water and served with no milk in very small cups.

Nutritional status. This diet, characterized by a low meat consumption, high intake of complex carbohydrates with an emphasis on grains, legumes, vegetables and fruits, is low fat with high monounsaturated fats from olive oils, and moderate alcohol consumption. In general, the traditional Mediterranean diet, particularly that of southern Italy, reflects a health-promoting diet to reduce cardiovascular disease and promote weight loss.

European—German.

Traditional values. In many American cities, huge populations of German immigrants have settled hundreds of years ago so that the German diet has been modified and assimilated in American foods. As a result, a great deal of German cooking has been incorporated into American cuisine with the "meat and potatoes" philosophy of the Germans forming the base of many American meals.

Common American foods such as pretzels, hamburgers and frankfurters have been derived from German immigrants. Most people do not realize that the tradition of the Christmas tree was derived from the Germans when the tree was decorated with cookies and candies.

Cultural foods. The rich cuisine of German food incorporates the use of heavy organ meats, sausages, dairy products, dumpling soup and smoked meats. In addition, consumption of the traditional salted pickles such as **sauerkraut**, followed by heavy bouts of beer drinking, makes it one of the heaviest ethnic diets. Food often is preserved by being dried, pickled and fermented.

In Germany, wheat is difficult to grow in the cold temperature so bread often is made with rye and other grains, resulting in darker colors and hardier breads. There are numerous varieties of bread. German breads are made from healthy whole grains using no preservatives and little or no sugar. They include hearty, dark nutritious bread high in protein such as pumpernickel, whole grain rye and muesli which is a mixture of toasted grains, e.g. oats, wheat, millet, barley, whet germ, dried fruits, nuts and seeds.

Traditional German cuisine is rich in game, venison, roebuck and rabbit, with goose and duck being the favorites. However beef, pork and lamb are used more commonly today. They often are lightly breaded and fried, and then called **schnitzel**.

Germans are famous for pork and its by-products and for various sausages prepared in different ways, especially in smoked forms. **Knackwurst** is made of pork and beef seasoned with garlic and cumin while **wiener** is a smoked mixture of lean pork and bacon fat. In North America, **bratwurst** sausage, cured pork and beef that is air dried and smoked, is very popular for grilling.

The most common seasonings used include vinegar, mustard, horseradish, black pepper and honey. Germans use dairy products such as butter, sour cream and buttermilk widely with eggs and cheese often is eaten as a main dish. Mashed potatoes, a mainstay of German fare, often are mixed with apples. Other common vegetables include asparagus, cabbage, carrots and green peppers.

Although Germans traditionally ate five meals a day, nowadays they tend to eat three meals a day with a lighter lunch and heavier dinner. Desserts usually are lavish pastries such as **strudel**, pastry that usually is stuffed with ground apples, and **black forest cake**, layered chocolate cake with cherries, served with **espresso**. Another popular dessert is **marzipan**, a paste of ground almonds and sugar sold in coffee houses and bakeries. Guests usually are not invited for dinner, but may come for dessert and wine later on in the evening. Of course, German wines and beers must not be forgotten. **Octoberfest** is an ethnic festival that is celebrated in many large German communities annually and people drive very far to attend the traditional suckling pig meal and beer drinking.

Nutritional status. German food is rich in flavor and texture and must be carefully evaluated. The German diet is high in saturated fats and cholesterol, sodium, smoked foods, and limited in vegetables and fruits. This diet may carry a high risk for developing heart disease and colon cancer.

European—British and Irish.

Traditional values. English and Irish immigrants formed the basis for the typical American family and are distributed all over North America. The British always believed that a good education is an investment in the future and, if they could afford it, they sent their children to private schools. The traditional family has the father at the head of the family and the mother controlling the social and domestic responsibilities. There are very large Irish populations in the United States and traditional Irish, who are mainly Catholics, have assimilated into American society with many of them marrying outside their religion.

Both British and Irish believe that a "proper" attitude is important in daily life and prefer formality in communication. When addressing English clients, it may be better to address them formally and not by their first names, particularly the older ones. However, that properness seems to be disappearing with the influence of Americanization in their society. The proximity of France to Great Britain and Ireland has led to many similarities in their cuisines.

In Britain, four meals—breakfast, lunch, tea and dinner—are served daily and Americans derived their hearty breakfast of bacon, ham and eggs, oatmeal and toast with ham from the British.

Cultural foods. In addition to dairy products, both Great Britain and Ireland traditionally have used animal products in most meals. Roast beef and lamb are common meats with the traditional **Yorkshire pudding**, a popover cooked in meat drippings. **Fish and chips**, battered deep fried fish served with fried potatoes and seasoned with salt and malt vinegar, commonly are served at pubs and fast food outlets. **Bangers**, or pork sausages, and bacon are the hallmarks of the British menu for breakfast. Smoked fish known as **kippers** and smoked salmon often are served at breakfasts or as appetizers.

Dairy products, particularly eggs and cheeses, are common features of English culture. English cheeses include the **stilton**, a blue cheese, and **clotted cream**, slightly fermented thick cream, often used on scones, or biscuits made with baking powder.

English tea or "high tea" is a favorite of the English culture, particular the upper class, and many fine hotels all over the world still offer the traditional English high tea where scones, jams and dainty cucumber sandwiches are served.

The English do not drink coffee like the Americans, but prefer strong black tea served with milk and sugar. **Soda bread**, made with baking soda instead of yeast, traditionally is prepared daily, especially in Ireland. **Biskcake** are biscuits such as bread, cake, cookies and crackers. Potatoes are the mainstay of the Irish and British fare and are stewed or incorporated into meat pies. Mashed potatoes often are referred to as "mash".

The influence of the Indian community in Great Britain led to chutneys, highly spiced fruit and vegetable pickles that are very popular and served with meals. **Plum pudding** is a traditional Christmas dish of suet, dried, candied fruit and other ingredients, and **trifle**, a layered dessert made from custard, pound cake, jams, whipped cream, sherry and almonds, originated from England.

The most common beverages in Great Britain are tea, beer and whiskey. A favorite of the Irish is **stout**, a dark rich beer high in calories, while the British favor **bitters**, a rich amber-colored beer that is flavored strongly with hops.

Nutritional status. Researchers believe that the American cuisine of high cholesterol and fats, low fiber and complex carbohydrates was influenced by the British and French culture. The diet would be healthier if Americans ate more fish and less meat.

Pub drinking is a very popular social habit and gluten intolerance, **celia sprue** or **celiac disease**, appears to be prevalent among the Irish, reported to have a high rate of alcoholism. The cold, damp weather of Great Britain is unfavorable to the growth of many fruits and vegetables, and there is a limited variety available. This may result in deficiency of vitamins, minerals and fiber in the British diet. Dietary supplements should be considered to offset these deficiencies.

European—Judaism.

Traditional values. It is appropriate to briefly discuss the Jewish religion and its effects on food because so many clients are of this faith, and in many cities, they form the majority of residents. It is beneficial to know about their dietary laws and the different terms used in their food preparation to prevent ignorance and embarrassment.

The Jewish culture is very complex and, if you have a large Jewish clientele, it will be worthwhile to research their culture in order to develop a better understanding of their beliefs and values, and communicate more effectively with them.

In the early 19th century, a huge number of Jews, primarily from Germany, immigrated to North America to seek economic opportunities. The following centuries found more Jews migrating from other countries, settling mainly in New York, Chicago and Los Angeles in the United States, and Toronto in Canada.

The cornerstone of the Jewish religion is the Hebrew Bible, particularly the *Torah*, the first five books of the Bible. Many Jews belong to a **synagogue**, or temple, led by a *rabbi*. Jews can be of different groups, **Orthodox**, which is very strict, **Reform**, which is not as strict, and **Conservative**, which lies between Orthodox and Reform.

Cultural foods. Many people think of Jewish food as dill pickles, bagels, *lox*, or smoked salmon, and chicken soup. However, most Jews in the United States follow a diet from Germany and Eastern Europe where their families originated. All Orthodox and some Conservative Jews follow the **kashrut** laws set down in the Torah.

Kosher means "fit" and is a term used to describe dietary laws among Jews. The Jewish dietary restrictions have been postulated to be a form of spiritual health, not physical. To follow the kosher dietary laws is to express their sense of obligation to God, their fellow Jews and to themselves. The following describes the dietary laws of Judaism.

1. "Clean" animals and their by-products are permitted. This refers to any mammals with a completely cloven foot—five toes that chews the cud so that digestive enzymes continue to work, including cattle, deer, goats, oxen and sheep. Clean birds must have a crop, gizzard and an extra talon such as chickens, ducks, turkey and geese. Fish with fins and scales are permitted. In addition, the meat of the animal can be eaten only if its life was taken by a special process where the jugular vein and trachea are cut simultaneously for a quick, painless death, and most of the blood drained. In addition, the person who kills the animal must be trained and licensed to perform the killing. The animal must be examined afterward for any blemishes in the meat, and then certified to be fit for consumption. **Kosher** refers to the preparation of the meat where the **heleb**, the layer of solid fat that is not mixed with the flesh, blood, blood vessels and sciatic nerve are removed, usually by a Jewish butcher. The heleb only applies to four-footed animals. The meat then is soaked in water and covered with kosher salt. After the blood has been drawn out, the meat is rinsed many times with water.
2. "Unclean" animals such as swine, carnivorous animals and rabbits are prohibited for consumption. Fish that are not allowed include catfish, eels, rays, shark, shellfish, reptiles, amphibians and invertebrates. Blood from any animal, even an egg with a small bloodspot in the yolk, is forbidden. The only exception to the rule of unclean animals is honey, because is believed that it does not contain any parts from the insect.
3. In addition to the above dietary laws, meat and dairy products may not be eaten together. Furthermore, one must wait six hours after eating meat before any dairy products can be consumed. However if dairy products are taken first, only one hour is necessary.

Many Jews are lactose intolerant and do not drink milk but they do consume other dairy products such as cheese, sour cream and yogurt. They use separate sets of utensils for preparing and eating meat and dairy products. Eggs, fruits, vegetables and grains are neither considered meat nor dairy products and therefore can be eaten with both. A processed food product is considered kosher only if it is certified by a rabbi, the most common insignia is a "K" permitted by the FDA.

Many businesses that depend on a large Jewish clientele are affected by the numerous Jewish holidays throughout the year. The Jewish Sabbath is the day of rest and is observed before sundown starting on Friday until after nightfall on Saturday. Therefore, all cooked meals must be prepared before sundown on Friday since no fires can be used on the Sabbath. For the Friday meal, fish, chicken or **cholet**, a bean and potato dish, often is served with **challah**, a braided bread and **kugel**, a pudding often made with noodles.

Rosh Hashanah is the Jewish New Year which marks ten days of penitence that ends with **Yom Kippur**, the holiest day of the year. Yom Kippur is a complete fast day, meaning no food or water except for medications, and the meal to break the fast is usually a light one. This date varies annually because the Jewish calendar is based on lunar months counted according to biblical customs. **Hanukkah**, the festival of lights, is celebrated for eight days in December, similar to the Christian Christmas, during which traditional potato pancakes called **latkes** are eaten and candles are lit. The **Purim** is celebrated in February or March when traditional cookies filled with fruit preserves or poppy seeds are eaten. **Passover** is an eight-day festival of spring signifying the anniversary of the Jewish exodus from Egypt and takes place in March or April. During this time, no leavened food such as wheat, barley, rye or oats can be eaten. Wheat flour can be eaten only in the form of **matzah**, a white flour cracker, the descendant of the unleavened bread. In addition, no pulse foods such as beans, peas, lentils, maize, millet, mustard and no leavening agents such as beers or malt liquors are to be consumed.

Nutritional status. It must be noted that the health practitioner should not criticize any diet with religious underpinnings.

Enhance relationships

Each culture defines how an individual views life based on traditional values, beliefs and attitudes of their ethnic group. How food habits are affected and changed depends a great deal upon perception and the process of acclimation within a new society. After reviewing the above ethnic cuisines, some of their traditional foods, and their cultural outlook on health and beauty, hopefully providing some insight into the various cultures will prove to be beneficial in enhancing the relationship and understanding with members of the multicultural society that currently exists in the 21st century.

APPENDIX I

Fat Soluble Vitamins

Remember that that the Recommended Daily Allowance (RDA) was set to meet the needs of almost all healthy individuals in a particular stage or gender group. The Dietary Reference Intake (DRI), representing the most current nutrition information, is the new set of recommendations for daily nutrient intakes used by both American and Canadian health scientists for individual counseling. DRIs are the new harmonized values for micronutrients such as vitamins and minerals that are replacing the RDAs and the Canadian Recommended Nutrient Intakes (RNIs). Many health care providers use DRIs for assessing a patient's nutrient intakes, planning diets and developing appropriate nutrition education materials for individuals or population groups.

In the following tables, the DRIs are given for adults in general, unless specified for a specific age group or gender. The Upper Level (UL) values represents the highest levels of daily nutrient intake that is least likely to pose any risk of adverse health effects to almost all individuals. Unless indicated, the UL represents total intake from food, water and supplements. The following table lists the characteristics of fat soluble vitamins, the latest DRIs, main functions, deficiencies, toxicity and significant sources. In some cases, the poor absorption or enhanced absorption of each vitamin may be given.

Note: For vitamin A conversions:

- 1 (Retinol Activity Equivalent) RAE = 1 ug retinol; 2 ug beta carotene in supplements
- 12 ug beta carotene; 24 ug from other precursors of carotenoids
- 1 (International Unit) IU = 0.3 ug retinol; 0.6 ug beta carotene in supplements
- 3.6 ug beta carotene; 7.2 from other precursors of carotenoids

Dietary Reference Intakes (DRIs 2000-01) of Fat Soluble Vitamins

Vitamin A

Also known as retinol, retinal and retinoic acid. Precursors are carotenoids such as beta carotenoids.

DRIs (19–50 years old):

- *DRIs:* 900 ug/d for men and 700 ug/d for women.
- *Upper levels:* 3,000 ug/d.

Main functions:

- Antioxidant.
- Good vision.
- Maintenance of healthy skin, hair, bones and nails.
- Improves acne.
- Immunity.

Deficiency:

- Poor night vision.
- Hyperkeratosis, or dry rough skin with plugged hair follicles with keratin, itchy peeling skin.
- Reduced immunity.
- Poor growth.

Toxicity:

- Usually occurs from excess intake of dietary supplements.
- Nausea and vomiting.
- Dry, cracked lips.
- Hair loss, brittle nails.

Significant sources:

- *Retinol*—milk and milk products, liver, eggs.
- *Beta carotene*—yellow-red vegetables such as sweet potatoes, carrots and squash, dark orange fruits such as cantaloupe and apricots, dark green leafy vegetables such as broccoli and spinach.

Vitamin D

Also known as calciferol and cholecalciferol.

DRIs (19–50 years old):

- *DRIs:* 5 ug/d (19–50 years old), 10 ug/d (51–70 years old), 15 ug/d (> 70 years old).
- *Upper levels:* 50 ug/d.

Main functions:

- Also functions as a hormone.
- Strong bones and teeth.
- Helps calcium absorption in intestinal tract.

Deficiency:

- Rickets, or soft bones in children.
- Osteomalacia, or soft bones in adults.
- Osteoporosis, or soft bones in older years.

Toxicity:

- Calcification of soft tissues such as kidney stones.

Significant sources:

- Sunlight.
- Fortified foods such as milk, butter and margarine.

Vitamin E

Also known as alpha tocopherol.

DRIs (19–50 years old):

- *DRIs:* 15 mg/d.
- *Upper levels:* 1,000 mg/d.

Main functions:

- Most important antioxidant as it protects poly unsaturated fats (PUFA) and vitamin A.
- Strengthens immunity.

Deficiency:

- Rare.

Dietary Reference Intakes (DRIs 2000-01) of Fat Soluble Vitamins *(cont.)*

Vitamin E (cont.)

Toxicity:
- Rare.

Significant sources:
- Vegetable oils such as wheat germ and safflower.
- Nuts and seeds.
- Leafy green vegetables.
- Readily destroyed by heat, such as in deep fried foods, and air.

Vitamin K

Also known as phytomenadione.

DRIs (19–50 years old):
- *DRIs:* 120 ug/d for men and 90 ug/d for women.

Main functions:
- Blood clotting.

Deficiency:
- Uncontrolled bleeding.
- Deficiency can occur when taking antibiotics.

Toxicity:
- Red blood cell hemolysis, or separation of red blood cells from hemoglobin.

Significant sources:
- Synthesized in gastrointestinal tract by bacteria flora.
- Green leafy vegetables, nails, hair and all cellular structures.
- Source of energy, although the body uses carbohydrates and fats first.
- Blood clotting—manufactures blood proteins such as fibrin.
- Maintains acid/base balance, essential for health.

Sources: www.dialadietitian.org/resources, Whitney & Rolfes, Understanding Nutrition, 9th ed., 2002, The National Academies Press, 2002.

APPENDIX II

Water Soluble Vitamins

Water soluble vitamins are not stored by the body so toxicity is rare. Deficiencies of a single B vitamin are seldom because foods contain a mixture of them. The skin and tongue appear to be most sensitive to vitamin B deficiencies. Unless indicated, the following values for Dietary Reference Intakes (DRIs) are from 1998.

Unless indicated otherwise, recommendations refer to adults 19 years and over. If Upper Levels (UL) are given, they refer to the highest continuing daily intake of a nutrient that is least likely to pose any risks of adverse health effects for almost all individuals. If the daily intake exceeds ULs, the risk of adverse effects increases.

Dietary Reference Intakes (DRIs) of Water Soluble Vitamins

Vitamin B-1

Also known as thiamin.

DRIs 1998 (19–50 years old):

- *DRIs:* 1.2 mg/d for men and 1.1 mg/d for women.

Main functions:

- Essential for function of healthy nervous system.
- Part of coenzyme in energy metabolism.

Deficiency:

- Beri-beri, or wet/dry edema.
- Muscle weakness.
- Paralysis.
- Fatigue, irritability, poor short-term memory, weight loss.
- Heavy alcohol consumption reduces absorption.

Toxicity:

- Unknown.

Significant sources:

- All yeast products such as whole grains.
- Pork and pork products.
- Legumes.

Vitamin B-2

Also known as riboflavin.

DRIs 1998 (19–50 years old):

- *DRIs:* 1.3 mg/d for men and 1.1 mg/d for women.

Main functions:

- Healthy skin, eyes.
- Coenzyme to release energy from foods.

Deficiency:

- Inflamed skin lesions with greasy scales.
- Inflamed eyes, cracked, dry lips.

Toxicity:

- Unknown.

Vitamin B-2 *(cont.)*

Significant sources:

- Milk products.
- Enriched grains.
- Meat, fish, poultry, liver.

Vitamin B-3

Also known as niacin, precursor is amino acid tryptophan.

DRIs 1998 (19–50 years old):

- *DRIs:* 16 mg/d for men and 14 mg/d for women.
- *Upper levels:* 35 mg/d for adults.

Main functions:

- Healthy skin, nervous and digestive systems.
- Coenzyme to release energy from foods.

Deficiency:

- Pellagra symptoms—diarrhea, dermatitis, dementia.
- Skin rash, painful flush, hives, rash.
- Depression and fatigue.

Toxicity:

- Blurred vision.
- Nausea.
- Liver damage.

Significant sources:

- All proteins.
- Whole grains.
- Nuts.

Dietary Reference Intakes (DRIs) of Water Soluble Vitamins *(cont.)*

Vitamin B-6

Also known as pyridoxine.

DRIs 1998 (19–50 years old):

- *DRIs:* 1.3 mg/d (19-50 years old) 1.7 mg/d (51+ men) 1.5 mg/d (51+ women).
- *Upper levels:* 100 mg/d (adults).

Main functions:

- Manufacture of red blood cells (rbcs).
- Coenzyme role.

Deficiency:

- Anemia (small rbc's).
- Scaly dermatitis.
- Nerve degeneration.

Toxicity:

- Fatigue, depression, headaches.
- Skin lesions.

Significant sources:

- Animal sources: meat, fish, poultry, soy, liver.
- Plants: legumes, fortified cereals, potatoes.

Vitamin B-12

Also known as cobalamin.

DRIs 1998 (19–50 years old):

- *DRIs:* 2.4 ug/d for adults.

Main functions:

- DNA synthesis and red blood cells.
- Essential to convert folate to its active form.
- Maintains function of myelin sheath.
- Necessary for homocysteine metabolism.

Deficiency:

- Usually from poor absorption and not poor intake.
- Occurs most likely among vegans.

Vitamin B-12 *(cont.)*

- Hypersensitive skin.
- Pernicious anemia.
- Elevated homocysteine levels in body.

Toxicity:

- None reported

Significant sources:

- All animal products such as meat, fish, poultry, milk, cheese and eggs.

Folate

Also known as folic acid.

DRIs 1998 (19–50 years old):

- *DRIs:* 400 ug/d for adults.
- *Upper levels:* 1,000 mg/d in addition to above DRIs for women capable of getting pregnant.

Main functions:

- DNA synthesis and cell formation.
- Helps to fight heart disease by metabolism of homocysteine.

Deficiency:

- Anemia-impaired cell division.
- Neural tube defects such as spina bifida in fetus of young pregnant female.
- Elevated homocysteine levels.

Toxicity:

- Hides symptoms of B-12 deficiency.

Significant sources:

- Leafy green vegetables.
- Fortified foods.
- Legumes, seeds.
- Eggs, liver.

Dietary Reference Intakes (DRIs) of Water Soluble Vitamins *(cont.)*

Pantothenic acid

DRIs 1998 (19–50 years old):

- *DRIs:* 5 mg/d for adults.

Main functions:

- Helps release energy.

Toxicity:

- None reported.

Significant sources:

- All foods.

Biotin

DRIs 1998 (19–50 years old):

- *DRIs:* 30 ug/d for adult.

Main functions:

- Energy metabolism.

Deficiency:

- Red, scaly rash around eyes, nose and mouth.
- Hair loss.
- Depression, lethargy.
- Digestive disorders.

Toxicity:

- None reported.

Significant sources:

- Widespread in foods such as organ meats, avocados, mushrooms and whole grains.

Vitamin C

Also known as ascorbic acid.

DRIs 2000:

- *DRIs:* 90 mg/d for men and 75 mg/d for women. Add extra 35 mg/d for smokers.
- *Upper levels:* 2,000 mg/d for adults.

Main functions:

- Helps absorb iron.
- Collagen formation.
- Anti-inflammatory effect.
- Antioxidant.

Deficiency:

- Easily bruised, blotchy skin, broken capillaries.
- Poor skin/wound healing.
- Bleeding gums, loosened teeth.
- Prone to infections.
- Anemia.
- Fragile bones.
- Antioxidant function.

Toxicity:

- From excessive intake of dietary supplements.
- Nausea, diarrhea.
- Hot flashes, rashes.

Significant sources:

- All citrus fruits.
- Cruceriferous dark green vegetables.
- Potatoes, tomatoes, mangoes, papayas.

Dietary Reference Intakes (DRIs) of Water Soluble Vitamins *(cont.)*

Vitamin P

Also known as bioflavonoids.

Main functions:

- Work together with vitamin C.
- Antioxidant.
- Anti-inflammatory.
- Strengthens capillary walls of blood vessels.

Deficiency:

- Bruises easily.
- Broken capillaries.

Toxicity:

- Unknown.

Significant sources:

- White rinds of citrus fruits such as lemons, oranges and grapefruits.
- Cherries and apricots.

Sources: www.dialadietitian.org, Whitney & Rolfes, 9th ed., 2002, The National Academies of Sciences, 2000.

APPENDIX III

Minerals

These inorganic elements form electrolytes in the body's solutions to regulate fluid balance. Deficiency results in various abnormalities or diseases. Like vitamins, minerals vary in their absorption and toxicity effects. Fibers in certain foods such as legumes, grains and spinach may affect their absorption by binding with specific minerals such as calcium, iron and zinc that carry them out of the body together with wastes. Calcium and phosphorus are the main minerals that are essential to form the molecule calcium phosphate—the main structural material for bone and teeth. Other important minerals are potassium, sulfur, sodium chloride and magnesium. The name of each mineral is followed by its chemical symbol.

Minerals required in large doses are called macrominerals and are measured in milligrams (mg), while those needed in tiny doses are referred to as microminerals measured in micrograms (ug). The terms mg/d or ug/d refers to the recommended Dietary Reference Intakes (DRIs) for age group and gender. Please note that the recommendations for DRIs are undergoing dramatic changes at this time of research and will be updated completely in the near future, therefore the values given here vary according to the data available at the present time with some data is as old as 1997 unless otherwise indicated. The following table shows the DRI recommendations for minerals in adults 19–50 years, their main functions, deficiencies, toxicity in the body and significant sources.

Dietary Reference Intakes of Minerals

Calcium (Ca)

Adult DRIs (19–50 years old):

- *DRI (1997):* 1,000 mg/d and 1,200 mg/d for those 51 or older.
- *Upper level:* 2,500 mg/d for adults.

Main functions:

- Strong bones and teeth.
- Muscular contraction.
- Blood clotting.
- Blood pressure.
- Nerve functioning.
- Energy production.

Deficiency:

- Tetany.
- Stunted growth in children.
- Bone loss, or osteoporosis.

Toxicity:

- Stiffness.
- Constipation.
- Urinary stones.

Significant sources:

- Milk and milk products.
- Small fish with bones such as sardines.
- Tofu.
- Greens such as broccoli, chard and bok choy.
- Legumes.

Phosphorus (P)

Adult DRIs (19–50 years old):

- *DRI (1997):* 700 mg/d.
- *Upper level:* 4,000 mg/d (51–70 years old) 3,000 mg/d (over 70 years old).

Main functions:

- Part of all cells (DNA).
- Helps to form bones and teeth.
- Part of phospholipids.

Phosphorus (P) *(cont.)*

Deficiency:

- Weakness.

Toxicity:

- Low blood calcium levels.

Significant sources:

- All animal tissues such as meat, fish, poultry and eggs.

Potassium (K)

Adult DRIs (19–50 years old):

- *DRI:* 2,000 mg/d.

Main functions:

- Main cation in intracellular fluid.
- Maintains normal fluid balance therefore controls blood pressure.

Deficiency:

- Muscular weakness.
- Dehydration.
- Diarrhea.

Toxicity:

- High blood pressure.

Significant sources:

- All whole foods such as meats, legumes, vegetables and milk.

Sulfur (S)

Adult DRIs (19–50 years old):

- *N/A.*

Main functions:

- Constituent of all proteins.

Deficiency:

- Unknown.

Toxicity:

- Unknown.

Significant sources:

- All protein foods.

Dietary Reference Intakes of Minerals *(cont.)*

Sodium (Na)

Adult DRIs (19–50 years old):

- *DRI:* 2,400 mg/d.

Main functions:

- Main cation in extracellular fluid.
- Maintains fluid and electrolyte balance-nerve transmission.

Deficiency:

- Muscle cramps.
- Appetite loss.

Toxicity:

- Edema, acute hypertension.

Significant sources:

- Table salt, salty foods, soy, processed foods.

Chloride (Cl)

Adult DRIs (19–50 years old):

- *DRI:* 750 mg/d.

Main functions:

- Main anion in extracellular fluids.
- Maintains fluid and electrolyte balance.

Deficiency:

- None normally.

Toxicity:

- Vomiting.

Significant sources:

- Table salt, soy sauce, processed foods.

Magnesium (Mg)

Adult DRIs (19–50 years old):

- *DRI:* 400 mg/d for men 19–30, 310 mg/d for women 19–30, 420 mg/d for men over 31, 320 mg/d for women over 31.
- *Upper level:* 350mg/d nonfood source daily.

Magnesium (Mg) (cont.)

Main functions:
- Strong bones and teeth.
- Muscular contraction.

Deficiency:
- Muscular weakness.
- Extreme deficiency results in convulsions of eye and face muscles.

Toxicity:
- Only from supplements: diarrhea, alkalosis, dehydration.

Significant sources:
- Nuts, legumes, vegetables, whole grains.
- Seafood.

Iron (Fe)

Adult DRIs (19–50 years old):
- *DRI 2001:* 8 ug/d for men,18 mg/d for women, 8 mg/d for those over 51.

Main functions:
- Hemoglobin formation.

Deficiency:
- Main cause is poor nutrition.
- Skin itching.
- Anemia, paleness of skin and eyes.
- Pale concave nails.
- Tiredness, fatigue.
- Intolerance to cold.

Toxicity:
- Skin pigmentation.
- Hair loss.
- Nausea.
- Vomiting.
- Lethargy.

Significant sources:
- All protein foods.

Dietary Reference Intakes of Minerals *(cont.)*

Zinc (Zn)

Adult DRIs (19–50 years old):

- *DRI 2001:* 11 mg/d for men, 8 mg/d for women.
- *Upper level:* 40 mg/d.

Main functions:

- Part of many enzymes and proteins.
- Growth and development.
- Wound healing.
- Increases immunity.

Deficiency:

- Stunted growth.
- Poor wound healing.
- Rough dry skin.
- Skin lesions.
- Hair loss.

Toxicity:

- Vomiting, diarrhea.
- Raised low density lipoproteins (LDL), low high density lipoproteins (HDL).

Significant sources:

- All protein foods.
- Whole grains, vegetables.

Iodine (I)

Adult DRIs (19–50 years old):

- *DRI 2001:* 150 ug/d.
- *Upper level:* 1.1 mg/d.

Main functions:

- Manufacture of thyroxine hormone that regulates growth, development and metabolic rate of body.

Deficiency:

- Goiter, cretinism.
- Weight gain.
- Dry, cool skin.

Toxicity:

- Goiter.

Significant sources:

- Iodized salt, seafood.
- Dairy products, bread.

Copper (Cu)

Adult DRIs (19–50 years old):

- *DRI 2001:* 900 ug/d.
- *Upper level:* 10 mg/d.

Main functions:

- Necessary for iron absorption.
- Formation of collagen, hemoglobin.

Deficiency:

- Anemia.

Toxicity:

- Vomiting, diarrhea.

Significant sources:

- Seafood, nuts.
- Whole grains, seeds, legumes.
- Drinking water.

Dietary Reference Intakes of Minerals *(cont.)*

Selenium (Se)

Adult DRIs (19–50 years old):

- *DRI 2000:* 55 ug/d.
- *Upper level:* 400 ug/d.

Main functions:

- Antioxidant
- Regulates body metabolism.

Deficiency:

- Reduced skin elasticity.
- Premature skin aging.

Toxicity:

- Loss of hair, nails.
- Skin lesions.
- Disorders of digestive systemm.

Significant sources:

- Seafood, meat, whole grains, vegetables.

Fluoride (F)

Adult DRIs (19–50 years old):

- *DRI 1997:* 4 mg/d for men, 3 mg/d for women.
- *Upper level:* 10 mg/d.

Main functions:

- Forms bone and teeth.
- Prevents teeth decay.

Deficiency:

- Tooth decay.

Toxicity:

- Tooth discoloration.
- Nausea.

Significant sources:

- Fluoridated drinking water.
- Tea, seafood.

Chromium (Cr)

Adult DRIs (19–50 years old):

- *DRI 2000:* 35 mg/d for men, 25 mg/d for women.

Main functions:

- For release of energy from glucose.

Deficiency:

- Diabetes-like condition.

Toxicity:

- Unknown.

Significant sources:

- Meat, fats.
- Unrefined foods.
- Vegetable oils.

Sources: www.dialadietitian.org., Rolfes & Whitney, Understanding Nutrition, 2002 and The Academies of Science, 2001

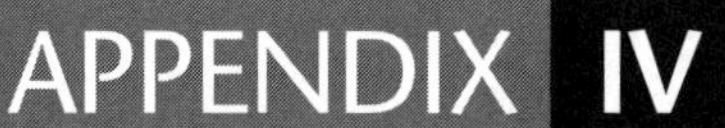

Ideal Body Weight and BMI

Ideal Body Weight

Height	Small frame	Medium frame	Large frame
1.42 m / 4'8"	39-42 kg–86-92 lb.	41-46 kg–90-101 lb.	44-51 kg–98-113 lb.
1.47 m / 4'10"	41-44 kg–91-98 lb.	44-49 kg–96-107 lb.	47-54 kg–104-120 lb.
1.52 m / 5'0"	44-47 kg–96-104 lb.	46-52 kg–102-114 lb.	50-57 kg–110-126 lb.
1.57 m / 5'2"	46-50 kg–102-110 lb.	49-55 kg–108-121 lb.	53-60 kg–116-133 lb.
1.65 m / 5'5"	50-54 kg–111-119 lb.	53-60 kg–116-131 lb	57-65 kg–126-143 lb.
1.76 m / 5'9"	57-61 kg–126-135 lb.	60-68 kg–133-149 lb.	65-73 kg–143-160 lb.

Estimating Body Mass Index (BMI)

Look for your height on the left column and correlate it with the closest number for your weight across the column. Check below the column to identify your BMI.

Age	18	19	20	21	22	23	24	25	26	27	28
Height					Body Weight (lb)						
4'10"	86	91	96	100	105	110	115	119	124	129	134
4'11"	89	94	99	104	109	114	119	124	128	133	138
5'0"	92	97	102	107	112	118	123	128	133	138	143
5'1"	95	100	106	111	116	122	127	132	137	143	148
5'2"	98	104	109	115	120	126	131	136	142	147	153
5'3"	102	107	113	118	124	130	135	141	146	152	158
5'4"	105	110	116	122	128	134	140	145	151	157	163
5'5"	108	114	120	126	132	138	144	150	156	162	168
5'6"	112	118	124	130	136	142	148	155	161	167	173
5'7"	115	121	127	134	140	146	153	159	166	172	178
5'8"	118	125	131	138	144	151	158	164	171	177	184
5'9"	122	128	135	142	149	155	162	169	176	182	189
5'10"	126	132	139	146	153	160	167	174	181	188	195
5'11"	129	136	143	150	157	165	172	179	186	193	200
6'0"	132	140	147	154	162	169	177	184	191	199	206
6'1"	136	144	151	159	166	174	182	189	197	204	212
6'2"	141	148	155	163	171	179	186	194	202	210	218
6'3"	144	152	160	168	176	184	192	200	208	216	224
6'4"	148	156	164	172	180	189	197	205	213	221	230
6'5"	151	160	168	176	185	193	202	210	218	227	235
6'6"	155	164	172	181	190	198	207	216	224	233	241
	Underweight (<18.5 years old)			Healthy Weight (18.5–24.9 years old)						Overweight (25–29.9 years	

29	30	31	32	33	34	35	36	37	38	39	40
					Body Weight (lb)						
138	143	148	153	158	162	167	172	177	181	186	191
143	148	153	158	163	168	173	178	183	188	193	198
148	153	158	163	168	174	179	184	189	194	199	204
153	158	164	169	174	180	185	190	195	201	206	211
158	164	169	175	180	186	191	196	202	207	213	218
163	169	175	180	186	191	197	203	206	214	220	225
169	174	180	186	192	197	204	209	215	221	227	232
174	180	186	192	198	204	210	216	222	228	234	240
179	186	192	198	204	210	216	223	229	235	241	247
185	191	198	204	211	217	223	230	236	242	249	255
190	197	203	210	216	223	230	236	243	249	256	262
196	203	209	216	223	230	236	243	250	257	263	270
202	209	216	222	229	236	243	250	257	264	271	278
208	215	222	229	236	243	250	257	265	272	279	286
213	221	228	235	242	250	258	265	272	279	287	294
219	227	235	242	250	257	265	272	280	288	295	302
225	233	241	249	256	264	272	280	287	295	303	311
232	240	248	256	264	272	279	287	295	303	311	319
238	246	254	263	271	279	287	295	304	312	320	328
244	252	261	269	277	286	294	303	311	319	328	336
250	259	267	276	284	293	302	310	319	328	336	345
					Obese (30 years old)						

APPENDIX V

Practical Diet Assessment

a. 3-day food diary

Use this form to record the complete food intake for three individual days, preferably two weekdays and one day of the weekend. Be as accurate as possible in recording serving sizes such as slices, cups, ounces and small versus large fruit.

In addition, remember to record how the food was prepared such as raw, boiled or fried, since the kcal and nutrient values change with different food preparation. You can photocopy this page and carry it around with you since it is best to record the information immediately after eating. On completion of this diary, transfer the number of servings that were recorded on to the appropriate daily Food Guide Plan, form b.

Quantity	Type of food/how prepared (boiled, raw, fried)
Monday	
Tuesday	

a. 3-day food diary *(cont.)*

Quantity	Type of food/how prepared (boiled, raw, fried)
Wednesday	
Thursday	
Friday	
Saturday	
Sunday	

b. Balancing of Daily Food Groups

Use the following charts to help you decide if your client's daily food intake complies with the Daily Food Guide Plan. Choosing the relative Food Guide Plan depends on whether your country uses a four-group or a five-group plan, so choose the appropriate one on these pages for your use. You can photocopy this page for your diet analysis. The average number of servings for three days from each food group can be compared with the Daily Food Guide Plan as indicated. It is very important to remember that insufficient servings in one food group can imply deficiencies in certain nutrients. For example, insufficient servings in bread, whole grains or cereals may indicate a diet that is low in fiber and vitamin B complex, while insufficient meat or alternative meat products may imply a deficiency in iron. On the other hand, excess consumption in meat servings may indicate a higher fat and iron content. If your client is low in fruits and vegetables, she may be deficient in vitamins and minerals, while insufficient servings in milk or milk products may indicate a deficiency in calcium. Remember that a diet rich in milk products may be low in iron and that postmenopausal and nursing women require more servings of milk products. It also is important to check the miscellaneous column for hidden fats if the client is overweight, as well as the amount of fluids, especially water. Based on your analysis, you can make suitable recommendations to rectify the client's daily food intake.

b. Balancing of Daily Food Groups (cont.)

A five-group plan.

Indications for daily servings (United States)

- **Milk group** (cheese, milk, yogurt): 2–3 servings: each may be 1 cup of milk or 2-oz. processed cheese; 1 1/2-oz. cheese.
- **Meat/meat alternatives** (chicken, fish, beans): 2–3 servings: each may be 2–3-oz. lean cooked meat; 1 egg; 1/2 cup legumes; 2 tsp peanut butter.
- **Fruits** (juices, fruits): 2–4 servings: each may be 1 medium fruit, 1/2 grapefruit, 3/4 cup juice; 1/2 cup chopped or canned fruit; 1/4 cup dried fruit.
- **Bread, cereals, whole grains:** 6–11 servings: each may be 1 slice bread; 1/2 cup cooked cereals, rice, pasta; 1-oz. ready-to-eat cereals; 1/2 bun/bagel; 2 large crackers.
- **Vegetables:** 3–5 servings; each may be 1/2 cup cooked/raw vegetables; 3/4 cup vegetable juice; 1 cup leafy raw vegetables; 1/2 cup cooked legumes.

Day	Bread/whole grains 6-11 servings	Meat products 2-3 servings	Vegetables 3-5 servings
M T W T F S S			
M T W T F S S			
M T W T F S S			
M T W T F S S			
M T W T F S S			
M T W T F S S			
M T W T F S S			
M T W T F S S			
M T W T F S S			
M T W T F S S			
M T W T F S S			
M T W T F S S			
M T W T F S S			
M T W T F S S			
M T W T F S S			
M T W T F S S			
M T W T F S S			
M T W T F S S			
M T W T F S S			
M T W T F S S			
Total Servings:			

Fruits 2-4 servings	Milk products 2-3 servings	Miscellaneous (including water)

b. Balancing of Daily Food Groups (cont.)

A four-group plan.

Examples of one serving:

- **Milk/milk products**: 2 servings (adults), 3–4 servings (pregnant/nursing/menopausal women): 250 ml (1 cup) milk; 3/4 cup yogurt; 50 g cheese; 50 g processed cheese, 1/2 cup cottage cheese.
- **Meat/fish/alternatives**: 2–3 servings: approximately 50–100 g (2–3-oz.) cooked lean meat, fish, poultry; 30 ml (2 tsp) peanut butter; 250 ml (1 cup) cooked dried legumes; 125 ml (1/2 cup) nuts or seeds; 100 g (1/2 cup) tofu; 1–2 eggs.
- **Bread/grains/cereals**: 5–12 servings: approximately 1 slice bread, 175 ml (3/4 cup) cooked cereals; 1 small roll/muffin, 1/2 bagel or hamburger bun; 1/2 to 3/4 cup cooked pasta, rice.
- **Fruits/Vegetables**: 5–10 servings: approximately 125 ml (1/2 cup) vegetables/fruits either fresh, frozen, or canned; 125 ml (1/2 cup) juice; 1 medium sized vegetable/fruit.

Day	Milk/milk products 2-4 servings	Meat/fish/alteratives 2-3 servings
M T W T F S S		
M T W T F S S		
M T W T F S S		
M T W T F S S		
M T W T F S S		
M T W T F S S		
M T W T F S S		
M T W T F S S		
M T W T F S S		
M T W T F S S		
M T W T F S S		
M T W T F S S		
M T W T F S S		
M T W T F S S		
M T W T F S S		
M T W T F S S		
M T W T F S S		
M T W T F S S		
M T W T F S S		
Total Servings:		

reads/grains/cereals 5-12 servings	Fruits/vegetables 5-10 servings	Miscellaneous (including water)

c. Diet Analysis

Food (serving)	Weight (g)	Energy (kcal)	Protein (g)	Carbohydrate (g)	Fiber (g)	Fat (g)	Sat (g)
Day 1							
Day 2							
Day 3							
TOTALS							
3 Day Average TOTALS							
RDA/DRIs							

Formulas

- ***BMR*** = Gender (0.9 women/1.0 men) x weight (kg) x 24 (hrs/day)
- ***BEN*** = BMR x activity level (example: 1274 x 1.6 (moderately active female) = 2033 (kcal/day)

Formula for Protein/Carbohydrate and Fat Intake

	% of BEN
Proteins	15-20
Carbs	50-55
Fats	<30
Sat Fats	<10

Cholesterol (mg)	Calcium	Iron (mg)	Zinc (mg)	Sodium (mg)	Potassium (mg)	Vitamin A (IU)	Vitamin C (mg)	Vitamin B-6 (mg)	Folate (mg)	Thiamin (mg)	Riboflavin (mg)

d. Nutrition Guidance/Counseling

Now that you have finished the Diet Analysis, the last step is to give nutrient counseling. The following form can be used to do so. Any deficiencies or excess can be noted from the Diet Analysis sheet and can be brought forward to this form. Check the Appendices for the RDA/DRIs; the client's daily nutrient intake can be compared to them. Deficiencies or excess of macronutrients and micronutrients can be listed and the 3-Day Food Diary can be checked to trace the foods that are too high or too low when compared with RDA or DRI values. Possible symptoms then are noted and the most significant sources given to guide the client to make better food choices. An example is shown below.

Sample

Nutrient	Client's nutrient intake (mg/ug/d)	RDA or DRIs	Deficiency	Excess
Fiber			✔	
Iron			✔	
Calcium			✔	

Possible symptoms	Most significant sources
ncreased risk of colon cancer rregular bowel movements Risk of diverticulitis Risk of high blood cholesterol	• Fruits and vegetables • Legumes • Whole grains • Cereals
'ale skin and eyes asily fatigued	• Lean red meat and liver • Legumes • Soy products
etany)steomalacia	• Milk and milk products • Soy products

d. Nutrition Guidance/Counseling (cont.)

Working Sheet

Nutrient	Client's nutrient intake (mg/ug/d)	RDA or DRIs	Deficiency	Excess

Possible symptoms	Most significant sources

REFERENCES

American Board of Anti-aging Medicine study materials.

Apgar B, "Comparison of Common Calcium Supplements," *American Family Physician*, p 2-3 (2000).

Associated Press, "Health and Science," *The Orange County Register* (January 9, 2000).

Barnhart K et al, *A Clinical Guide to the Premenstrual Syndrome in Office Gynecology*, 79: 6, pp 1457-8 (1995).

Bhathena SJ and Velasquez M, "Beneficial role of dietary phytoestrogens in obesity and diabetes," *American Journal of Clinical Nutrition*, 76, pp 1191-1194 (December 2002).

Bidlack W, et al, "Developing Claims for New Phytochemical Products," *Phytochemicals – a New Paradigm*, (1998).

Bloch A and Thomson C, "Phytochemicals and Functional Foods," *Journal of the American Dietetic Association*, 95: 4, pp 493-96 (April 1995).

Boelsma E et al, "Nutritional skin care: health effects of micronutrients and fatty acids," *American Journal of Clinical Nutrition*, 73: 5 pp 853-64 (May 2001).

Boyle M, *Personal Nutrition, 4th Edition*, pp 14, 68, 103-105, 114-118, 242-249 (2000).

Brand-Miller J, "Diets with a Low Glycemic Index: From Theory to Practice," *Nutrition Today*, (March 1999).

Canada's Food Guide to Healthy Eating, 1992.

Chabner D, *The Language of Medicine*, p 48 (1996).

Clark N, *The Physician and Sportsmedicine*, 7, p 29 (July 1992); 24: 2, pp 45-46 (February 1996); 24: 10, pp 15-16 (October 1996).

Conner M et al, "Why do women use dietary supplements? The use of the theory of planned behavior to explore beliefs about their use," *Social Science and Medicine*, 52: 4, pp 621-33 (February 2001).

Cousiner J and Hartman G, *Food Technology*, p 77 (July 1996).

Dattner AM, "Nutritional dermatology," *Clinics in Dermatology* 17: 1 pp 57-64 (1999).

Deurenberg P et al, "Body mass index and percentage body fat: a meta-analysis among different ethnic groups," *Int. J. Obes Relat Metab Disorder*, 22: 12 pp 1164-71 (December 1998).

Dieticians of Canada

e.antiaging.com, "Proven Secrets to Longevity," p 12.

FDA, HHs," "Food labeling: trans fatty acids in nutritional labels nutrient content claims and health claims," *Fed. Regis 2003*, Final rule 68: 133 414-33-1506.

Fernandez JR et al, "Is percentage body fat differentially related to body mass index in Hispanic Americans, African Americans and European Americans?" *American Journal of Clinical Nutrition*, 77 p 71 (January 2003).

Fitness Ontario, Leadership Program, The BASICS, 1989. Ministry of Culture, Tourism and Recreation.

Flavelle D, "Food industry targets consumers' taste for wellness," *Toronto Star* (October 28, 2003).

Food and Nutrition Board (FNB), Institute of Medicine (IOM), The National Academies Press, "Dietary Reference Intakes: Recommended Intakes for Individuals," p 770 (2002).

Gallant A, *Body Treatments and Dietetics for the Beauty Therapist*, p 177, (1978).

Giacomoni P et al, *Skin Aging: Mechanisms and Possible Interventions in the Science of Anti-aging Medicine*, p 159 (1996).

Grandjean AC, *Dietary strategies for modifying weight or body composition in strength and conditioning*, No. 3, p 7-17 (June 1995).

Galuska D et al, "Are Health Care Professionals Advising Obese Patients to Lose Weight?" *Journal of the American Medical Association*, 282 pp 1576-78 (October 1999).

Hakim I, "Some Aspects of the Mediterranean Diet in Vegetables," *Fruits and Herbs in Health Promotion*, p 221-222 (2001).

Haas E, *www.healthworld.com*, pp 2-13 (July 1999).

Heart and Stroke Foundation, "Living with cholesterol," Cat. 50020, p 16-17 (1997).

Heasman M and Mellentin J, *The Functional Foods Revolution*, pp 5-11 (2001).

Heber D and Bowerman S, "Applying Science to Changing Dietary Patterns," *American Institute for Cancer Research 11th Annual Research Conference on Diet, Nutrition and Cancer Journal of Nutrition*, 131: 3078s-3081s (2001).

Hegarty V, *Nutrition and the Environment*, pp 80-133 (1995).

Hellmich N, "Obesity Predicted for 40% of America," *USA Today*, p 7D (October 14, 2003).

Herbert V and Subak-Sharpe GT, *The Mount Sinai School of Medicine Complete Book of Nutrition*, pp 600-10, 753 (1990).

Hoppe P, Kramer K and Packer L, "Nutraceuticals: The Link between Nutrition and Medicine," *Nutraceuticals in Health and Disease Prevention*, pp 7-10 (2001).

Hoppe P, Kramer K and Packer L, *Nutraceuticals in Health and Disease Prevention*, pp 7-10, 37-42 (2001).

Hyman PM, "Legal Developments in Marketing Foods with Health Claims in USA," *Vegetables, Fruits and Herbs in Health Promotion*, pp 320-324 (2001).

Johnson RK and Frary C, "Choose Beverages and Foods to Moderate Your Intake of Sugars," *American Society for Nutritional Sciences*, 131, p 276s-67 (2001).

Hunt JR, "Vitamin and mineral supplementation–position of ADA," *Journal of American Dietary Association*, 96: 1 pp 73-77 (January 1996).

Kirwan JP et al, "Effects of a moderate glycemic meal on exercise duration and substrate utilization," *Medicine and Science in Sports Exercise*, 33: 9 pp 1517-23 (September 2001).

Kittler P et al, *Food and Culture in America*, pp 1-36, 152-83, 200-202, 259-90, 322-337, 439-471 (1998).

Klatz R and Goldman R, *Stopping the Clock*, pp 13-25 (1996).

Klatz R and R Goldman, *Anti-aging Secrets*, pp 43-45, 71, 118-119, 140 (1996).

Kleiner S *The Physician and Sports Medicine*, 23: 2, pp 15-16 (February 1995); 20: 8, pp 15-16 (August 1992); 23: 4, pp 21-22 (April 1995); 23: 9, pp 7-8 (September 1995); 23: 12, 15-16 (December 1995).

Kreipe R, Forbes G, "Osteoporosis: A 'new morbidity' for dieting female adolescents," *Pediatrics*, 86:3, pp 478-80 (September 1990).

Kurtzweil P, "Taking the Fat out of Food," *FDA Consumer Magazine* (July-August 1996).

Lam lecture notes, Lam School of Advanced Esthetics, Toronto, Canada (2003).

Lee J and Watson R, "Nutrients and Vegetables in Skin Protection," *Fruits and Herbs in Health Promotion*, pp 99-104 (2001).

Maffetone P "In Fitness and in Health, Everyone is an Athlete," David Baremore Productions, Board of Anti-aging Medicine study materials.

Mason P," *Handbook of Dietary Supplements: Vitamins and Other Health Supplements*, pp 4-20, 107 (1995).

Meschino J, *Standards in Natural Solutions*, (1998, 1999).

Meschino J, *The Building Blocks of Wellness*, Super Wellness Seminar, (1998).

Meschino J, *Adeeva Supplementation in Vitamin Supplements for Healthy Skin*, (2003).

Messina M and Messina V, *The Simple Soybean and Your Health*, pp 72-77 (1994).

Michalun N and M, *Skin Care and Cosmetic Ingredients Dictionary*, p 17-19, 191 (2004).

Mokdad A et al, *Journal of American Medical Association*, 286: 10, pp 1195-1200, (2001).

Moller P et al, "Oxidative stress associated with exercise, psychological stress and lifestyle factors," *Chemi-Biol. Interact*, 102 p17 (1996).

National Academics Press, Washington DC, Institute of Medicine, Food and Nutrition Board (1998). Dietary Reference Intakes for Thiamin, Riboflavin, Niacin, Vitamin B6, Folate, Vitamin B12, Panthothenic acid, Biotin, Choline.

Murray M and Pizzorno J, "Nutritional Medicine," *Textbook of Natural Medicine, Second Edition*, 2, pp 247, 369-79, 474-84, 545-49, 582, 652, 733-48, 837, 1008, 1161-64, 1322-25, 1392-94 (1999).

National Academy of Sciences, *Estimating Daily Energy Expenditures at Various Levels of Physical Activity*, (1999).

National Health and Nutrition Examination Survey (NHANES III), 1988-94.

National Institute of Health, *Understanding Adult Obesity*, p 1(6) (November 1993).

Nesheim MC, "What is the research base for the use of dietary supplements?" *Public Health Nutrition* 2:1 pp 35-38 (1999).

Omaye S and Zhang P, "Phytochemical Interactions: Beta Carotene, Tocopherol and Ascorbic Acid," *Phytochemicals – a New Paradigm*. p 59 (1998).

O'Neill K et al, "Fruits and Vegetables and the Prevention of Oxidative DNA Damage in Vegetables," *Fruits and Herbs in Health Promotion*, pp 140-141 (2001).

Ontario Soybean Growers' Marketing Board

Oosting C, *www.bodybuilding.com*, Body Types, pp 1-4.

Per B, *The Lancet*, 350: 9075 p 423-4 (1997).

Passwater R, "The Metabolic Energizer," *Lipoic Acid: The Metabolic Antioxidant*, pp 15, 20 (1998).

Perricone N, Lecture at Skin and Aging Symposium (2002).

Personal Interviews with various ethnic community leaders, 2003.

Pizzorno J and Murray M, *Textbook of Natural Medicine*, pp 65-69, 165, 653, 1387 (1999).

Pugliese P, *Physiology of the Skin II*, pp 13, 80-81 (2001).

Purves W et al, *Life: The Science of Biology*, 4: 1, p 257 (1995).

Rimm EB et al, "Vitamin E consumption and risk of coronary heart disease in men," *New England Journal of Medicine*, 328, pp 1450-56 (May 20, 1993).

Roberts S, *Nutrition Reviews*, 58: 6 pp 163-69 (2000).

Robbins SP, "Women's Self-Conception of Nutrition, Societal Influences on Eating Behaviors," *Nutritional Concerns of Women*, pp 16, 25-30 (1996).

Roe D, *Nutrition and the Skin*, p 269 (1999).

Russell L, "The importance of patients' nutritional status in wound healing," *Br. J. Nurs.*, 10:6, Suppl. S42, S44-9 (March 2001).

Scholl D, Langkamp-Henken B, "Nutrient recommendations for wound healing," *J. Intraven Nurs.* 24: 2, pp 124-32 (March-April 2001).

Scott B, "The Vegetarian Resource Group 1991 Survey Results," *Vegetarian Journal*, 10: 6, pp 14-17 (1991).

Shapiro A et al, "Guidelines for Responsible Nutritional Counseling on Complementary and Alternative Medicine," *Nutrition Today*, 36: 6 p 291 (November/December 2001).

Sutherford K, "Deciphering Food Labels," *http://kidshealth.org*, (2001).

Simeon DT et al, "Effects of missing breakfast on cognitive functions of school children of differing nutritional status," *Am. J. Clin. Nutrition*, 49, p 646 (April 1989).

Solomon E and Phillips G, *Understanding Human Anatomy and Physiology*, p 61 (1987).

Sparling M, Anderson J, "Modified Foods in the Marketplace," *Nutrition Today*, 3: 4, p 213 (July/August 2001).

Stampter MJ et al, "Vitamin E Consumption and Risk of Cardiovascular Disease in Women," *New England Journal of Medicine*, 329, pp 1440-44 (1993).

Stannard S et al, "The effect of glycemic index on plasma glucose and lactate levels during incremental exercise," *International Journal of Sport Nutrition and Exercise Metabolism*, pp 10, 51- 61, (2000).

Starr M et al, "Health Benefits of Cranberries and Related Fruits in Vegetables," *Fruits and Herbs in Health Promotion*, p 2264 (2001).

Taylor S et al, "Food Allergies and Avoidance Diets," *Nutrition Today*, 34: 1, p 18 (January/February 1999).

The Journal of the American Medical Association, 292: 16 (Oct. 1999).

Tryfoods International, 1997.

Uhl S, *Food Technology*, pp 61-84 (July 1996).

USDA, *Food Guide Pyramid*, (1992).

U.S. Food and Drug Administration, Center for Food Safety and Applied Nutrition, pp 1-10 (June 2000); (July 9, 2003).

USA Today Magazine, 130: 12675, p 1 (Aug. 2001).

U.S. Department of Health and Human Services, NIH Publication 97-4063 (September 1997).

Virgilli F et al, "Plant Phenols and Cardiovascular Diseases: Antioxidants and Modulations of Cell Response," *Nutraceuticals in Health and Disease Prevention*, pp 187-97 (2002).

Watson R, "Herbal Remedies that promote Health and Prevent Disease in Vegetables," *Vegetables, Fruits and Herbs in Health Promotion*, pp 180-197 (2000).

Wein D, "Glycemic Index," *IDEA Personal Trainer* (November-December 2001).

Weiss RF, Fintelmann V, *Herbal Medicine, 2nd Edition*, p 283, (2000).

Whitney E and Rolfes S, *Understanding Nutrition, 9th Edition*, pp 12-13, 54, 48, 72, 234, 246-47, 253-55, 355-68, 396-411, 563 (2002).

Wise J, "Health Benefits of Fruits and Vegetables, The Protective Role of Phytonutrients," *Vegetables and Herbs in Health Promotion*, p 152 (2001).

Wood RJ et al, "Mineral Requirements of Elderly People," *American Journal of Clinical Nutrition*, 62, pp 493-505 (September 1995).

www.dialadietitian.org, "Nutrition Recommendations," (May 28, 2003).

www.hc-sc.gc.ca, "A Consumers Guide to the DRIs."

www.sentara.com, "Healthy Living," pp 3-4.

www.ttfit.com, "What Body Type are You: Endomorph, Mesomorph or Ectomorph?"

www.nlm.nih.gov, Medline Plus, Medical Encyclopedia, "Food labeling," (December 2, 2001).

www.fsis.usda.gov, "Basis for handling food safely," Food and Safety Facts (April 2002).

www.cfsan.fda.gov, "Food Safety for You," (September 1998).

www.mayoclinic.com, Organic foods, "New options with growing differences," (October 2003).

www.mayoclinic.com, "What's for breakfast? Healthy choices can give your day a boost," (May 2003).

www.foodallergy.org, (September 21, 2003).

www.fda.gov, "FDA warns milk producers to remove 'hormone free' claims from the labeling of dairy products," News (2003).

www.unescape.org, "Table 2.12: Life Expectancy at Birth and Average Number of Years Women Outlive Men."

Young VR, "Soy protein in relation to human protein and amino acid nutrition," *Journal of American Dietetic Association*, 94: 7, pp 739-43 (1991).

Ziebart E, "The Ethnic Food Lover's Composition," *Understanding the Cuisines of the World*, pp81-85, 166, 195-206, 318-340, 393-397 (2001).

GLOSSARY

A

abduct movement Drawn away from the midline.

acesulfame potassium (acesulfame-k) An FDA approved sweetener that doesn't add extra calories.

acetic acid The simplest fatty acid with a two carbon chain is responsible for the sour taste in vinegar.

acidosis Excess acids in blood.

ackee A peapod containing yellow flesh that looks like scrambled eggs when cooked, but has a lemony flavor. A signature dish of Jamaicans.

acquired immunity As a result of receiving flu or vaccine shots, the body develops a powerful immunity against foreign agents such as viruses and toxins.

actinic keratoses Flat hyperpigmented lesions that appear dry and hard with a reddish color giving the skin a rough texture. Commonly found in sun-exposed areas among middle-aged individuals, especially among blondes and redheads and those who are always in the sun.

added sugars Sugars that are eaten separately or found in processed foods.

additives Nutrients that have been added to enhance or fortify food such as calcium to milk, folic acid to fruit juices and omega-3 fatty acids to eggs.

adduct movement Drawn toward the midline.

adenosine triphosphate (ATP) A compound of high energy.

adrenocorticotropic hormone (ACTH) This hormone secreted by the pituitary gland stimulates the adrenal cortex to produce its steroid hormones, primarily cortisol.

allergens A substance that is capable of inducing allergic reactions or hypersensitivity.

allergy An abnormal hypersensitivity from exposure to an antigen.

aloe vera A substance secreted by the leaf of the aloe plant; it is employed by the cosmetic industry to soften the skin.

alpha hydroxy acids (AHAs) The family name for a variety of acids including glycolic acid from sugar cane, citric acid from citrus fruits, lactic acid from sour milk and tartaric acid from apples. AHAs are used as peeling agents for acneic, aging and hyperpigmented skins. They also have been found to have moisturizing properties.

alpha-tocopherol The most active form of vitamin E found in the body providing powerful antioxidant effects.

amenorrhea Absence or abnormal stoppage of menses.

amino acid The basic building block of protein.

anchovies Small herring-like fish often served with Italian dishes.

anion A negatively charged ion that progresses from a negative pole to a positive pole.

anorexia nervosa A serious psychological problem that affects young people, particularly females who believe that they are too fat and take drastic measures in dieting. They starve themselves to be thin leading to serious medical problems.

antacids Medications that neutralize excess acidity in the stomach, relieving indigestion.

anterior Front half of the body. Also known as frontal view.

anthocyanins The pigments that give the rich red colors to berries such as cranberries and grapes.

anthropometric measurements The most common methods used to measure the physical characteristics of the body and compare against a similar individual specific for that age and gender.

anti-aging A term used to describe any form of preventive care to slow down the aging process. Aging is viewed not as an inevitable process, but as a disease that can be prevented.

antibodies Proteins released by the lymphatic system rendering antigens harmless.

antigen A foreign substance that enters the body.

antioxidants Such as vitamins A, C and E combat oxidation.

antipastas Italian appetizers, can be served cold or warm.

apple-shaped A term used to refer to those men and women who have excess fat in the chest and abdomen, and are at a higher risk for cardiovascular diseases. More commonly found among middle-aged men due to poor lifestyle habits such as unhealthy dietary intake, alcohol and smoking.

arachidonic acid Found in animal products such as meat and vegetable oils.

aracidis oil Also known as peanut oil.

artesian water Contains high mineral concentration—comes from a well that taps into a rock formation.

atherosclerosis The hardening and thickening of arterial walls characterized by plaque buildup implicated in cardiovascular diseases.

antibodies Protein substances made by white blood cells to destroy foreign antigens present in the body.

antigen Any foreign substance that causes antibodies to be produced in response to its entrance into the body.

arugula Leafy salad greens with a unique peppery sweetness.

asanas Poses of Hatha yoga that involve deep breathing, stretching and meditation.

aspartame An FDA approved sweetener that doesn't add extra calories.

assimilation The occurrence when individuals from a culture sheds their ethnic identity and fully merge with the mainstream culture, adopting most beliefs and behavioral patterns.

atom The smallest part of any matter that can exist and retain its chemical property. It is neutral in electrical charge.

B

bad cholesterol Low density lipoproteins (LDL).

baklava The most famous Greek dessert, a phyllo pastry drenched in sugar, syrup and nuts.

balance Maintaining equilibrium while exercising.

bangers Pork sausages, frequently served as part of an English breakfast.

basal energy needs (BEN) The estimated amount of energy required for daily activities calculated from the BMR multiplied by a percentage of activity level.

basal metabolic rate (BMR) The amount of energy output or calories required when the body is at complete rest, not asleep, approximately 12 hours after a meal so no digestion is taking place and in a warm room so no energy is required to keep warm. BMR varies according to age, gender and activity levels.

basic metabolism Internal processes within the body that are unnoticed such as breathing, digestion and excretion.

beri-beri A disease that affects the nervous and muscular system and occurs from a deficiency of thiamine, or vitamin B-1. First observed in Asia when thiamin was removed in the process of polishing rice.

bioflavonoids Found in mostly citrus fruits and together with vitamin C have an anti-inflammatory action on tissues by reducing the effects of histamines. They are not as powerful as quercetin, but help in strengthening capillary walls and reducing skin bruising.

biological age The functional ability of an individual is what counts and not the chronological age. For example, a 60-year man may look younger than his chronological age because of lifestyle, both physiologically and functionality.

biological stressors Adverse physiological conditions such as malnutrition, illness and trauma.

biomarker A significant biological mark of a health condition such as high blood cholesterol, a biomarker for cardiovascular disease.

biskcake Irish biscuits.

bitters A British favorite, a rich amber-colored beer that is flavored strongly with hops.

black forest cake A popular German dessert, chocolate cake with cherries.

blood cholesterol Cholesterol manufactured by the liver.

body alignment Refers to the proper positioning of body parts in relation to one another.

botanicals Plant extracts containing active ingredients that can elicit certain biological responses when applied to the skin. Botanicals were used by ancient societies as remedies for a variety of external and internal disorders. They have not undergone any chemical processing so there are no government regulations about their usage.

bran The fibrous protective part of the grain, rich in nutrients and the main source of fiber.

bratwurst sausage Popular in North America, cured pork and beef that is air dried and smoked, and is very popular for grilling.

bromelain An enzyme from pineapple used as a skin exfoliant. It may cause skin irritation.

bruschetta A popular Italian appetizer.

bulimia An impulsive behavior where there is an excessive concern with body image. Those with bulimia lack control in eating and binge followed by purging. This disease is not as visible as anorexia nervosa and is difficult to detect.

butylated hydroxyanisole (BHA) An additive used in processed food.

butylated hydroxytoluene An additive used in processed food.

C

cacciatore Chicken stewed in wine with onions and tomatoes. A popular Italian dish.

calalloo A Creole soup containing salted meats and a wide variety of vegetables. Also known as pepperpot.

calciferol Also known as Vitamin D.

calcitonin An endocrine hormone produced by the thyroid gland to lower blood calcium when levels are too high.

calories Units of measurement for energy. Food energy is measured in kilocalories (kcal) that equals 1,000 calories and is used in metabolic studies to measure the amount of heat required to raise the temperature of one kilogram of water to one degree Celsius.

cannelloni Rolled tubular pasta stuffed with chicken.

carbohydrate substitutes These include dextrins, fiber, gums and starches that are used as emulsifiers and stabilizers.

carnivores Those who eat mainly meat.

carotenoids As pigments commonly found in plants and animals, some of them act as precursors for vitamin A.

catalase A natural antioxidant enzyme that keeps free radicals under control and minimizes cellular damage.

catechins A group of flavonoids that act as powerful free radical scavengers and antioxidants. Significant sources are found in green and black tea.

cation A positively charged ion, carrying a positive charge from a positive pole to a negative pole.

celiac disease Also known as gluten intolerance, it is a genetic disorder experienced by many people of different cultures, particularly in Northern Europe. They must consume a wheat-free diet.

celia sprue See celiac disease.

cellular metabolism Cellular metabolism refers to the expenditure of energy within each individual cell.

cellulase An enzyme supplement now available in predigested foods to improve digestion and prevent digestive disorders.

cellulose The chief constituent of a plant's cell wall, it is a polysaccharide composed of glucose molecules that do not branch out. Found in all vegetables, fruits and legumes, it is indigestible and an excellent source of fiber.

ceramides A glue-like cement in the epidermal layer that bind cells together.

challah A braided Jewish bread.

chapatti Flat, pita-like bread used in Eastern Indian cooking.

chi Vital energy force which flows along meridian lines in the body.

cholesterol A sterol fat produced in the liver and found only in animal foods.

cholet A Jewish bean and potato dish.

chorizo A spicy unsmoked pork sausage of Mexican origin.

chronological age Age by date of birth.

chylomicrons The largest and least dense lipoproteins that carry lipids from the intestinal cells to the rest of the body.

coenzymes Small organic molecules that assist the main enzyme's function. Most coenzymes are made from water-soluble vitamins.

collagen tightening Part of the repair process after laser skin resurfacing, resulting in smoother, tighter and more youthful looking skin.

complementary proteins Two or more protein foods used by vegetarians to combine plant protein foods in such a way that all twenty amino acids are balanced to support health. An example would be black beans and rice.

complete proteins Those foods that contain all twenty amino acids and usually are found in foods from animal sources such as meat and dairy products. Also known as first class proteins.

complex carbohydrates Also called polysaccharides, they are composed of many monosaccharides linked together to form starch or fiber. Diets high in complex carbohydrates tend to be low in fat and high in fiber, vitamins and minerals.

concentric Movement that bends or flexes a limb at a joint. Muscle fibers shorten and become thicker.

coordination The ability to integrate body movements involving several muscle groups at the same time during exercise.

core strength The deep postural muscles of the body, the abdominal and lower back muscles are considered the powerhouse of the body in the fitness regime developed by Joseph Pilates. In developing core strength, a contraction between the abdominal and back muscles will help to stabilize the torso.

coronal plane The vertical plane that divides the body into the anterior (front) and posterior (back) sections. Also known as the frontal plane.

clotted cream A slightly fermented thick cream, often used on scones, a British dish.

culture The beliefs, attitudes, values, customs, rituals and habits accepted and practiced by a community.

D

daily values (DVs) These standards developed by the United States Food and Drug Administration for food labels show recommendations for important nutrients relating to health and help consumers make informed decisions about the food they are purchasing. The information gives the consumer some idea of the percentage of the nutrient's contribution towards the total daily dietary intake and is usually based on a "normal" man or woman's daily calorie intake. It helps keep track of how much more of that particular nutrient one will need for the rest of the day making it easy to compare the values of different foods.

dal The different kinds of lentils that are usually pureed or stewed, sometimes with potatoes and peas, that are very popular in Indian cuisine.

denaturation A change in the usual structure of a substance.

dermis The layer of skin immediately below the epidermis and above the subcutaneous layer, also called the true skin because it contains nerve endings and blood vessels.

detoxification Elimination of toxins either by direct neutralization or excretion in the form of urine, feces, or other areas such as lungs or skin.

dietary cholesterol Cholesterol found in foods.

dietary reference intakes (DRIs) The collaborative efforts of researchers in United States and Canada have resulted in this set of values that can be used in planning and assessing dietary nutrient intakes of healthy people in both countries.

dietary supplements Nutrients in the form of pills, gels or powder meant to be in addition to a person's diet, not be to be used in place of dietary intake.

dipeptide Two amino acids are bonded to one another by chemical bonds forming protein chains of varying lengths.

disaccharides Double sugars that contain glucose that is bonded with one of the other monosaccharides.

distal The furthest to a point of reference.

distilled water Water that has been vaporized and condensation has taken place to produce water without minerals.

diuretics Drugs that increase the production of urine and reduce water retention in the body.

diverticulitis Inflammation of the intestinal walls caused by improper elimination of waste products resulting in small pockets that leads to infection. It commonly is caused by a low dietary fiber intake.

DNA Deoxyribonucleic acid—the genetic blueprint of the cell.

Dowager's Hump A condition affecting the dorsal bones in the vertebrae that become wedged-shaped giving rise to extreme pain and an overall reduction in height.

E

eccentric Movements where limbs are straightened or stretched and muscle fibers lengthen.

edamame Soybeans, served fresh in their pods, usually are lightly salted as appetizers or snacks.

electrolytes Substances that dissociate into ions fused in solution and capable of conducting electricity. They are essential to life.

electron A negatively charged particle that revolves on the orbits of the atom. Electrons give an atom its ability to bond with other atoms to create molecules.

emulsifiers Ingredients that binds both water soluble and oil soluble substances to create a homogenous substance or emulsion.

endosperm The soft, inner part of the grain that is eaten, and contains starch and protein.

endothelial cells The thin inner layer of arterial walls.

enema A solution that is inserted into the rectum and colon to stimulate a bowel movement and empty the large intestine.

enriched Nutrients are added to certain foods after they have become lost during the manufacture of refined foods.

enzyme An organic catalyst made from protein that causes a chemical reaction without itself being affected. They break down and build up substances, as well as transforming one substance into another one. The body cannot function without enzymes.

ephedrine The chemical form of the Chinese plant, ephedra in supplemental form and used for treatment of certain conditions such as asthma, hay fever and rhinitis. It also has been marketed to promote weight loss but there can be several side effects such as increased blood pressure and heart rate, insomnia and anxiety. The FDA recently banned its usage.

ephinehrine A hormone secreted by the adrenal gland in response to the stress stimulus. Also known as adrenaline.

epidermis The top layer of the skin that has many protective functions.

ergogenic Substances or treatments claimed to enhance physical performance. For example, ergogenic aids such as whey protein are aimed primarily at athletes.

errector pili muscles Tiny muscles attached to the skin and hair follicle that contract involuntarily when the body is cold to maintain homeostasis of body's temperature.

escarole Leafy salad greens with a touch of bitterness.

espresso Strong Italian coffee.

essential amino acids The nine amino acids that must be provided in daily dietary intake to form complete proteins.

essential fatty acids Fatty acids that have to be taken into the body through diet.

eversion Involves the limb turning outward away from the midline.

extrinsic factors Factors associated with aging caused by environmental influences.

F

fat replacers Provide less than half of the nine calories per gram of regular fat with the exception of olestra, which has no calories.

feta cheese A sharp, salty, semi-soft cheese commonly used in salads. Used in Greek cooking.

fiber Fibers form the structures of plants and are non-starchy and indigestible.

fibrin A blood clotting protein.

fibrinogen A polypeptide chain found in the blood that promotes blood clotting.

fibromas Benign tumors that are either flat, raised, small or large. They either sit on the skin's surface or are found attached by a short thin neck. An example is a skin tag.

fish and chips Battered deep fried fish served with fried potatoes and seasoned with salt and malt vinegar. Originated in British pubs.

flan A popular Mexican dessert.

flavonoids A group of water-soluble plant pigments with biological activity responsible for the colors of many fruits and flowers. They have been found to be effective in treatment and prevention of many health conditions by acting as potent antioxidants. More than 4,000 flavonoid compounds have been documented. Also known as polyphenols.

flexibility The range of motion (ROM) at joints. The greater the ROM, the better the flexibility.

foam cells Scavenger cells from the immune system adopt the appearance of sea foam after they have ingested the LDL cholesterol particles in the arteries. They eventually burst leaving the accumulated cholesterol on the arterial walls resulting in plaque accumulation and leading to atherosclerosis.

focaccia bread A thick crust often used in Italian cooking for pizza or sandwiches.

fontina An Italian soft cheese.

fortified The process where a nutrient that was not sufficiently present is added to certain foods to either increase or prevent that nutrient deficiency in a population.

free radicals By-products of cellular metabolism that cause cellular aging and eventual destruction.

free-range poultry Considered the healthier form of poultry to eat, this term refers to poultry brought up on a farm where they can run around freely developing muscular tissues.

frontal plane The vertical plane that divides the body into the anterior (front) and posterior(back) sections. Also known as the coronal plane.

fructose Naturally occurring sugars in fruits, honey and table sugar—the sweetest of the three monosaccharides.

functional foods Any food or food ingredient that has modified ordinary foods by being incorporated in order to provide particular health benefits beyond the traditional nutrients it contains. For example, any dietary supplements such as fiber that has been added to orange juice. Also known as nutraceuticals.

fusilli Spiral-shaped pasta.

fusion foods Refers to new cuisine that results from the combination of two or more cuisines.

G

galactose A monosaccharide derived from milk and milk products. Lactose contains both galactose and glucose.

gastrocnemius Calf muscles.

gastroplasty Also referred to as stomach stapling, a drastic measure in which surgery is performed to remove part of the gastrointestinal tract forcing the person to eat less.

germ The nutritious inner part of the grain where cells develop and grow.

ghee Clarified butter that is boiled, the surface fat skimmed off then filtered, resulting in a finer, smoother form of butter.

glucoasmine sulfate A compound that is available commercially for the treatment of osteoarthritis.

glucose This monosaccharide appears in all plant sugars. It is the building block of carbohydrates and is used as quick energy by the body.

glutamine In sickle cell anemia, a blood disease typically found in people of African descent, the normal position of the amino acid glutamine in the side chain is replaced by valine during its formation.

glutathione peroxidase An enzyme produced by the body to deactivate free radicals.

glycemic index A method of measuring how fast carbohydrate foods are digested and show up in the blood stream.

glycoaminoglycans (GAG) A polysaccharide consisting of amino sugars credited with moisturizing and firming qualities in the skin. Hyaluronic acid is the most well known GAG and is one of the newest cosmetic ingredients.

glycogen The form in which excess glucose is stored in the liver and skeletal muscles.

gnocchi Italian dumplings made from semolina wheat.

good cholesterol High density lipoproteins (HDL).

gorgonzola A fine blue cheese often used in Greek cuisine.

growth hormone (hGH) A hormone produced by the pituitary gland that regulates growth and development of the body tissues.

guacamole Mashed and seasoned avocado popular with Mexican cuisine.

guar gum Found in sticky gums in certain plants. It often is used as a thickener or emulsifier in cosmetics and as added fiber in certain foods.

gum arabic Gummy parts that exude from plants when cut, used as additives in foods.

H

hatha yoga The most popular form of yoga in North America with a focus on physical health and mental well-being. This involves deep breathing, stretching and meditation.

heart disease The leading cause of death today.

heleb The layer of solid fat in meat that is not mixed with the flesh, blood, blood vessels and sciatic nerve are removed, usually by a Jewish butcher, during the preparation of kosher foods.

hemangiomas Benign minor vascular abnormalities of the skin appearing as blood spots in a cavity or under the skin. Cherry angiomas are bright red to purple dots of blood usually found on the upper trunk such as the neck while strawberry hemangiomas during childhood appear raised, red and soft in the shape of a strawberry, but usually disappear in adulthood.

heme The part of hemoglobin that holds iron and is found in animal derived foods.

hemicellulose The main fibers in cereals with branching side chains of monosaccharides.

hemoglobin The oxygen-carrying pigment of the erythrocytes developed in the bone marrow and made up of four polypeptide chains. Cells low in hemoglobin appear to be pale in color.

hemorrhoids Dilation and painful swelling of the veins in the rectum.

high density lipoproteins (HDL) Protein carriers taking remnants of cholesterol from the blood back to the liver for disposal. It is known as the good cholesterol.

histamine A substance produced by cells of the immune system in response to the entrance of an allergen into the body and resulting in inflammation.

homeostasis Equilibrium or constancy in the internal environment of the body, such as blood pressure and temperature.

homocysteine Increased level of this substance in blood are linked with heart disease. During protein metabolism, sufficient amounts of certain B vitamins are necessary to convert homocysteine into the amino acid methionine. Lack of these nutrients result in high homocysteine levels in the blood.

horizontal plane Runs across the body parallel to the ground, dividing the body into superior (upper) and inferior (lower) portions. Also known as the transverse plane.

hormone replacement therapy (HRT) Scientists have determined that the body's level of hormones are reduced dramatically as the body ages reducing its functionality. Many believe that using synthetic HRTs can increase the levels of growth, sex and other hormones to rejuvenate the body and by restoring these levels, the healthy functioning of the body systems would be maintained.

huevos reales A popular Mexican dessert.

humoral immunity Immune response in which B cells transform into plasma cells and secrete antibodies.

hummus A Greek dish of cooked, pureed chickpeas, popularly used as a dip or appetizer.

husk The part of the grain that is not used for human consumption, only for animal feed.

hyaluronic acid A component of glycosamionoglycans (GAGs) that occurs naturally in the dermis. It has a strong ability to hold water due to its negatively-charged ability and is used to lubricate the joints to enable smooth movement. Its ability to retain water gives immediate smoothness to rough, dry skin leading to significant improvement in the skin's appearance.

hydrogenation The process of adding hydrogen to monounsaturated or polyunsaturated fats to make a more solid form such as margarine or shortening resulting in the production of trans fatty acids.

hydrogen peroxide A bleaching and oxidizing ingredient, detergent and antiseptic used in cosmetics. If not diluted, it can damage the skin's surface.

hydroquinone A depigmentation chemical used to lighten the skin. Also used as an antioxidant in bleaching creams and hair products.

hydroxyl radical One of the most potent oxidants known to science because it can react with any compound in the body. They act on lipids causing lipid peroxidation and causing proteins to cross link and damage the DNA leading to premature skin aging.

hydroxlysine A polypeptide chain.

hydroxyproline A polypeptide chain formed during collagen formation consisting of approximately 1,000 amino acids.

hyperextension Joint movement is beyond the midline.

hyperglycemia Excess of sugar in the blood.

hyperplasia The increase of cells in number and size.

hypertrophy The growth of muscles in response to use.

hypoglycemia Abnormal low blood glucose.

I

incomplete proteins Those proteins that do not contain all the essential amino acids and are not derived from animal sources such as most vegetables, legumes or wheat and rye. Also known as second class proteins.

inferior The lower section of the body.

inorganic Not containing carbon or pertaining to living things, such as minerals.

insertion One of the two points of attachment, where the muscle attaches to another muscle or bone causing movement at the joints. Origin is the other point of attachment.

insoluble fiber Mostly found in whole grains, cereals and vegetables, these indigestible fibers contribute toward weight loss, relieve constipation and help prevent intestinal disorders.

insulin resistance The body's reduced ability in regulating the metabolism of glucose.

intrinsic factors Genetic factors associated with chronological age.

inversion Involves the limb turning inward toward the midline.

isoflavones The largest subcategory of isoflavonoids. They are believed to have health benefits in reducing the incidence of cancer and other health problems.

isometric Refers to the toning of a muscle without any change of length. No movement occurs and no calories are burnt.

isotonic Refers to any free activity where muscles change in length becoming shorter to bring about movement.

isotretinoin A derivative of retinoid used for the treatment of severe acne skin conditions.

K

kashrut Dietary laws set in the Torah, followed by all Orthodox and some Conservative Jews.

kebabs Greek style of cooking where meat is marinated and then grilled or roasted on a spit.

ketone bodies When glucose is not available in the blood, the body turns to burning fat. But it is not broken down completely and ketone bodies are formed in the blood and urine.

ketosis A condition where a high level of ketone bodies is found in the blood and urine.

kippers Smoked fish often served at English breakfasts or as appetizers.

knackwurst sausage A German sausage made of pork and beef seasoned with garlic and cumin.

kosher Dietary laws followed by many Jewish people.

kugel A Jewish pudding often made with noodles.

kypholordosis A combination of kyphosis and lordosis.

kyphosis Convex curvature of the upper back noticeably in old age.

L

lactase An enzyme that acts on lactose, or milk sugar, in the stomach for digestion.

lactic acid A multipurpose ingredient used as a preservative, exfoliant and moisturizer. Added to products for its acidic pH, it is an alpha hydroxy acid from fermentation from sour milk and other foods, and is a component of the skin's natural moisturizing factor. Also known as sodium lactate.

lacto-ovos People who avoid meat but eat animal-derived foods such as milk products and eggs.

lactose Lactose is the main sugar in milk and is a disaccharide comprised of both glucose and galactose.

lactose intolerant Refers to the inability to digest milk sugars—lactose—usually caused by the lack of the enzyme lactase, resulting in lactose molecules remaining undigested. Symptoms include bloating, gas, abdominal discomfort and diarrhea.

lacto-vegetarians Those who avoid red meat and eggs but consume dairy products.

Langerhans cells These cells, found in the upper layers of the skin, travel to the lymphatic nodes in the immune response and histamine is released in the tissues.

laser A surgical device using a beam of intensive light that acts as the energy source to literally burn the skin's surface layers. The healing of the skin after the trauma causes the collagen fibers in the dermis to contract and tighten leading to a smoother, tighter and more youthful looking skin.

lateral plane Vertical plane that divides the body into left and right sections. Also known as the saggital plane.

latkes Traditional potato pancakes served during Hanukkah, the festival of lights, celebrated by the Jewish faith.

legumes High quality plant protein such as peas and beans that are used commonly as complementary proteins.

lentigines Small macules that are uniform in color appearing on sun-exposed areas particularly during middle age.

leptin A protein produced by an obesity gene in fat cells that is believed to decrease appetite. Although it acts as a hormone to inhibit fat storage, it has not proven to be effective in treating obesity.

lignins Tough, woody parts of vegetables and seeds of fruits.

line of gravity An imaginary line that runs down the middle of the body to divide the body into two halves. Any deviation from this line can be used to indicate abnormalities in posture and body alignment.

linolenic acids Also known as omega-3 fatty acids, they consist of 18 carbons and three double bonds and are necessary to manufacture certain compounds that are important for the health of the body. They have been found to have protective factors in strengthening the immune system, lowering blood cholesterol levels and reducing tissue inflammation.

lipase An enzyme that catabolizes fats in the small intestine.

lipid peroxidation Lipids, particularly LDL cholesterol, are highly susceptible to oxidation or lipid peroxidation. This leads to plaque formation in blood vessels.

lipoproteins Special transport vehicles that distribute triglycerides and fatty acids to body tissues via the lymphatic system.

lordosis A concave lumbar curve that may be associated with shortened hip flexors and anterior pelvic tilt. More likely found among tall, thin individuals.

low density lipoproteins (LDL) Protein carriers that mainly transport cholesterol from the liver to the cells of the body. It is referred to as the bad cholesterol.

lysine An essential amino acid.

M

macronutrients A term referring to large amounts of food such as proteins, carbohydrates and fats measured in grams required for health and maintenance of the body.

Ma Huang The Chinese plant from which ephedrine is derived.

maki Rolled sushi.

maltose Consists of two glucose units and is produced from the final breakdown of carbohydrates such as wheat, barley or oats. When fermented, maltose can yield alcohol.

manicotti Square pasta with a filling.

marzipan Another popular German dessert, a paste of ground almonds and sugar.

matzah A white flour cracker, the descendant of the unleavened bread, popular in the diet of Jewish people.

maximum heart rate (MHR) The highest heart rate that a person attains during the height of consistent aerobic exercise. It decreases with age about one beat per minute per year after age 20.

melasma Also known as cholasma or pregnancy mask. A patchy brown hyperpigmentation found on the forehead, cheeks, upper lip and chin. It occurs primarily in females who are pregnant or may be using birth control pills or hormone replacement therapy. With pregnancy, it may fade after birth of the child, but may remain permanent if using hormone supplementation or birth control medication.

melting pot The term used to infer that numerous cultural groups have "melted" into a mainstream group.

metabolic effect A chain of reactions set off by enzymes that speed up reactions in cells without themselves being affected.

metabolism The process of life—burning blood sugar to produce energy.

microdermabrasion: A non-invasive skin resurfacing procedure where inert crystals are propelled across the skin's surface to exfoliate dead cells.

micronutrients A term that refers to smaller units of food such as vitamins and minerals measured in milligrams and micrograms required for health and maintenance of the body.

midline An imaginary line that passes through the middle of the body.

milk allergy The most common food allergy caused by milk resulting in production of antibodies for protection.

minerals Inorganic elements found mainly in plants.

mineral water Drawn from an underground source and contains at least 250 parts per million of dissolved solid mineral salts.

miso A paste of fermented soybean, often used during fasting.

mitochondria A small rod-shaped organelle in the cytoplasm. Known as the powerhouse of the cell where metabolic processes occur to produce energy.

monosaccharides Single sugar molecules in simple carbohydrates. There are three types of monosaccharides, each one having the same number of atoms, but because they are arranged differently, have different physical and chemical properties accounting for varying amounts of sweetness. The three types are fructose, glucose and galactose.

monounsaturated fatty acid (MUFA) A fatty acid lacking two hydrogen atoms and one double bond between carbons such as oleic acid found in olive and canola oils.

moussaka A Greek casserole made from eggplant or potatoes.

movement In fitness terminology, movement occurs when muscles contract.

mozzarella An Italian soft cheese.

multicultural The term used to depict that different ethnic groups can exist peacefully alongside on another and still carry on their individual cultural norms without restrictions.

N

naan A flaky leavened bread used in Asian-Indian cooking.

natural immunity A natural protective ability to easily resist certain allergens.

natural moisturizing factors (NMF) Found in the corneum layer of the skin, it is composed of hygroscopic and water soluble substances that control and bind the water content in the skin. The NMF is composed of free amino acids and other substances such as urea and lactose. Many modern moisturizers use NMF in their ingredients for holding moisture in the skin.

nigiri Bite-sized roll of seasoned rice used in sushi.

non-essential amino acids Eleven non-essential amino acids are produced in the body by other amino acids and, together with the nine essential amino acids, form a complete protein.

non-heme Iron from plants.

noradrenaline The hormone produced by the adrenal gland in response to the higher amount levels of energy required by the brain and muscles in dealing with duress experienced.

nori sheets Dark green paper made from algae rolled into logs, then sliced to make maki, or rolled sushi.

nutraceuticals A term used to describe the biological activity of any food or food ingredient that may not necessarily be a nutrient, but when isolated from other nutrients, provide protective health benefits. For example, lycopene in tomatoes has been found to maintain prostrate health and prevent heart disease. Also known as functional foods.

O

obesity Excess amount of body fat relative to height.

Octoberfest An ethnic festival that is celebrated in many large German communities.

omnivores Those who eat all foods from animals and plants.

organic A substance containing the element carbon found in living organisms. The term also is used to describe agricultural products where natural fertilizers and feed are used instead of chemicals, and crops are rotated to manage weeds instead of using pesticides.

origin One of the two points of attachment, the fixed point of a muscle where no movement occurs. Insertion is the other point of attachment.

orlistat A drug used in treatment of obesity by inhibiting fat absorption in the intestines.

osteoblast Bone forming cells for growth and repair.

osteoclast Cells inside bone cavity that reabsorb bone cells back into soluble calcium which then enters the blood helping to keep the bone hollow and preventing it from getting too heavy.

osteomalacia A condition of soft bones in adults from a vitamin D deficiency.

osteoporosis A brittle bone disease that affects older adults, particularly women in menopause due to hereditary or lifestyle factors. The porous bone structures develop from deficiency of minerals and often lead to fractures in the limbs and hips.

overweight An excess amount of body weight including muscle, bone and water.

ovo-vegetarians Those who avoid milk products, meat, poultry, fish and seafood but consume eggs.

oxidants See free radicals.

P

papain An enzyme from papaya used as a skin exfoliant in cosmetics.

parathormone An endocrine hormone produced by the parathyroid gland to control homeostasis of blood calcium levels.

parmesan An Italian hard cheese.

pear-shaped Used to describe body types found mainly among post-menopausal women who have more body fat in the trunk area. Associated with a sedentary lifestyle.

pectins Found in apples, they commonly are used as thickeners, and stabilizers in foods and cosmetics.

pellagra A deficiency of niacin, or vitamin B-2, that was prevalent in the early 1900s when many people lived on a low-protein diet. Characterized by diarrhea, dermatitis and dementia.

penne Angle-shaped tubular pasta.

pepperpot A Creole soup containing salted meats and a wide variety of vegetables. Also known as calalloo.

peptides Amino acids are bonded to one another by chemical bonds forming protein chains of varying lengths called peptides.

pesto An Italian paste made from a cheese base.

phospholipids One of the three main forms of lipids, similar to tryglycerides but containing phosphorus. They are important constituents of cell membranes. Lecithin, the best known phospholipids, is a popular emulsifier in cosmetics and foods.

photosynthesis A chemical process by which plants containing chlorophyll manufacture carbohydrates utilizing carbon dioxide from the air, water from the soil and sunlight.

phytic acid Although it is not fiber, it is often found in fiber foods. It has been found that a high fiber diet may risk losing certain minerals through the feces because phytic acid is capable of binding with them and taking them out of the body.

phytochemicals Specific compounds in plant foods that have been shown to exert biological activity by acting as antioxidants with other protective effects such as anti-inflammatory, anti-viral, anti-allergic and anti-cancerous.

phytosterols Plant seeds such as pumpkin seeds, soy, rice and yams that are used for health benefits in herbal therapy.

Pilates Originated by Joseph Pilates in 1920s, this popular form of fitness focuses on developing deep core strength, balanced flexibility, endurance and movement coordination.

pita bread A thin, round Arabic bread with a hollow center.

plane An imaginary flat surface in relation to a reference point such as the midline. It is used to divide the body into parts such as front and back, upper and lower, left and right parts.

platelets In heart disease, platelets become stickier forming clots that grow into arterial walls clogging the width of the artery.

plum pudding Traditional British Christmas dish of suet, dried, candied fruit and other ingredients.

polychlorinated biphenyls (PCBs) Environmental toxins found in herbicides and pesticides. When taken into the body, they are stored in the fat cells. They are believed to contribute to health problems.

polypeptide Many amino acids are bonded to one another by chemical bonds forming protein chains of varying lengths.

polyunsaturated fatty acid (PUFA) "Poly-" means *many*—this is a fatty acid lacking four or more hydrogen atoms, and two or more double bonds between carbons such as linoleic acid—two double bonds, found in vegetable oils, and linolenic acid—three double bonds, found in fish oils.

posterior Back half of the body. Also known as ventral view.

preventive approach The belief that if one follows certain dietary practices and lives a healthy lifestyle, a wide range of diseases can be prevented, or lessened in severity.

proanthocyanidins One of the most beneficial groups of flavonoids that provide antioxidant properties, protect collagen integrity, strengthen capillaries and notably are found in plants with red wine pigments such as all berries, grape seed extracts, red wine and pine bark. Also known as procyanidins.

procollagen The precursor of collagen manufactured in the ribosomes of cells before going on to be modified by enzymes to form the tropocollagen.

procyanidins See proanthocyanidins.

probiotics A functional food constituent cultivated from microbes that have therapeutic health benefits such as improving immune function, protecting against colon cancer and lowering blood cholesterol.

product One of the three parts of an enzyme reaction along with enzyme and substrate. For example, in the digestive process, the substrate can be fats, the enzyme, lipase, and the resulting product, fatty acids and glycerol.

proline One of the main amino acids in collagen formation.

proscuitto An Italian raw, salted, air-cured ham that is a popular antipasta.

proteases Enzymes that break down protein.

protein The second most abundant substance in the body.

protein replacers Are made from whey, milk or egg protein. They contain only 1–2 calories and taste like the real thing.

proteolytic enzymes They break down proteins into amino acids, each one working on a specific protein.

prothrombin An inactive protein that is converted to thrombin, an enzyme in the process of blood coagulation.

proximal The nearest to a point of reference.

psychological stressors Adverse conditions affecting the psyche such as low self-esteem, fear and guilt.

purified water Denotes that all minerals have been removed.

Q

quercetin The most active flavonoid giving anti-inflammatory, anti-viral and anti-cancer effects. It gives most medicinal plants their high potency.

R

R-group: This is the side chain above the central carbon atom in the chemical structure of an amino acid. It varies in composition and is the deciding factor that determines the type of protein formed.

radicchio Leafy salad greens with a touch of bitterness.

range of motion (ROM) The flexibility or possible movement of muscles at a joint.

recommended dietary allowance (RDA) This is used by health care professionals as a goal for dietary intake of individuals and is the recommended daily average amount of nutrients considered adequate to meet the nutritional needs of groups of most healthy individuals in a population. These guidelines had been designed to reduce or prevent certain severe nutritional deficiencies such as scurvy that were prevalent during a specific era. However, recently it has been criticized because those diseases no longer exist and few people fall within the criteria. It was believed to be inadequate for individuals since important lifestyle and environmental factors such as smoking and drinking were not considered.

recommended nutrient intakes (RNIs) A set of daily nutrient values similar to the Recommended Dietary Allowance (RDA) recommended for the majority of healthy Canadians.

recommended optimal nutrient intakes (RONIs) These are a set of dietary values developed over twenty years ago by some American researchers to be used as a preventive measure for health by recommending optimal values of nutrients to maintain a healthy body and prevent diseases.

resting heart rate (RHR) The number of heartbeats recorded upon awakening and before you start moving.

Retin A A derivate of vitamin A used for acne and other skin disorders such as deep wrinkles and hyperpigmentation. Manufactured by Ortho-McNeill Corporation, Raritan, NJ.

retinol equivalents (RE) The new measurement for vitamin A activity.

retinoids This is a collective term for the three active forms of vitamin A—*retinol, retinal* and *retinoic acid,* each having specific functions in the body.

reverse osmosis Water is forced by faucet pressure through a semi-permeable membrane to remove most heavy metals, parasites and most microscopic particles.

riboflavin Vitamin B-2. Essential for healthy skin and eyes.

ribosome The manufacturing plant in the cytoplasm of the cell where various amino acids are brought by the tRNA to build the desired protein.

ricotta An Italian soft cheese.

rigatoni Grooved pasta.

risotta A creamy Italian rice dish cooked in butter and chicken stock.

romaine Long, leafy salad greens.

romano A hard Italian cheese.

rosacea A chronic disease of the skin of the nose, forehead and cheeks, marked by flushing and followed by redness caused from dilated capillaries with acne-like pustules. It usually appears during middle age and occurs worse among men but more common in women.

rotation Fitness movement referring to turning on a long axis such as the shoulder rolls at the shoulder joint.

rotelle Spiral-shaped pasta.

S

saccharin An FDA approved sweetener that doesn't add extra calories.

saggital plane Vertical plane that divides the body into left and right sections. Also known as the lateral plane.

St. John's Wort An herb that reduces mild to moderate depression by enhancing the release of the serotonin hormone. It is sometimes used to suppress the appetite in weight loss.

sake Japanese wine.

samosas Deep fried turnovers filled with spicy lamb, potatoes or vegetables. A popular Asian-Indian dish.

sashimi Plain raw seafood and seaweed.

saturated fats Composed of triglycerides in which most of the fatty aids are saturated. They are found mostly in animal derived foods and certain plant oils such as coconut and palm.

sauerkraut German cabbage salted and fermented in its own juice.

schnitzel In German cooking, schnitzel described meat that is lightly breaded and fried.

scoliosis A deviation of the spine results in uneven shoulder positions, scapular deviations, slight horizontal rotation of the pelvis and uneven lengths of legs.

scurvy A vitamin C deficiency that was prevalent in the early part of the century with symptoms of tissue inflammation and bleeding gums.

sebaceous hyperplasia Small skin lesions in the shape of a doughnut or cauliflower appearing on the forehead and cheeks on oily and asphyxiated skins. They have a soft, yellowish color and usually appear solitary, giving a rough texture to the skin.

sebaceous keratoses Small plugs of lipids covered with skin commonly found on the facial area where there is poor skin exfoliation.

secretagogues Dietary supplements formulated from 191 amino acids like endogenous human growth hormones. They are precursors to growth hormones to stimulate the hGH from the pituitary gland and are used as an alternative to hormone injections.

semi-vegetarian Avoiding the consumption of red meat and opting for poultry, fish and dairy products instead.

serotonin A hormone that initiates sleep.

set point A controversial unproven theory that refers to a certain point that determines satiety therefore helping to regulating homeostasis in the body.

sibutramine A drug used to treat obesity by suppressing appetite.

sickle cell anemia An abnormal protein formed in the body that is found frequently among people of African descent. The normal sequence of hemoglobin is changed when one amino acid is replaced by another one, changing the characteristic and shape of the protein so much that the hemoglobin loses its ability to carry oxygen effectively and the red blood cells collapse forming sickle or crescent shaped cells instead of their normal disc shape.

simple carbohydrates Include naturally occurring sugars found in fresh fruits, vegetables.

soba Japanese buckwheat noodles.

social stressors Adverse conditions caused outside the body such as relationships, finance and war.

socioeconomic status The relationship between financial status and different levels of social class. Studies suggest that the higher the economic status, the higher the social class, while the lower the economic status, the lower the social class.

soda bread An Irish bread made with baking soda instead of yeast, prepared daily.

solar keratoses Also known as actinic keratosis or sunspots, are flat skin-colored macules with scaling patches, commonly found on sun-exposed areas of the body. They are caused by cumulative sun damage to the skin over many years and have the potential of developing into skin cancer. Commonly found on redheads, blondes and those who freckle easily.

soluble fiber Water soluble fiber found in mostly fruits, oats, barley and legumes have been found to give health benefits such as reducing blood cholesterol and helping with weight loss.

souvlaki A Greek kebab.

soy isoflavones Plant estrogens or phytoestrogens that are believed to provide protection against breast cancer.

soy protein Considered to be the only plant protein that contains the essential amino acids and therefore falls under complete proteins. Soybeans and its constituents have been found to have beneficial effects in the prevention or reduction of cardiovascular diseases, certain cancers and osteoporosis.

sparkling water Mineral water with carbonation.

spider naevi Dilated capillaries with radiating legs resembling a spider. Commonly found on the facial area, especially on the nose, cheeks or décolleté.

spina bifida A deficiency of folate in the diets of child-bearing females can result in an infant who develops neural tube defects. Adequate levels must be taken before and during the first few weeks of pregnancy to prevent this disease.

spring water has been collected from an underground spring that flows to the Earth's surface.

starch Various enzymes in the GI tract break down the starch molecules into glucose units for absorption.

stearic acid A common example of a long chain fatty acid chain, composed of 18 carbons. It commonly is used as an emulsifier or stabilizer in the manufacture of cosmetics.

sterols One of the three groups of lipids or fats.

stilton An English blue cheese.

stout A dark rich high-caloric beer, popular in Great Britain.

stress An abnormal reaction in response to a stressor.

strudel A German dessert pastry that usually is stuffed with ground apples.

subcutaneous layer The layer of skin lying under the dermis composed primarily of fat cells. It helps protect the bones and underlying structures of the body.

substrate One of the three parts of an enzyme reaction along with enzyme and product. For example, in the digestive process, the substrate can be fats, the enzyme, lipase, and the resulting product, fatty acids and glycerol.

sucralose An FDA approved sweetener that doesn't add extra calories.

sucrose Commonly known as table sugar, it is a double sugar composed of glucose and fructose, and is refined from cane sugar. Found in fruits, vegetables and grains.

sukiyaki Thinly-sliced Japanese meat stew.

superoxide dismutase (SOD) An enzyme produced in the body that acts as an antioxidant.

superoxide radicals The most common free radicals formed in the body.

sun salutation The most common yoga pose.

superior The upper section of the body.

sushi A Japanese dish consisting of thin slices of fresh fish or seaweed wrapped around a cake of cooked rice.

Syndrome X A term used to describe a set of cardiovascular risk factors associated with apple-shaped individuals.

T

tandoori cooking Asian-Indian style of cooking using a special clay oven heated with charcoal.

telomerase The enzyme responsible for repairing and replacing telomeres in germ and cancer cells, and is the cause of cell proliferation.

telomeres Sequences of amino acids found at the tips of chromosomes that are lost every time the cell divides. The Hayflick Hypothesis proposes that the cell dies at the 50th cell division.

tempura Japanese style of fried foods.

tensing The isometric toning of a muscle without any change in length. No movement occurs.

tetany A condition caused by calcium deficiency where severe twitching by skeletal muscles occurs involuntarily.

thermogenesis The chemical process that burns fat to release heat. It is believed that impaired thermogenesis can contribute to weight gain.

thiamin Vitamin B-1. Essential for healthy nervous system.

thrombin An enzyme that converts the plasma protein fibrinogen to fibrin during blood coagulation.

tolerable upper intake The maximum amount of a nutrient that is least likely to pose any risk in healthy people when consumed daily. This figure is higher than the RDA and was designed because more people are taking dietary supplements. It is intended to help people determine when an excessive amount of a nutrient taken over a long time may pose harm.

tortellini Stuffed ring pasta.

toxin Any compound that may have a detrimental effect on cellular function or structure.

trace elements Minerals that occur in tiny doses.

trans fatty acids A type of fatty acid created when an unsaturated fat such as a vegetable undergoes the process of hydrogenation to form a firmer state, such as margarine. During the chemical process a new chemical configuration is formed where hydrogen atoms of fat lie on the opposite sides of the point of unsaturation in the carbon chain. Trans fatty acids have been linked to heart disease. Some foods also list "partially hydrogenated vegetable oils" on the Nutrition Fact Panel. Trans fatty acids are found primarily in margarines, shortenings, commercial frying fats and baked goods.

transverse plane Runs across the body parallel to the ground, dividing the body into superior (upper) and inferior (lower) portions. Also known as the horizontal plane.

trifle A layered dessert made from custard, pound cake, jams, whipped cream, sherry and almonds, originated from England.

triglycerides The main form of fat in the diet, stored as fat in the body. Composed of three fatty acids bonded to a glycerol molecule.

tripeptide Three amino acids are bonded to one another by chemical bonds forming protein chains of varying lengths.

tRNA Special RNA molecules in the cell that gather basic building materials in the cytoplasm and brings them to the ribosomes.

tropocollagen Three polypeptide chains wrapped around one another to give rigidity and firmness form the collagen molecule. Once formed it is secreted into the intercellular space where it is worked on by enzymes to form polymers of collagen fibrils.

tyrosinase The enzyme that converts the amino acid tyrosine to melanin, the pigment formed in the melanocytes found in the epidermis.

U

udon Soft, fat and plain Japanese noodles.

uncoupling protein (UCO) Another protein component of brown fat that helps to burn the white fat to release energy.

unsaturated fats These fats are composed of triglycerides in which most of the fatty acids are unsaturated and can be found in both plant and animal foods. They either can be monounsaturated fats (MUFA) or polyunsaturated fats (PUFA).

V

valine An essential amino acid that is necessary to form complete protein in the body.

vegans Strict vegetarian diet where all animal-derived foods are excluded. Also called pure or total vegetarians.

very low density lipoproteins (VLDL) These protein carriers leave the liver carrying mainly triglycerides packaged by the liver to body tissues where they are needed. As the triglycerides are given out, the lipoprotein becomes denser, carrying more cholesterol than triglycerides, and becomes LDL.

vitamins Minute organic substances found in living foods, both plants and animal that are essential for the good health and maintenance of the body.

W

wasabi A hot green Japanese paste that tastes like horseradish.

water The most important nutrient for the body since it forms part of every cell.

whole grain Wheat that is milled but not refined.

wiener sausage A German sausage made from a smoked mixture of lean pork and bacon fat.

X

xanthalasmas Soft yellowish plaques of lipids usually found around the eye area. They are tiny to medium in size and some may be raised.

Y

yang Hot, should balance with yin (cold) to create harmony.

yin Cold, should balance with yang (hot) to create harmony.

yoga A system of living designed to promote both mental and physical health with increased awareness of the body using deep breathing, stretching and different poses.

Yorkshire pudding A traditional British dish, a popover cooked in meat drippings.

Yo-Yo Syndrome The viscous cycle in which the obese individual is always losing and gaining weight. When the obese starves to lose weight by going on low calorie diets, the body responds by reducing its metabolic rate to survive, so when even if little food is consumed, it is metabolized very slowly. When the dieter eventually resumes regular dietary habits, the metabolism remains low and weight gain reoccurs.

INDEX

Symbols

A

B

C

D

E

F

G

H

I

K

L

M

N

O

P

Q

R

S

T

U

V

W

Y